# Navigating Swallowing Disorders - From Symptoms to Solutions

*Edited by Hardip Singh Gendeh*

Published in London, United Kingdom

Navigating Swallowing Disorders - From Symptoms to Solutions
http://dx.doi.org/10.5772/intechopen.1000419
Edited by Hardip Singh Gendeh

Contributors
Aleksandar Včev, Bojana Simovic Markovic, Bojan Stojanovic, Djordje Kralj, Donnette Alicia Wright, Dusan Popovic, Dusan Radojevic, Emmanuel Ocheli, Hardip Singh Gendeh, Hee-Young Kim, Irfan Corovic, Isidora Stanisavljevic, Ivan Jovanovic, Karol Myszel, Liam D. Hyland, Lilamani Rajthala, Ljiljana Širić, Marina Jovanovic, Marinela Rosso, Mawaddah Azman, Mladen Maksic, Nghiem H. Nguyen, Nur Simsek Yurt, Piotr Henryk Skarzynski, Piyush Kumar, Prachi Upadhyay, Ronik Kothari, Sabir Sagdati, Samir Alsalek, Samir Vucelj, Shayan U. Rahman, Tijana Veljkovic



First published in London, United Kingdom, 2025 by IntechOpen
IntechOpen is the global imprint of INTECHOPEN LIMITED, registered in England and Wales, registration number: 11086078, 167-169 Great Portland Street, London, W1W 5PF, United Kingdom

For EU product safety concerns: IN TECH d.o.o., Prolaz Marije Krucifikse Kozulić 3, 51000 Rijeka, Croatia, info@intechopen.com or visit our website at intechopen.com.

British Library Cataloguing-in-Publication Data
A catalogue record for this book is available from the British Library

Navigating Swallowing Disorders - From Symptoms to Solutions
Edited by Hardip Singh Gendeh
p. cm.
Print ISBN 978-0-85466-023-0
Online ISBN 978-0-85466-022-3
eBook (PDF) ISBN 978-0-85466-024-7

If disposing of this product, please recycle the paper responsibly.

# Meet the editor

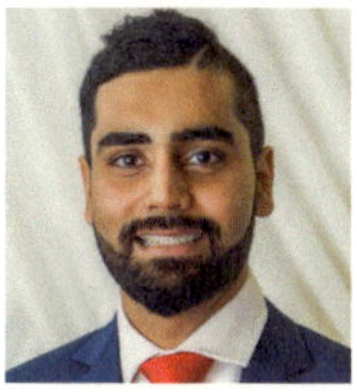

Dr. Hardip Singh Gendeh is a lecturer at the Faculty of Medicine, Universiti Kebangsaan Malaysia (UKM), Kuala Lumpur, Malaysia. He serves as a specialist Otorhinolaryngologist and Head and Neck Surgeon at the Hospital Canselor Tuanku Muhriz, UKM, in Kuala Lumpur. He obtained his Bachelor of Medical Science (BMedSci) and Bachelor of Medicine, Bachelor of Surgery (BMBS) at the University of Nottingham, United Kingdom, in 2009 and 2011, respectively. Dr. Gendeh served as a junior house officer at the Nottingham University Hospitals in England before returning to Malaysia in 2012. He obtained his Doctor of Otorhinolaryngology, Head and Neck (Dr ORL-HNS) specialty training from UKM in 2019. Dr. Gendeh is pursuing subspecialty training in Rhinology and is currently researching rhinosinusitis and nasal valve collapse of the nose.

# Contents

# Preface

Swallowing is one of the most fundamental physiological processes, yet it remains underappreciated until a disorder arises. As a medical professional, I have witnessed the challenges patients and healthcare providers face in diagnosing and managing swallowing disorders. This book was born out of a desire to bridge the gap between theory and practice, offering a clear, comprehensive resource for understanding swallowing and its complexities.

In producing this book, I sought to bring together insights from multiple disciplines—including speech and language therapy, gastroenterology, otolaryngology, and nutrition—highlighting the importance of a multidisciplinary approach. Researchers and scientists in the field also provided specific insights on swallowing and its disorders. The goal is to provide a structured, evidence-based guide that aids in both diagnosis and treatment, focusing on current insights and ensuring that knowledge is accessible to clinicians, therapists, researchers, and anyone interested in the science of swallowing.

I have divided the book into two sections: "Swallowing Fundamentals" and "Swallowing Disorders". The fundamentals section encompasses the background, anatomy and physiology of swallowing. Chapter 1 provides a broad overview of the various aetiology of swallowing disorders. Chapters 2 and 3 discuss oesophageal motility and how this intricate mechanism can be disrupted, resulting in swallowing problems. Chapter 4 shares a physiological process relevant to all of us: ageing. Ageing is a phenomenon that, while being termed as a disease, impacts our swallowing. Meanwhile, Chapter 5 covers various radiological assessments, highlighting their benefits and limitations.

Swallowing disorders can be attributed to specific diseases or conditions that prevent swallowing or disrupt its process. These points are covered in the second section. In Chapter 6, my colleagues and I have dwelled on how cleft disorders of the lip and/or palate cause a significant impairment in swallowing. Following this, Chapter 7 explains in depth how swallowing disorders affect our Eustachian tube function, affecting our hearing and balance. Both chapters exemplify the need for a multidisciplinary approach to managing swallowing disorders. Following this, Chapter 8 discusses how the cervical spine, located just posterior to the oesophagus, may disrupt our swallowing process. Chapter 9 depicts a common cause of dysphagia, which is neoplasms or tumours of the oesophagus. These are often overlooked as they usually require endoscopy or imaging to detect abnormalities within the lumen of the upper gut. Laryngectomy, a process of surgically removing one's voice box, does affect swallowing as the posterior glottis, pharynx, and part of the cervical oesophagus share the same anatomy. This is discussed in Chapter 10. Chapter 11 dives into radiation, a treatment for many malignancies and its sequel in causing dysphagia, and how technological advancements have helped in reducing it. Chapter 12 provides good background knowledge on nutrition, its substitute for oral feeding, and the energy requirement for patients with swallowing disorders.

I want to extend my deepest gratitude to my colleagues, mentors, and contributors whose expertise and support have enriched this book. Special thanks to my parents, Dr. Balwant Singh Gendeh and Dr. Pritam Kor Mangat. My father, a retired professor of Otorhinolaryngology, has been a constant source of encouragement, guiding me in my writing journey. My mother, a dedicated dentist, has spent her life ensuring her patients maintain proper dental function. She has constantly reminded me of the critical role dentition plays in the early stages of mastication.

I am also grateful to Mr. Manjit Singh Mangat from Alor Setar, Kedah, for his unwavering encouragement to strive for excellence. My sister, Dr. Manvin Kaur Gendeh, a physician in Atlanta, United States, has nurtured my artistic side, inspiring me to illustrate various books over the years.

My heartfelt appreciation goes to the Faculty of Medicine at Universiti Kebangsaan Malaysia, which has enriched my research and academic writing environment. Lastly, I thank IntechOpen and its team, including Maja Bozicevic, for offering a platform to disseminate knowledge and make it easily accessible to all.

To my readers, whether you are a healthcare professional, clinician, researcher, or student, I hope this book serves as a valuable resource in your journey of understanding and managing swallowing disorders. If you are a patient looking for answers to swallowing disorders, may this book shed some light and be a source of betterment.

With appreciation,

**Hardip Singh Gendeh**
Faculty of Medicine,
Lecturer at the Department of Otorhinolaryngology, Head and Neck Surgery,
Universiti Kebangsaan Malaysia,
Kuala Lumpur, Malaysia

Specialist Otorhinolaryngologist, Head and Neck Surgeon,
Otorhinolaryngology, Head and Neck Surgery Clinic,
Hospital Canselor Tuanku Muhriz,
Kuala Lumpur, Malaysia

Section 1

# Swallowing Fundamentals

Chapter 1

# Medical Conditions Associated with Concurrent Dysphagia and Dysphonia

*Karol Myszel and Piotr Henryk Skarzynski*


## Abstract

Swallowing and voice production are important processes enabling a comfortable life. For appropriate alimentation, effective passage of food and fluids through a digestive system is necessary. Interpersonal communication depends on good voice and speech. Conditions associated with swallowing and speech problems leads dysfunctions and seriously affect the patient's comfort of living. This chapter is a review of medical conditions associated with concurrence of dysphonia and dysphagia. There are a large number of medical conditions leading to the simultaneous occurrence of swallowing problems and hoarseness. The diversity of disorders is a serious interdisciplinary issue. Diagnostics of concurrent dysphagia and dysphonia is complicated and requires a holistic interdisciplinary approach. The reasons include functional and organic dysfunctions, neurological conditions, tumors, vascular disorders, autoimmune inflammations, post-operative complications, post-COVID complications, and others. Our research was conducted by reviewing PubMed and Scopus network using key words "dysphagia", "dysphonia", "hoarseness." We found 966 publications, then narrowed the search to 99 articles describing medical conditions and case reports, which present with dysphagia and dysphonia occurring together. Detailed analysis enabled us to categorize the disorders into groups, depending on characteristics and body region involved in the pathological process. Finally, the description of the medical conditions was done systematically according to those groups.


**Keywords:** dysphagia, dysphonia, swallowing, voice, disorders

## 1. Introduction

Swallowing and voice production are both coordinated by a nervous system. From anatomical and physiological standpoint, these two acts have a lot in common. Appropriate swallowing takes place with the larynx closed by the epiglottis, which is a protective mechanism for the lower part of the respiratory system against aspiration of food and fluids.

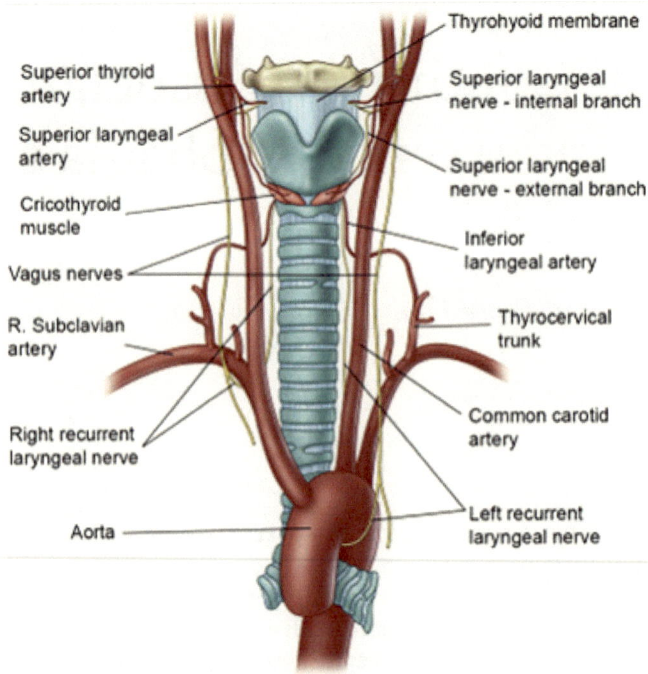


**Figure 1.**
*Recurrent laryngeal nerve path (description in the text) (source: [1]).*

Swallowing is a highly complex neuromuscular process modulated by the central nervous system. It requires a timely coordination of laryngeal and pharyngeal muscles. When swallowing begins, food and fluids are pushed from mouth to pharynx and then down to esophagus. To protect the food from accessing the airway, this needs vocal cords to close timely and the epiglottis to cover the glottis. A short apnea appears. Muscles involved in the process are innervated by superior and recurrent laryngeal nerves (RLN) (**Figure 1**), which on both sides are the branches of the vagus nerve. Left RLN leaves the vagus right after it enters the chest. It bends around the aortic arch and then around the subclavian artery. Further, the RLN of both sides go together upward along the trachea, in the tracheoesophageal sulcus and reach the posterior wall of the thyroid gland. Any condition that leads to discoordination of the above process causes the risk of aspiration. When it happens, the cough reflex is activated by the initiation of intercostal, abdominal and diaphragm muscles.

Voice production is also a complex process involving several physiological mechanisms. Laryngeal muscles are responsible for tensioning and closing the vocal cords as well as for relaxing the cords and opening the glottis. They are innervated respectively, by the superior laryngeal nerve (cricothyroid muscle) and by the recurrent laryngeal nerve (all remaining muscles). Specific vibrant movements of vocal folds also need a subglottic air pressure to begin and thus to initiate phonation [2]. The frontal section of the larynx structure is presented below (**Figure 2**).

Different pathologies may lead to discoordination of swallowing and voicing physiology and be causative factors for dysphonia and dysphagia. A whole group of medical conditions may be reasons for both of them to occur at the same time.

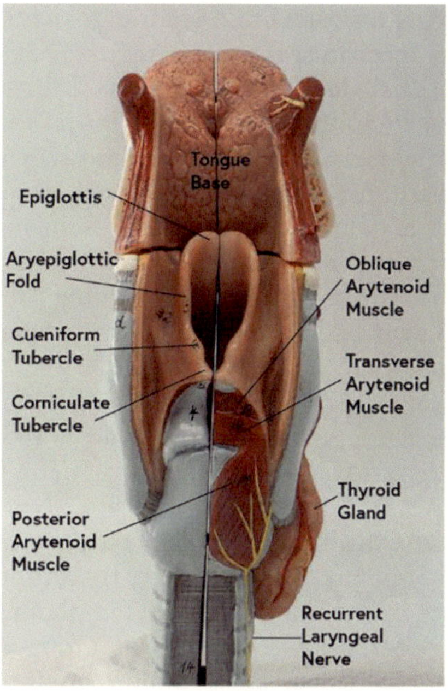


**Figure 2.**
*The structure of larynx (source: University College of London Hospitals, NHS Foundation Trust).*

Depending on the type and location, pathologies causing coexistence of swallowing and voice production can be differentiated according to the location of the basic disorder. They include disorders in the central nervous system, peripheral nerves, cervical spine, larynx, neck, mediastinum, muscles, connective tissue, and COVID infection complications.

## 2. Central nervous system

Central nervous system control over swallowing and phonation is a superior mechanism ensuring appropriate function of those two acts. Centers in the brain responsible for efferent signal transmission to peripheral parts of IX, X, XI, and XII cranial nerves need to be supplied with blood and oxygenated in an appropriate way to keep their function. It is assumed that the brain uses approximately 20% of all blood. Therefore, every condition leading to ischemia, hypoxia, or mechanical damage disrupts the function, which may seriously affect both the brain itself and the effector organs.

Lesions that cause dysphagia and hoarseness may localize in different areas in the central nervous system. Cerebral cortex sends signals to nuclei of IX and X cranial nerves (CN). The signals are also sent to them through corticobulbar tracts located in the medulla. Therefore, both lesions localized in cerebral hemispheres and those in the brainstem, may lead to dysarthria by disrupting the nerve conduction. On the other hand, damages to the peripheral nervous system may lead to dysarthria and dysphagia, as they affect the function of motor neurons and cause neuropathies, dysfunctions of the neuromuscular junction or pharyngeal, and laryngeal myopathies. Finally, they also lie behind disturbances in motility of the esophagus.

Dysphagia and dysphonia together often occur in patients after stroke. Both ischemic and hemorrhagic mechanisms cause brain tissue dysfunction. Brain stroke is number one cause of death in developed countries [3]. Vascular mechanisms of the stroke include thrombosis, embolism, and artery rupture. Thrombosis and clots lead to transient or permanent hypoxia, which may lead to brain infarct. Serious hypoxia of the whole brain may also occur in hypovolemic shock. Hemorrhagic stroke causes cell dysfunction as a result of damage and secondary ischemia. All the conditions above lead to the development of neurological symptoms, such as headache, face numbness, hemiplegia, dysarthria, difficulty swallowing, and dysphonia [4–6].

Similar effects of swallowing and voice production problems originated centrally may occur when the brain is mechanically pressed by the mass of edema, intracranial hematoma, or tumors. Swallowing and phonation dysfunctions occurring together are seen in post-traumatic patients when edema develops and leads to gomphosis. The same effect of mechanical pressure appears in those with brain neoplasms, including gliomas (astrocytoma, oligodendroglioma, and ependymoma). Prevailingly, gliomas spread as diffuse and infiltrating tumors (astrocytoma, oligodendroglioma), less as solid masses (ependymoma). Other primary tumors of the central nervous system causing mass effect are medulloblastomas, lymphomas or germ cell tumors. Secondary brain tumors, occurring as 25–50% of all intracranial tumors, include metastases from the lungs, skin (melanoma), kidney, or digestive system. Usually, they are formed as solid masses in between white and gray substances, well separated from the healthy tissues. Dysphagia and dysphonia, accompanied by headaches, were also described in patients with multiform glioblastoma in the cerebellopontine angle with trans-tentorial spread [7]. Similarly, vestibular schwannomas were described to cause swallowing and voice problems. The bigger the tumor size, the more intensity of symptoms were found. Vagal schwannoma occupying the left cerebellar-medullary cistern and extending from the pontomedullary junction to the jugular foramen was also reported to cause similar clinical effects [8].

Literature analysis shows that a whole variety of other conditions in the central nervous system may also affect swallowing and voice simultaneously. Meningitis cases were described in the course of a varicella zoster infection to cause dysphagia, dysarthria, and hoarseness. Sudden vomiting, dysphagia, dysphonia, and food regurgitation were found in the condition named neuromyelitis optica (NMO). This inflammatory disorder affects the spinal cord centers and optic nerves. The pathology has an autoimmune background and causes nerve demyelination. The set of above symptoms is referred to as acute brainstem syndrome [9].

Bulbar symptomatology (progressive dysphagia, dysphonia, and dysarthria) may also appear as a result of vascular brainstem compression in the course of intracranial arterial dolichoectasia (IADE). The condition is often a result of atherosclerosis that leads to local enlargement of the artery, which gets wider, longer, and more tortuous [10]. Dysphonia, dysphagia, and nasality were also reported in patients with isolated bulbar palsy as a result of neurosarcoidosis, a non-caseating granulomatous chronic inflammatory disease that can affect any organ, including the central nervous system [11].

Voice and swallowing impairments are common in movement disorders. The group of diseases is mainly represented by Parkinson's disease (PD), but also includes essential tremor (ET), dystonia, and other related syndromes named atypical Parkinsonian syndromes (APS). They may lead to disturbed voice production and speech, but often affect swallowing acts as well. Imbalance between breathing, vocal folds' biomechanics, and vocal tract function used in voicing may negatively affect the quality of voice. Discoordination of muscles activated during swallowing can result in dysphagia, or difficulty moving food or liquid from the mouth to the stomach [12–14]. In its two variants of spinal and bulbar onset, amyotrophic lateral sclerosis (ALS) affects muscle function and may lead to swallowing and voice problems and dysarthria. The pathology is caused by neurogenerative mechanism involving upper and lower motor neurons [15].

Other conditions in central nervous system were also reported to cause dysphagia and dysphonia together. Alexander's disease (AD), a progressive disorder of cerebral white matter caused by a heterozygous GFAP pathogenic variant, comprises nonspecific neurologic manifestations in adults. An additional symptom of muscle dysfunction in the disease is nasal speech [16]. Dysphagia, followed by dysphonia, diplopia, and ataxia were described in individuals suffering from Wernicke encephalopathy (WE) that develops as result of thiamine (vitamin B1) deficiency. The condition is seen mainly, but not only, in individuals prone to alcohol abuse [17].

## 3. Peripheral nervous system

Pathologies involving peripheral nerves include a whole variety of symptoms. They are caused by major mechanisms, including mechanical, inflammatory, degenerative, or neoplasmatic. Pathology disturbs nerve conduction, which results in improper function of effector organs. Therefore, muscles responsible for swallowing and voice may be seriously affected.

Guillain-Barré syndrome (GBS) is a neurological disease of inflammatory origin leading to demyelination and degeneration of nerve fibers. Usually preceded by infection, GBS develops in an autoimmune mechanism. The condition is sometimes seen as a vaccination side effect. Progressive fatigue, muscle weakness, dysphonia, dysphagia, and dysarthria were described in patients diagnosed for GBS weeks after covid infection [18]. Similarly, GBS was described as the cause of polyradiculoneuropathy leading to dysphagia, dysphonia, bilateral facial palsy, areflexia, and ataxia, which are characteristic of a bulbar palsy [19]. The same symptoms may be present in cases of wound botulism seen in heroin users. The symptoms result from a wound contamination with *Clostridium botulinum*, which produces neurotoxin that inhibits acetylcholine release by binding irreversibly to the presynaptic terminal. Usually, symmetrical cranial nerve palsies occur that lead to mouth dryness, blurry vision, dysphagia, dysarthria, dysphonia, and peripheral muscle weakness. In most serious cases, respiratory muscles are involved, which causes neuromuscular respiratory failure. Appropriate diagnosis and early treatment are crucial [20].

Dysphonia, dysphagia, muscle weakness, and fatigue may also occur in post-polio syndrome (PS), which is defined as a set of various symptoms in subjects who survived acute paralytic poliomyelitis. PS may develop a long time after recovery. The virus, transmitted with contaminated food and water or through the fecal-oral route, causes death of the lower motor neuron by damaging the cells of the anterior horn of the spinal cord [21].

The Varicella zoster (VZ) virus has been associated with a wide range of neurological complications. It usually affects upper cranial nerves (trigeminal and facial), but also lower cranial polyneuropathies resulting from Varicella zoster virus reactivation were seen [22]. Herpes zoster (HZ) infection involving cervical, vagus, and accessory nerves causing severe vocal paralysis, asymmetric palate, trapezius atrophy, and scalene muscle atrophy was described as another condition causing simultaneous dysphonia and dysphagia [23]. Varicella zoster is also recognized as the etiology for jugular foramen syndrome (JFS), alternatively named Vernet's syndrome (VS). Jugular foramen conducts glossopharyngeal and vagus nerves, as well as jugular vein. JFS may be caused by trauma, tumor, or vascular and infectious factors. The syndrome is characterized by paresis of the IX, X, and XI cranial nerves, which causes loss of taste at the posterior 1/3 of the tongue, vocal fold paresis, and weakened function of trapezius and sternocleidomastoid muscles. This ultimately leads to dysphonia and dysphagia.

Cases of Collet-Sicard syndrome (CSS), a rare disorder caused by cranial nerve compression at the skull base, were also identified to cause dysphagia, dysphonia, and a deviated tongue following an upper respiratory tract infection. The syndrome is associated with spontaneous carotid artery dissection leading to the formation of pseudoaneurysm as a result of persistent coughing. Delays in diagnosis could result in subsequent stroke or other morbidity associated with prolonged cranial nerve compression [24].

Transient cranial nerve palsies causing swallowing and voice disorders were observed as a complication of spinal anesthesia with a bupivacaine-fentanyl combination [25]. Dysphagia with dysphonia was also described in epileptic patients developing pharyngolaryngeal spasm as a side effect of vagus nerve stimulation therapy [26]. Progressive dyspnea, dysphonia, dysphagia for solids, and globus pharyngeus were reported in individuals with laryngeal schwannoma [27].

## 4. Cervical spine

Pathologies located within the cervical spine as well as surgical interventions in this region may lead to various multisymptomatic conditions. Diffuse idiopathic skeletal hyperostosis (DISH) known as Forestier's disease, is a common elderly disease of unknown etiology that leads to hardening of ligaments and entheses of the skeleton. Cases of DISH were reported to cause dysphonia, stridor, dysphagia, globus, and dyspnea as a result of mechanical compression of ossified tissues and DISH-related cervical osteophytes on the posterior wall of the respiratory and digestive tract [28, 29].

Patients diagnosed with cervical stenosis (spondylosis) are often treated surgically. Cervical spondylosis (CS) is a progressive disease of the cervical spine. It disturbs the cervical spine function as a result of pathological changes leading to stenosis. It is often associated with degeneration or herniation of the disc, the formation of osteophytes, and ligament hypertrophy (**Figure 3**). Patients may present with any combination of neck pain, radiculopathy, or myelopathy. Unsatisfactory preservative treatment may lead to the need for cervical disc replacement (CDR). This type of surgical procedure includes discectomy and, as a result, enables a disc space to be restored and the stenosis to be decompressed. As a complication of the treatment, dysphagia and dysphonia were also reported in many cases [31].

Dysphagia, dysphonia, and odynophagia were often reported to occur after surgical treatment of degenerative cervical myelopathy (DCM). Degenerative cervical myelopathy causes cord compression and is often treated surgically (ACDF, anterior cervical discectomy) to remove the compressive pathology, increase the space available for the spinal cord, and stabilize the spinal column. Dysphagia can occur during all three phases of swallowing. Dysphonia is most commonly caused by damage to the recurrent laryngeal nerve, which can appear during any of the operations involving the upper cervical region near C3-C4 [32, 33].

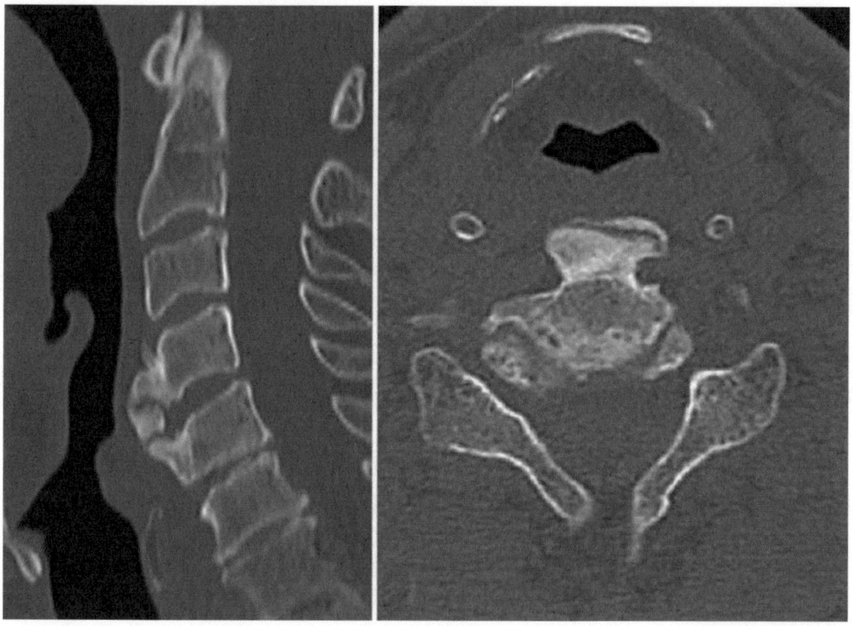

**Figure 3.**
*Anterior cervical osteophyte in CT scan (sagittal and axial view) (source: [30]).*

## 5. Muscular/connective tissue disorders

The literature review shows that pathologies of muscles leading to muscle weakness may be associated with swallowing and voice production problems.

Dermatomyositis (DM) is one of a few types of autoimmune inflammatory myopathy together with polymyositis, myositis overlap syndrome (including anti-synthetase syndrome), inclusion body myositis (IBM), and immune-mediated necrotizing myopathy (IMNM). It is a rare autoimmune condition that affects children and adults and is one of the many idiopathic inflammatory myopathies that predominantly affect the skin and muscles. DM is characterized by inflammation-related muscle weakness. Skin rash is often seen. As a result, pathological mechanisms of DM may finally lead to muscle dystrophic calcinosis. Muscle stiffness involves different groups of muscles, including those taking part in the swallowing process as well as voice emission. Therefore, dysphagia and dysphonia are often present in patients with advanced cases of DM [34, 35].

Mitochondrial myopathy (MM), a genetic condition related to nuclear gene TK2, which encodes the mitochondrial thymidine kinase, an enzyme involved in the phosphorylation of deoxycytidine and deoxythymidine nucleosides, leads to serious muscle dysfunction. Pathology mainly involves skeletal muscles. Childhood-onset TK2 deficiency typically causes a rapidly progressive proximal myopathy, which leads to mobility dysfunction and severe respiratory impairment. In some cases of slowly progressive mitochondrial myopathy, ptosis, hypoacusis, dysphonia, and dysphagia were described in the literature [36].

The Ehlers-Danlos syndrome (EDS) is a heritable disorder of connective tissue (HDCT), characterized by joint hypermobility, skin hyperextensibility, and tissue fragility. Hypermobile EDS (hEDS) is the most common subtype, representing more than 90% of cases. EDS presents with pain, fatigue, anxiety, gastrointestinal issues, autonomic dysfunction, temporomandibular joint disorder (TMJD), dysphagia, dysphonia, and LPR symptoms [37].

Inflammatory diseases of the muscles may also be caused by parasite infections. A rare case of myositis caused by Haycocknema perplexum characterized by progressive facial and limb weakness, dysphagia, and dysphonia was described by the researchers of Mayo Clinic [38].

Another group of muscular diseases are those related to dysfunction of the neuromuscular junction. Myasthenia gravis (MG) is an autoimmune disease affecting the function of the neuromuscular junction. Dysfunction of the junction disturbs nerve-muscle conduction, leading to muscle weakness. The pathology relates to various groups of muscles and may present as dysphonia, dysphagia, dysarthria, and weakness of skeletal muscles. Affecting muscles of the eyes and face, this may also lead to ptosis, diplopia, and difficulty in closing the eyelid. The body of an MG patient produces autoantibodies that bind to acetylcholine receptors on skeletal muscle, thus causing muscle weakness and fatigability. Bulbar symptoms, including dysarthria, dysphagia, and dysphonia due to IX and X cranial nerve dysfunction, occur in approximately 15% of patients [39, 40].

## 6. Mediastinum

Mediastinum is a large space located in the chest containing various anatomical structures and organs. Superiorly, it is connected with the neck through a superior thoracic aperture, also named a thoracic inlet. It is a space limited by the first thoracic vertebra, ribs, and the sternal manubrium. The space includes various anatomical structures, including the trachea and esophagus, as well as nerves, arteries, and veins. Due to the connection, some pathologies (i.e., inflammation) may include neck and mediastinum at the same time.

Variability and proximity of the structures makes the mediastinum vulnerable to diseases involving different organs and functions. Large mediastinal tumors may lead to dysphagia, dysphonia, coughing, chest pain, and dyspnea. An example of such a tumor is a posterior mediastinal liposarcoma causing compression on the esophagus, trachea, and carotid arteries [41]. Other tumors in the chest may cause similar symptoms.

Various cardiac conditions may influence the swallowing and voice. Ortner's syndrome (OS), also named cardiovocal syndrome, is a cardiac disease related condition presented with hoarseness as well as dysphagia, cough, and dyspnea. Pathophysiology underlying the syndrome is a dysfunction (or palsy) of the left laryngeal nerve, which results from its friction, stretching, pulling, or compression. The many reasons leading to OS include aortic aneurysm, pulmonary hypertension, arterial hypertension, or mitral stenosis [42, 43].

Dysphonia and dysphagia may also occur as complications after cardiac surgery. Tapia's syndrome (TS), a palsy of recurrent laryngeal nerve and hypoglossal nerve, is one of such conditions. The most probable background is considered a compression on X and XII cranial nerves a result of orotracheal intubation. This may occur after a variety of cardiac surgeries, such as aortal valve replacement (AVR), coronary artery bypass grafting (CABG), atrial septal defect closure (ASDC), or mitral valve repair (MVR) [44, 45].

Diverse symptoms that include a palpable neck mass, dyspnea to asphyxia, dysphagia, dysphonia, and superior vena cava syndrome may also be seen in large thyroid tumors. One of them is substernal goiter, a thyroid tumor trespassing the line of the thoracic inlet and entering the mediastinum. This can cause various symptoms due to the compression of adjacent anatomical structures [46]. The same symptoms can be observed in the presence of other types of masses in the chest, that is, enlarged lymph nodes, sarcoidosis, cancer, thymoma, or mid-esophageal diverticula. The superior vena cava syndrome occurs when masses compress the superior vena cava and occlude its lumen. The occlusion blocks the flow down of the blood from the veins of the head and neck, leading to an increase in pressure in the vessels. This increases the compression on the anatomical structures and on the recurrent laryngeal nerve. The symptoms, apart from dysphagia and hoarseness, include edema, head, neck, chest, and arms veins enlargement and face cyanosis (**Figures 4** and **5**) [48, 49].

The diverticula are often formed as result of mediastinal lymph nodes inflammation. They adhere tightly to the esophagus wall and pull it to form various sizes diverticula. Another diverticula type, named pulsion mid-esophageal diverticula, tend to be associated with esophageal motor disorders (**Figure 6**) [50].

Esophageal perforation (EP) is a critical clinical status. EP may occur in the cervical thoracic, or abdominal part of the esophagus. Depending on the perforation location, symptoms may present various characters and intensities. Cervical perforation is mainly associated with dysphagia and neck pain (**Figure 7**), while this in the thoracic part is characterized by dyspnea, epigastric, back, or chest pain, suggestive of mediastinitis. Abdominal pain as a result of developing peritonitis is present in perforation of abdominal esophagus. Dysphagia in such cases is usually caused by dysfunction of inflamed tissues and muscles and thus disturbed esophagus motility. In cases of anterior perforation leading to tracheoesophageal fistula, mediastinitis or aspiration pneumonia may develop. Dysphonia is then often caused by the palsy of the recurrent laryngeal nerve that runs in the tracheoesophageal groove, the sulcus formed by the trachea anteriorly and esophagus posteriorly. The mortality rate associated with esophageal perforation is high, as it may lead to the development of systemic inflammatory response syndrome (SIRS), accompanied by fever, hypotension, and tachycardia. Reasons for EP may differ, including surgical procedures, endoscopy, external trauma, scleroderma, neoplasms, inflammation, achalasia, esophageal stricture, or

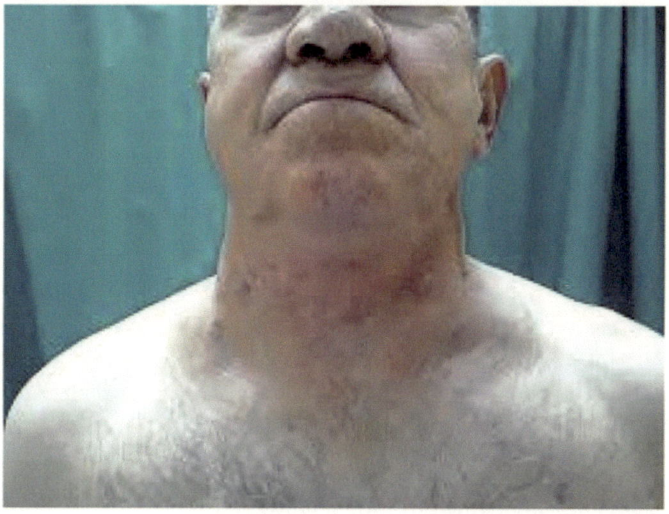

**Figure 4.**
*Images presenting the symptoms of superior vena cava syndrome, frontal view (source: [47]).*

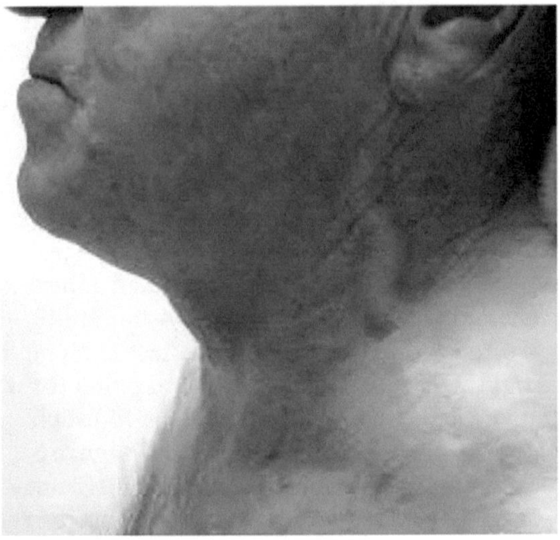

**Figure 5.**
*Images presenting the symptoms of superior vena cava syndrome, lateral view (source: [47]).*

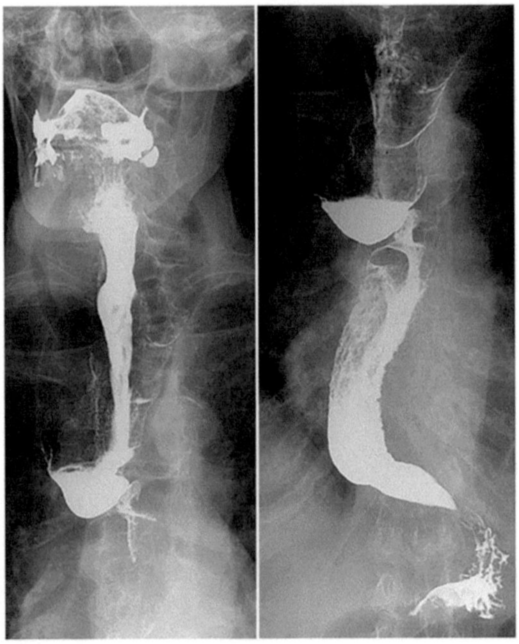

**Figure 6.**
*A barium swallow test showing esophagus dilatations (diverticula) (source: [50]).*

hiatal hernia. EP can also be a complication of bariatric procedures, mostly related to the intraoperative use of bougie. Laparoscopic sleeve gastrectomy (LSG) may be associated with emphysema, cervical pain, dysphagia, dysphonia, and fever [51, 52].

Dysphagia, dysphonia, and subcutaneous emphysema together, with pain in the back or neck were described as symptoms accompanying a condition called pneumomediastinum, also referred to as mediastinal emphysema (ME). Usually caused by trauma, barotrauma (mechanical ventilation), or happening spontaneously, it leads

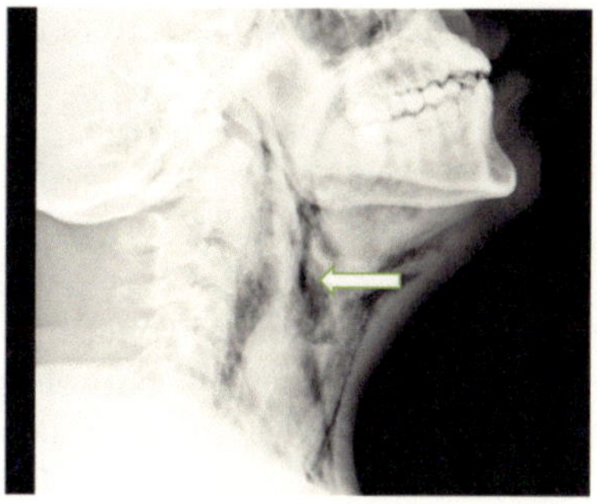

**Figure 7.**
*Radiograph image of cervical emphysema post-esophageal perforation (source: [51]).*

to air accumulation in the mediastinal space. This can also be induced by vigorous coughing or esophagus rupture as a result of intense vomiting. Underlying factors increasing the risk of mediastinal emphysema are respiratory diseases affecting the lungs and smoking (**Figure 8**) [53, 54].

Postpneumonectomy syndrome (PPS) is a condition occurring in some cases after pneumonectomy. In such condition, mediastinum with its organs gets shifted into the additional space created in result of pneumonectomy. Trachea and bronchus are compressed, which leads to dyspnea, dysphonia, and wheezing. In the long course, recurrent infections are also seen [55].

Mediastinal lipomatosis (ML) is presented with fatty tissue accumulation in mediastinum or pleura. Cases were described with manifestation of dyspnea, thoracic pain, cough, dysphonia, dysphagia, supraventricular tachycardia, and persistent pneumonia. In such cases an association of lipomatosis with myotonic dystrophy type 1 (MD1) was found. MD1 is the most prevalent myopathy in adults. The phenotypic spectrum of MD1 is highly variable and depends on the mutation load (homozygote and heterozygote) [56].

Swallowing problems associated with dysphonia were reported as complications of heart and lung transplantation procedure. The etiology of voice and swallowing complications in these patients can involve compromised respiratory function, prolonged intubation, trauma to the recurrent laryngeal nerve (RLN),

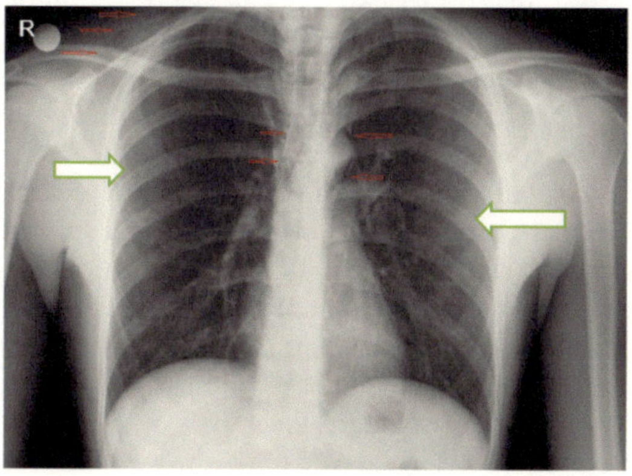

**Figure 8.**
*PA chest X-ray showing diffuse subcutaneous emphysema in neck and chest with pneumomediastinum (source: [53]).*

intensive care unit acquired weakness, alterations to neurological status, and chronic gastro-esophageal reflux [2].

## 7. Larynx

Pathologies of the larynx that lead to voice dysfunction may be of functional or organic origin. Dysphonia is a key symptom of the pathologies; however, some of them may also be associated with dysphagia. Literature data shows that dysphagia occurs in about 5–10% of patients with voice disorders [57–59].

Functional voice disorders include hyperfunctional, hypofunctional, and mixed dysphonia. The background of the disorders is inappropriate voice emission with hypertension or hypotension of internal and external muscles of the larynx. The muscle tension abnormalities in some cases also lead to swallowing problems referred to as muscle tension dysphagia (MTD). Literature data shows that some researchers confirmed tension abnormalities by laryngeal electromyography (LEMG) and superficial electromyography (SEMG) results [60].

Hoarseness and swallowing problems are also seen in functional voice disorders in the elderly. Due to muscle weakness progressing with age, glottal insufficiency appears (presbyphonia). This is linked to reduced ability to produce effective glottal closure and difficulty in expectoration. As glottal closure is needed to increase subglottal pressure, allowing effective coughing, glottal incompetence in the elderly also gives a higher risk of aspiration and pneumonia [61]. Apart from functional insufficiency, incomplete glottic closure can also be a result of vocal fold paresis (VFP) due to neck and chest pathologies, lung cancer, complications of thyroid, and mediastinal operations or idiopathic [62].

Bilateral vocal fold paresis (BVFP), a serious life-threatening condition, apart from breathing difficulties, leads to dysphonia and swallowing problems. BVFP is often seen in the course of various conditions including cancer (of lungs, larynx, and brain), infectious diseases (tuberculosis, *Treponema pallidum*, poliomyelitis, and Lyme disease), autoimmune conditions, neurological disorders (myasthenia gravis, Parkinsons disease, multisystem atrophy, motor neuron disorders, encephalopathy, and cerebrovascular lesions), intoxications (pesticides), bilateral cricoarytenoid joint fixation or laryngeal amyloidosis, and others [63]. Failure of abduction of bilateral vocal cords may lead to an insufficient airway passage resulting in stridor or decrease in exercise tolerance, often requiring intervention (**Figure 9**).

Chronic cough, throat clearing, pain, dysphagia, and hoarseness were described in patients with laryngopharyngeal reflux (LPR). LPR is a multisymptom syndrome which appears as gastroduodenal contents moves backward from the stomach into the larynx or pharynx. The etiopathology of LPR is still subject to further research; however, usually it is associated with the insufficiency of the lower esophageal sphincter. Acid fluids lead to irritation of the mucosa of the pharynx and larynx, causing globus and throat clearing. Ultimately, this may lead to swallowing problems [65]. LPR may lead to laryngeal edema and voice disorders. Apart from an irritation of the mucosa, the pathophysiology of dysphagia and dysphonia is also related to the stimulation of the vagal nerve by the backflow of gastric fluids, particularly at the lower part of the esophagus [66].

The whole variety of other laryngeal organic disorders and tumors were also described to cause voice problems and swallowing disorders. Lymphomas localized in the region of the head and neck may lead to dysphonia and dysphagia. They usually include lymph nodes, while those with extra nodal location (ENL) occur rarely.

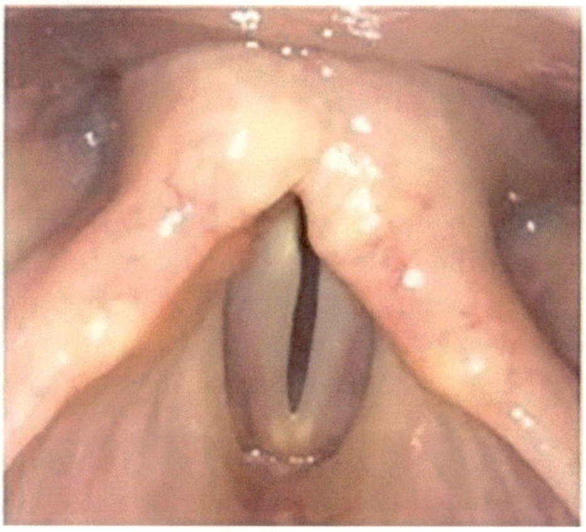

**Figure 9.**
*Bilateral vocal fold paralysis in adult (source: [64]).*

Some cases of non-Hodgkin lymphoma (NHL) of the larynx were described, usually occurring in the supraglottic region (**Figure 10**). They may present with dysphagia, dysphonia, snoring, and progressive respiratory distress [67]. Similarly, laryngeal cancer or neuroendocrine carcinoma (NEC) of the larynx, as well as laryngeal paraganglioma and paraganglioma of the recurrent laryngeal nerve, may lead to dysphonia with coexisting dysphagia. Paragangliomas are tumors of neuroendocrine origin that develop from the paraganglia in the head and neck. They originate from the chromaffin cells from the paraganglionic tissue of the autonomic parasympathetic nervous system. Among all paragangliomas, 65–70% occur within the head and neck, usually involving the carotid, jugular foramen, and vagal nerve. Some cases were described in the nasopharynx, nose and sinuses, larynx, thyroid gland, and orbit [68]. Other, non-neoplastic rare tumors of the larynx were also reported to produce swallowing and voice problems. One of them is adult laryngeal hemangioma (ALH), which usually involves the supraglottic or glottic region. It appears as a result of vocal abuse, cigarette smoking, or laryngeal trauma from intubation [69].

Tuberculosis of the larynx is a rare disease with laryngeal symptoms in the absence of constitutional symptoms. Cases of isolated laryngeal tuberculosis were reported as a reason for dysphonia with coexisting dysphagia [70]. Dysphonia,

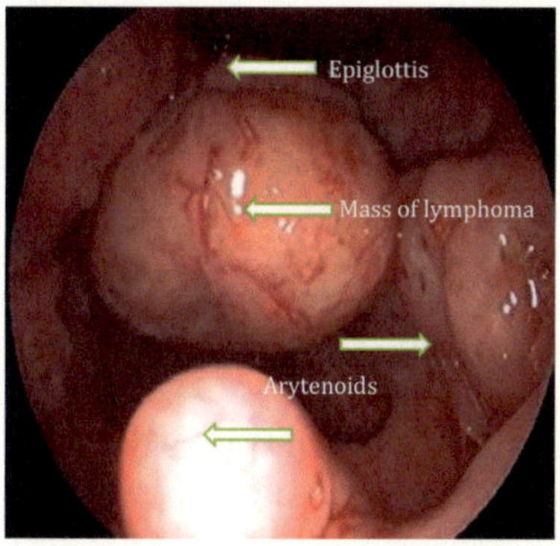


**Figure 10.**
*Video laryngoscopy showing laryngeal lymphoma (source: [67]).*

dysphagia, and respiratory distress occurred in patients with bullous pemphigoid (BP), an autoimmune condition with laryngeal manifestations. BP primarily affects skin, however, it may also be seen in the mucosa of the upper respiratory tract, larynx or esophagus [71].

Other cases described in the literature include multiple dermoid cysts of epiglottis [72], postradiotherapy laryngopharyngeal edema [73], traumatic laryngocele as a result of blunt trauma of the neck [74] or interarytenoid tumor-like lesions and ulcerative inflammatory lesions of the larynx in laryngeal leishmaniasis [75]. Hoarseness, voice fatigue, dysphonia, and dysphagia were also seen as complications of injection laryngoplasty, causing subchordal cysts containing non-degraded hyaluronic acid [76].

Blunt laryngeal trauma (BLT) is a serious, potentially life-threatening condition that leads to damages that may affect voice production, swallowing, and breathing. BLT results may vary, however, symptoms spectrum usually includes laryngeal edema, hoarseness, dysphagia, stridor, subcutaneous crepitus, vocal fold(s) immobility, and anterior neck pain [77].

## 8. Neck

Deep neck infection (DNI) is a complex infectious condition developing and spreading in the tissue spaces of the neck (intermuscular and fascial). It may ultimately lead to the formation of an abscess. Years ago, most DNIs originated from tonsillar and peritonsillar infections. Currently, most cases are odontogenic (38–49%) [78]. The tissues involved in an inflammatory process get swollen and cause a compression to surrounding organs. Dysphagia and dysphonia are usually present, and the symptoms may be accompanied by trismus, dyspnea, and infection symptoms. Dysphonia and complete dysphagia were also reported in patients with parapharyngeal and retropharyngeal space abscess with or without mediastinal emphysema [79]. High-grade fevers, dysphonia, dysphagia, anterior neck, and facial swelling may be present in Ludwig's angina. The condition progresses rapidly, causing edema and soft tissues gangrenous infection of the neck and floor of the mouth. A more aggressive course may end up with infection transmission to mediastinum (**Figure 11**) [81, 82].

Lemierre's syndrome (LS) is a disease characterized by thrombophlebitis of the internal jugular vein. As a result of bacterial infection, it is often preceded by oropharyngeal infection and often associated with *Fusobacterium necrophorum*. It was also reported to occur after surgical procedures within the neck (for example, transoral approach in a cervical osteophyte operation). Clinical presentation includes acute pharyngitis, high fever, dysphagia, dysphonia, and neck pain [83].

Hematomas can also be present in the neck tissues, leading to dysphonia and dysphagia occurring together. Reports were published in the literature describing such symptoms in spontaneous cervical hematoma caused by hemorrhage from a parathyroid carcinoma [84] and retropharyngeal hematoma appearing under rivaroxaban therapy for other reasons [85]. Commonly reported sites of spontaneous bleeding in patients treated with warfarin are the sublingual and retropharyngeal spaces. Hematomas occurring in these regions usually lead to sore throat, dysphagia, odynophagia, dysphonia, neck swelling, and dyspnea (**Figure 12**) [86].

Tumors of the neck region causing voice and swallowing problems together may represent the whole variety of histological and morphological types. Retropharyngeal liposarcoma can lead to neck swelling accompanied with dysphagia, orthopnea, and

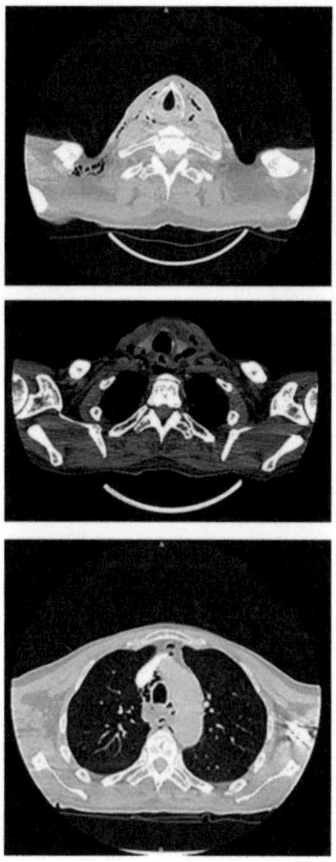

**Figure 11.**
*CT scans showing left parapharyngeal abscess with tracking into the prevertebral space and significant progression of air pockets in mediastinal and cervical soft tissue extending to the right axillary region (source: [80]).*

dysphonia [87]. Head and neck squamous cell carcinoma and head and neck low-grade chondrosarcoma were described in the literature to cause dysphonia and dysphagia as well as pain and neck mass sensation [88, 89]. Other tumors, like rhabdomyomas (RM), are benign and rare mesenchymal tumors made up of striated muscle cells. Extracardiac rhabdomyomas occur mostly in elderly men, prevailingly in the head and neck region like the oral cavity, larynx, pharynx, and soft tissue. Dysphagia, dysphonia, and stertor

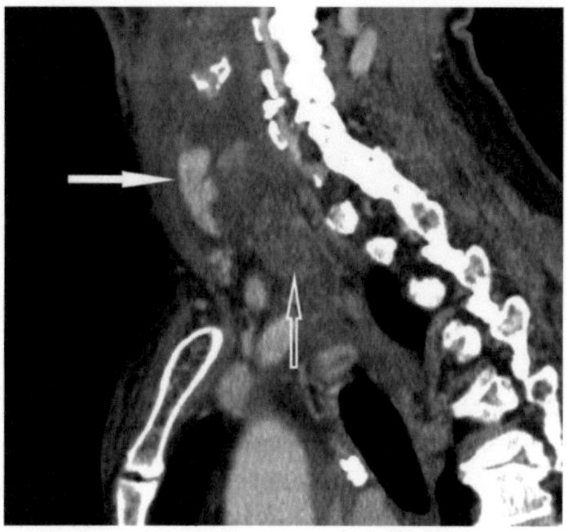

**Figure 12.**
*Contrast CT scan, sagittal plane, showing the thyroid gland (solid arrow) displaced anteriorly by a dense collection (open arrow) in keeping with a hematoma (source: [84]).*

are common symptoms [90]. A large sublingual dermoid cyst may become a reason for swallowing and voice problems [91] and so can an epidermal cyst of the thyroid gland with swelling in the anterior neck [92]. Similarly, Zenker diverticulum (ZD) or pharyngeal pouch, a structural or functional abnormality of the cricopharyngeal muscle, may cause dysphagia, dysphonia, cough, and regurgitation, while dysphonia is more frequent among patients with rather small pouches [93].

The thyroid gland, apart from its usual location in the anterior part of the neck, can also be seen in any place when remains of the thyroglossal duct (TGD) occur. In embryonic life, TDG comes down from the tongue to the diaphragm. Thyroid ectopia is commonly found at the base of the tongue in 90% of the reported cases. As such, it causes dysphagia and dysphonia at the same time [94].

Post-thyroid surgery hypocalcemia (PTSH) may occur after total thyroidectomy. Low calcium levels lead to neuromuscular instability and muscle numbness. The most severe cases may end up with laryngospasm and bronchospasm leading to breathing difficulties and stridor. Dysphonia and dysphagia are often in such cases [95].

A mass effect in the neck leading to swallowing problems and voice dysfunction with a weight loss was described in necrotizing sialo-metaplasia (NSM). This is a benign tumor of the salivary gland that occurs as a result of injury, chemical or traumatic metaplasia [96].

## 9. COVID complications

COVID infection was reported to have caused different clinical conditions with a whole variety of clinical manifestations. Many patients treated for COVID in intensive care units often suffered from dysphagia and dysphonia, laryngeal injuries as a result of prolonged intubation and neuropathies [97]. Post-extubating dysphagia and dysphonia were often described in COVID patients [98]. COVID patients often presented with dysphagia, dysphonia, middle airway disorders, such as chronic cough and hypersensitive larynx syndromes. The symptoms are multifactorial and wide ranging in pathophysiology, including medical interventions, tissue, and neurological injury [99].

Prolonged endotracheal intubation (also for non-COVID related reasons) may lead to some complications associated with dysphonia and dysphagia. Laryngeal granuloma

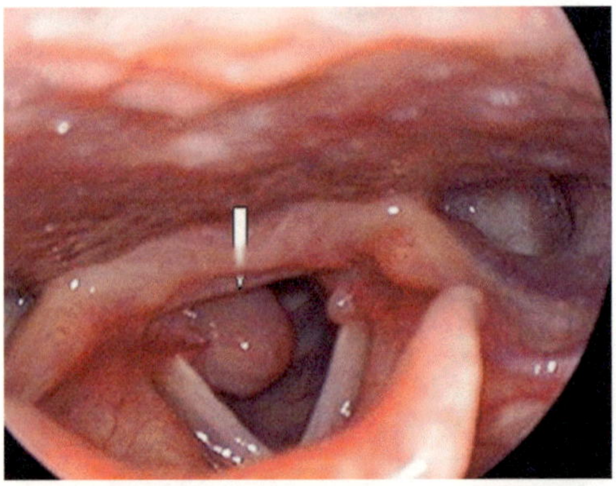

**Figure 13.**
*Laryngoscopic view of right-sided vocal cord granuloma. The granuloma appears lower than the level of the vocal cords (source: [100]).*

(LG) is a late complication of intubation and results from a trauma of the mucosa which ends up with granuloma formation (**Figure 13**). Compression of mucosa by an intubation tube may also lead to edema, ischemia, or damage to laryngeal mucosa and ultimately cause recurrent laryngeal nerve palsy. Dysphonia and dysphagia occur [100–102].

The post-COVID condition (PCC) is a disabling syndrome affecting at least 5–10% of subjects who survive COVID infection. As the main pathogenetic background of the condition, a SARS-CoV-2-mediated vagus nerve dysfunction is considered. The vagus nerve innervates the larynx, pharynx, lungs, heart, and gastrointestinal tract. PCC is therefore presented with dysphonia, dysphagia, dyspnea, dizziness, tachycardia, orthostatic hypotension, and gastrointestinal disturbances [103].

## 10. Treatment

Depending on the reason, dysphagia and dysphonia in cases described above, require multidisciplinary treatment. Due to complex etiology and possible life-threatening character, every medical condition associated with swallowing and voice problems needs a detailed, individual approach. As the causes are complex and vary, some cases may need medication; others are subjects to complicated operations and a systematic follow-up.

## 11. Conclusions

The above review is a detailed analysis of medical conditions and case reports described in the literature. Different pathologies leading to dysphonia and dysphagia need a complex approach both in diagnostics and treatment. It is a serious clinical problem and relates to various medical specialties. Due to this fact, concurrent dysphagia and dysphonia lie not only within the interest spectrum of otolaryngologists and phoniatricians but also neurologists, spine surgeons, chest surgeons, dental surgeons, oncologists, speech pathologists, rheumatologists, gastrologists, specialists in infectious diseases, and others. Effective diagnosis and treatment need the close cooperation of various specialists. Many cases may present a chronic course in some acute cases, however, the dynamics may lead to serious systemic complications, and ultimately to death.

Below, a list of abbreviations and a summary of the causes of concurrent dysphagia and dysphonia are presented (**Table 1**).

## Conflict of interest

The authors declare no conflict of interest.

## Abbreviations

| | |
|---|---|
| RLN | recurrent laryngeal nerve |
| CN | cranial nerve |
| NMO | neuromyelitis optica |

| | |
|---|---|
| Central nervous system | Hemorrhagic cerebral stroke<br>Ischemic cerebral stroke<br>Cerebral oedema<br>Intracranial hematoma<br>Primary brain tumors<br>*Glioma*<br>*Glioblastoma*<br>*Medulloblastoma*<br>*Lymphoma*<br>*Germ cell tumors*<br>*Vestibular schwannoma*<br>*Vagal schwannoma*<br>*Other*<br>Secondary brain tumors (metastases)<br>*Lung cancer*<br>*Melanoma*<br>*Prostatic cancer*<br>*Renal cancer*<br>*Gastric cancer*<br>*Other*<br>Gomphosis<br>Meningitis<br>Neuromyelitis optica<br>Acute brainstem syndrome<br>Intracranial arterial dolichoectasia<br>Parkinson's disease<br>Essential tremor<br>Atypical Parkinsonian syndromes<br>Amyotrophic lateral sclerosis<br>Alexander's disease<br>Wernicke encephalopathy<br>Bulbar palsy<br>Cranial nerves palsy |
| Peripheral nervous system | Guillain-Barre syndrome<br>Botulism<br>Post-polio syndrome<br>Varicella zoster infection<br>Herpes zoster infection<br>Jugular foramen syndrome (Vernet's syndrome)<br>Collet-Sicard syndrome<br>Spinal anesthesia complications<br>Vagus stimulation therapy complications |
| Cervical spine | Diffuse idiopathic skeletal hyperostosis<br>Cervical osteophytes<br>Cervical spondylosis (stenosis)<br>Cervical disc replacement complications<br>Degenerative cervical myelopathy<br>Anterior cervical discectomy and fusion complications |
| Muscles/connective tissue | Dermatomyositis<br>Mitochondrial myopathy<br>Ehlers-Danlos syndrome<br>Haycocknema perplexum induced myositis<br>Myasthenia gravis |

| | |
|---|---|
| Mediastinum | Liposarcoma<br>Ortner's syndrome (cardiovocal syndrome)<br>Tapia's syndrome<br>Thymoma<br>Lymphoma<br>Substernal goiter<br>Sarcoidosis<br>Mid-esophageal diverticula<br>Esophageal perforation<br>Mediastinal inflammation<br>Laparoscopic sleeve gastrectomy Complications<br>Pneumomediastinum (mediastinal emphysema)<br>Post pneumonectomy syndrome<br>Mediastinal lipomatosis<br>Heart and lung transplantation complications<br>Gastro-esophageal reflux |
| Larynx | Functional voice disorders<br>Muscle tension dysphonia<br>Glottal insufficiency (presbyphonia)<br>Unilateral vocal fold paresis<br>Bilateral vocal fold paresis<br>Laryngopharyngeal reflux<br>Extra nodal lymphoma<br>Non Hodgkin lymphoma<br>Laryngeal cancer<br>Neuroendocrine cancer<br>Laryngeal paraganglioma<br>Paraganglioma of the recurrent laryngeal nerve<br>Adult laryngeal hemangioma<br>Tuberculosis of the larynx<br>Laryngeal bullous pemphigoid<br>Epiglottic cyst<br>Postradiotherapy laryngopharyngeal edema<br>Traumatic laryngocele<br>Laryngeal leishmaniasis<br>Injection laryngoplasty complications<br>Blunt laryngeal trauma |
| Neck | Deep neck infections<br>Para/retropharyngeal abscess<br>Ludwig's angina<br>Lemierre's syndrome<br>Cervical hematomas<br>Neck tumors<br>*Cancer*<br>*Retropharyngeal liposarcoma*<br>*Neck squamous carcinoma*<br>*Rhabdomyoma*<br>*Sublingual dermoid cyst*<br>*Epidermic cyst of the thyroid gland*<br>*Pharyngeal pouch (Zenker diverticulum)*<br>*Thyroid ectopia (tongue location)*<br>*Post thyroid surgery hypocalcemia*<br>*Necrotizing sialometaplasia* |
| Covid complications | Prolonged intubation<br>Covid neuropathies<br>Post covid condition (vagus nerve dysfunction) |

**Table 1.**
*Summary of conditions associated with concomitant dysphagia and dysphonia.*

| | |
|---|---|
| IADE | intracranial arterial dolichoectasia |
| PD | Parkinson's disease |
| ET | essential tremor |
| APS | atypical Parkinsonian syndromes |
| ALS | amyotrophic lateral sclerosis |
| AD | Alexander's disease |
| GFAP | glial fibrillary acid protein |
| WE | Wernicke encephalopathy |
| GBS | Guillain-Barre syndrome |
| PS | post-polio syndrome |
| VZ | varicella zoster |
| HZ | herpes zoster |
| JFS | jugular foramen syndrome |
| VS | Vernet's syndrome |
| CSS | Collet-Sicard syndrome |
| DISH | diffuse idiopathic skeletal hyperostosis |
| CS | cervical spondylosis |
| CDR | cervical disc replacement |
| DCM | degenerative cervical myelopathy |
| ACDF | anterior cervical discectomy and fusion |
| DM | dermatomyosistis |
| IBM | inclusion body myositis |
| IMNM | immune mediated necrotizing myopathy |
| MM | mitochondrial myopathy |
| EDS | Ehlers-Danlos syndrome |
| HDCT | heritable disorder of connective tissue |
| hEDS | hypermobile Ehlers-Danlos syndrome |
| TMJD | temporomandibular joint disorder |
| LPR | laryngo-pharyngeal reflux |
| MG | myasthenia gravis |
| OS | Ortner's syndrome |
| TS | Tapia's syndrome |
| AVR | aortal valve replacement |
| CABG | coronary artery bypass grafting |
| ASDC | atrial septal defect closure |
| MVR | mitral valve repair |
| EP | esophageal perforation |
| SIRS | systemic inflammatory response syndrome |
| LSG | laparoscopic sleeve gastrectomy |
| ME | mediastinal emphysema |
| PPS | post-pneumonectomy syndrome |
| ML | mediastinal lipomatosis |
| MD | myotonic dystrophy |
| MTD | muscle tension dysphagia |
| LEMG | laryngeal electromyography |
| SEMG | superficial electromyography |
| VFP | vocal fold paresis |
| BVFP | bilateral vocal fold paresis |
| LPR | laryngopharyngeal reflux |
| ENL | extra nodal lymphoma |

| | |
|---|---|
| NHL | non-hodgkin lymphoma |
| NEC | neuroendocrine carcinoma |
| ALH | adult laryngeal hemangioma |
| BP | bullous pemphigoid |
| BLT | blunt laryngeal trauma |
| DNI | deep neck infection |
| LS | Lemierre's syndrome |
| RM | rhabdomyoma |
| ZD | Zenker diverticulum |
| TGD | thyroglossal duct |
| PTSH | post-thyroid surgery hypocalcemia |
| NSM | necrotizing sialo-metaplasia |
| LG | laryngeal granuloma |
| PCC | post-COVID condition |

## Author details

Karol Myszel[1*] and Piotr Henryk Skarzynski[2,3,4]

1 Center of Hearing and Speech, Nadarzyn/Kajetany, Poland

2 Department of Teleaudiology and Screening, World Hearing Center, Institute of Physiology and Pathology of Hearing, Warsaw, Poland

3 Institute of Sensory Organs, Nadarzyn/Kajetany, Poland

4 Faculty of Dental Medicine, Heart Failure and Cardiac Rehabilitation Department, Medical University of Warsaw, Warsaw, Poland

*Address all correspondence to: karol@myszel.pl

## References


[1] McCullagh KL, Shah RN, Huang BY. Anatomy of the larynx and cervical trachea. Neuroimaging Clinics of North America. Nov 2022;**32**(4):809-829. DOI: 10.1016/j.nic.2022.07.011. PMID: 36244725

[2] Black R, Novakovic D, Plit M, Miles A, MacDonald P, Madill C. Swallowing and laryngeal complications in lung and heart transplantation: Etiologies and diagnosis. The Journal of Heart and Lung Transplantation. 2021;**40**:1483-1494

[3] Jones CA, Colletti CM, Ding MC. Post-stroke dysphagia: Recent insights and unanswered questions. Current Neurology and Neuroscience Reports. 2020;**20**(12):61

[4] Labeit B, Michou E, Hamdy S, Trapl-Grundschober M, Suntrup-Krueger S, Muhle P, et al. The assessment of dysphagia after stroke: State of the art and future directions. Lancet Neurology. 2023;**22**(9):858-870

[5] Pereira VC, Fontão L, Engenheiro G, Gouveia F, Pinto L, Leal J, et al. Post-stroke dysphagia: Clinical characteristics and evolution in a single primary stroke center. NeuroRehabilitation. 2023;**52**(3):507-514

[6] Vasan V, Hardigan TA, Ali M, Downes M, Devarajan A, Rossitto CP, et al. Dysphagia after ischemic and hemorrhagic stroke: A propensity-matched 20-year analysis of the national inpatient sample. Journal of Stroke and Cerebrovascular Diseases. 2023;**32**(9):107295

[7] Caramanti R, Moreira Aprígio R, Tognola W, Laurenti M, Rocha C, Góes M. Transtentorial spread of glioblastoma multiforme to cerebellopontine angle. A rare case report. Surgical Neurology International. 2022;**13**(5):1-4

[8] Lieber S, Nunez M, Tatagiba M. Lateral suboccipital approach in semisitting position for resection of vagal schwannoma: 2-dimensional operative video. Journal of Neurological Surgery. 2021;**82**(suppl. S1):S51-S52

[9] Haider Alshurafa Z, Alkhateeb M. Seronegative neuromyelitis optica spectrum disorder: An unusual presentation of acute brainstem syndrome. American Journal of Case Reports. 2020;**21**:e922590

[10] Younus O, Hampton T, Silber E, et al. Progressive bulbar symptomatology due to vascular brainstem compression. BML Case Reports. 2021;**14**:e238323

[11] Chaudhry HS, Ata F, Abdelghani M, et al. Isolated bulbar palsy: A rare presentation of neurosarcoidosis. Cureus. 2020;**12**(2):e7010

[12] Thijs Z, Dumican M. Laryngeal symptoms related to motor phenotypes in Parkinson's disease: A systematic review. Laryngoscope Investigative Otolaryngology. 2023;**8**:970-979

[13] Dumican M, Watts C. Self-perceptions of speech, voice, and swallowing in motor phenotypes of Parkinson's disease. Clinical Parkinsonism and Related Disorders. 2020;**3**:100074

[14] Finger M, Madden L, Haq I, McLouth C, Siddiqui M. Analysis of the prevalence and onset of dysphonia and dysphagia symptoms in movement disorders at an Academic Medical Center. Clinical Neuroscience. 2019;**64**:111-115

[15] AlMadan N, AlMajed A, AlAbbad M, et al. Dental management of patients with amyotrophic lateral sclerosis. Cureus. 2023;**15**(12):e50602

[16] Srivastava S, Waldman A, Naidu S. Alexander disease. In: Adam MP, Feldman J, Mirzaa GM, Pagon RA, Wallace SE, Bean LJH, et al., editors. GeneReviews® [Internet]. Seattle (WA): University of Washington, Seattle; 2002 [Updated 2020 Nov 12]. pp. 1993-2024

[17] Cornea A, Lata I, Simu M, Rosca EC. Wernicke encephalopathy presenting with dysphagia: A case report and systematic literature review. Nutrients. 2022;**14**:5294

[18] Sidoli C, Bruni A, Beretta S, Mazzola P, Bellelli G. Guillain-Barre syndrome AMSAN variant in a 90-year-old woman after COVID-19: A case report. BMC Geriatrics. 2023;**23**:114

[19] Dukkipati S, Zhou D, Powers A, Piccione E, Koh. Acute bulbar palsy-plus variant of Guillain-Barré syndrome in a 3-year-old girl. Child Neurology Open. 1 Aug 2022;**9**:2329048X221115476

[20] Neeki et al. Early diagnosis and critical management of wound botulism in the emergency department: A single center experience and literature review. International Journal of Emergency Medicine. 2021;**14**:56

[21] Oluwasanmi OJ, Mckenzie DA, Adewole IO, Aluka CO, Iyasse J, Olunu E, et al. Postpolio syndrome: A review of lived experiences of patients. International Journal of Applied and Basic Medical Research. 2019;**9**:129-134

[22] Jia F, Ting E, Ahn JH, Duggins A. Varicella zoster-associated progressive lower cranial and upper cervical polyneuropathy: A case report. Journal of Medical Case Reports. 2022;**16**:313

[23] Wang Z, Lotina T, Malaty J. Uncommon presentation and complications of herpes zoster infection involving the cervical, vagus and accessory nerves which caused a delay in diagnosis and treatment. BMJ Case Reports. 7 May 2021;**14**(5):e241881

[24] Evan J, Johansen M, Akst LM. Dysphagia, dysphonia and a deviated tongue: Diagnosing Collet-Sicard syndrome. BML Case Reports. 21 May 2021;**14**(5):e243154

[25] Akhaddar A, Salami M, Darouassi Y. Transient lower cranial nerve palsies following spinal anesthesia with bupivacaine-fentanyl combination for transurethral resection of the prostate. Pan African Medical Journal. 2020;**35**:62

[26] Castellani L, Chiesa V, Maccari A, et al. Pharyngolaryngeal spasm-induced dysphagia in an epileptic patient undergoing vagus nerve stimulation therapy. Clinical Case Reports. 2020;**8**:858-861

[27] Costa CC, Valter H, Ramos L, Alves W, Lamounier P, Castro Velasco L, et al. Partial laryngectomy and reconstruction with rotation of the epiglottis in the treatment of a rare laryngeal schwannoma: A case report. Journal of Medical Case Reports. 2020;**14**:229

[28] Zarei M, Golbakhsh M, Rostami M, Moosavi M. Dysphonia, stridor, and dysphagia caused by diffuse idiopathic skeletal hyperostosis: Case report and review of literature. Advanced Biomedical Research. 2020;**9**:47

[29] Kumar M, Shahi PB, Adsul N, Acharya S, Kalra KL, Chahal RS. Progressive dysphagia and dysphonia secondary to dish-related anterior cervical osteophytes: A case report. Surgical Neurology International. 2020;**11**:69

[30] Maiuri F, Cavallo LM, Corvino S, Teodonno G, Mariniello G. Anterior cervical osteophytes causing dysphagia: Choice of the approach and surgical problems. Journal of Craniovertebral Junction and Spine. Oct-Dec 2020;**11**(4):300-309. DOI: 10.4103/jcvjs.JCVJS_147_20. Epub 2020 Nov 26. PMID: 33824560; PMCID: PMC8019107

[31] Saral Jain N, Nguyen A, Formanek B, Alluri R, Buser Z, Hah R, et al. Cervical disc replacement: Trends, costs, and complications. Asian Spine Journal. 2020;**14**(5):647-654

[32] Tetreault L, Lange S, Chotai S, et al. A systematic review of definitions for dysphagia and dysphonia in patients treated surgically for degenerative cervical myelopathy. Global Spine Journal. 2022;**12**(7):1535-1545

[33] Alsoof D, Perry J, Yang ZA, et al. Risk of dysphagia and dysphonia in patients with prior thyroidectomy undergoing anterior cervical discectomy and fusion. Global Spine Journal. 2024;**14**(2):494-502

[34] Weinreb SF, Piersiala K, Hillel AT, Lee M, Akst LM, Best SR. Dysphonia and dysphagia as early manifestations of autoimmune inflammatory myopathy. American Journal of Otolaryngology. 2021;**42**(1):102747

[35] Okogbaa J, Batiste L. Dermatomyositis: An acute flare and current treatments. Clinical Medicine Insights: Case Reports. 2019;**12**:1-8

[36] Manini A, Meneri M, Rodolico C, Corti S. Case report: Thymidine kinase 2 (TK2) deficiency: A novel mutation associated with childhood-onset mitochondrial myopathy and atypical progression. Frontiers in Neurology. 2022;**13**:857279

[37] Williams HR, Wood G, Hakim AJ, Birchall M, Hirani SP. Self-reported throat symptoms in Ehlers–Danlos syndromes and hypermobility spectrum disorders: A cross-sectional survey study. Laryngoscope Investigative Otolaryngology. 2023;**8**:1259-1264

[38] Pritt BS, Mathison BA, Bradbury RS, Liewluck T, Nickolau S, O'Horo JC, et al. Imported haycocknema perplexum infection, United States. Emerging Infectious Diseases. 2022;**28**(11):2281-2284

[39] Balabbigari N, Purewal J, Sakul NFM, Purewal A, Kankanala V, Califano T. Cranial nerve IX and X weakness: An unusual initial presentation of myasthenia gravis. American Journal of Case Reports. 2020;**21**:e923750

[40] Torres-Barrera G, Herrera-Quiñones G, Scharrer SI, Benavides-Salgado DE, Maldonado-Garza HJ, Achem SR. High-resolution esophageal manometry in myasthenia gravis. ACG Case Reports Journal. 2020;7:e00340

[41] Portnoy R, Abbasi R, Yablonsky TM, Cohen EG, Widmann M. Mediastinal liposarcoma: Case report with radiology review. Radiology Case Reports. 2024;**19**:3294-3300

[42] Verma S, An T, Ab T, Khan S, Krishnasastry KV, Ar T. Ortner's syndrome: A systematic review of presentation, diagnosis and management. Intractable and Rare Diseases Research. 2023;**12**(3):141-147

[43] Subramaniam V, Herle A, Mohammed N, Thahir M. Ortner's syndrome: Case series and literature review. Brazilian Journal of Otorhinolaryngology. 2011;77(5):559-562. DOI: 10.1590/s1808-86942011000500004

[44] Steehler AJ, Rothman R, Sadhar B, Saran M, Lipman SP, Lipman RI. Tapia's syndrome after cardiac surgery: A case report and review of literature. Ear, Nose and Throat Journal. 13 Jul 2022:1455613221113807

[45] Nalladaru Z, Wessels A, DuPreez L. Tapia's syndrome--A rare complication following cardiac surgery. Interactive Cardiovascular and Thoracic Surgery. 2012;**14**(1):131-132. DOI: 10.1093/icvts/ivr056. Epub 2011 Nov 17

[46] Koulouris C, Paraschou A, Manaki V, Mantalovas S, Spiridou K, Spiridou A, et al. Cardiopulmonary arrest caused by large substernal goiter—Treatment with combined cervical approach and median mini-sternotomy: Report of a case. Medicina. 2021;**57**:303

[47] Rolski W, Kiprian D. Superior vena cava syndrome. Medycyna Paliatywna/Palliative Medicine. 2012;**4**(2):90-94

[48] Kumar V, Abbas A, Aster J. Robbins Basic Pathology. 9th ed. USA: Elsevier Urban and Partner; 2014. ISBN 978-1-4377-1781-5

[49] Zimmerman S, Davis M. Rapid fire: Superior vena cava syndrome. Emergency Medicine Clinics of North America. 2018;**36**(3):577-584. DOI: 10.1016/j.emc.2018.04.011. Epub 2018 Jun 12

[50] Mes SD, Kalkeren TA, Jacobs RJ, Coene IMJH, Langeveld APM, Locher H. Hiding in plain sight: An unusual case of progressive dysphagia, dyspnea and dysphonia. Dysphagia. 2021;**36**:754-757

[51] Tadayon SM, Moeinvaziri N, Amini M, Setoodeh M, Haghighat N. Esophageal perforation during laparoscopic sleeve gastrectomy: Complication of bougie insertion. International Journal of Surgery Case Reports. 2021;**81**(105793)

[52] Khaitan PG, Famiglietti A, Watson TJ. The etiology, diagnosis, and management of esophageal perforation. Journal of Gastrointestinal Surgery. 2022;**26**(12):2606-2615. DOI: 10.1007/s11605-022-05454-2. Epub 2022 Sep 22

[53] Yılmaz F, Zortuk O. Subcutaneous emphysema, pneumomediastinum and spinal epidural emphysema as complications of violent coughing: A case report. Acta Biomed. 2021;**92**(Suppl. 1):e2021141

[54] Chen YH, Lin PC, Chen YL, Yiang GT, Wu MY. Point-of-care ultrasonography helped to rapidly detect pneumomediastinum in a vomiting female. Medicina. 2023;**59**:394

[55] Rego E, Abdelmeguid A, Wang YK, Dewan K. An uncommon cause of dysphagia: Postpneumonectomy syndrome. In: Case Reports in Otolaryngology. 2021. p. e6658690

[56] Finsterer J, Scorza FA. Mediastinal and pleural lipomatosis as a manifestation of myotonic dystrophy type 1. Lung India. 2021;**38**:486-488

[57] Altman K, Atkinson C, Lazarus C. Current and emerging concepts in muscle tension dysphonia: A 30-month review. Journal of Voice. 2005;**19**:261-267

[58] Krasnodebska P, Szkiełkowska A, Jarzynska-Bucko A, Włodarczyk E, Miaskiewicz B. Characteristics of swallowing disorders in patients with dysphonia. Otolaryngologia Polska. 2020;**74**:17-22

[59] DePietro J, Rubin S, Stein D, Golan H, Noordzij P. Laryngeal manipulation for dysphagia with muscle tension dysphonia. Dysphagia. 2018;**33**:468-473

[60] Krasnodebska P, Jarzynska-Bucko A, Szkiełkowska A, Bartosik J. Clinical and electromyographic assessment of swallowing in individuals with functional dysphonia associated with dysphagia due to muscle tension or atypical swallowing. Audiology Research. 2021;**11**:167-178

[61] Tsunoda K, Hashimoto S, Kuroda H, Ishii T, Takazawa M. Exploring the relation between glottal closure and plasma substance P: A study protocol. The Tohoku Journal of Experimental Medicine. 2019;**249**:237-240

[62] Onwordi LN, Al Yaghchi C. Airway glottic insufficiency. In: StatPearls. Treasure Island (FL): StatPearls Publishing; 2024

[63] Usman H, Protts F, Fathers E, Chisholm E. Thinking beyond otorhinolaryngology in patients presenting with bilateral vocal cord paresis. Journal of Surgical Case Reports. 2023;**3**:1-3

[64] Tibbetts KM, Simpson CB. Adult bilateral vocal fold paralysis. Current Otorhinolaryngology Reports. 2021;**9**:365-372. DOI: 10.1007/s40136-021-00359-1

[65] Lin Y, Peng S. Current treatment of laryngopharyngeal reflux. Ear, Nose and Throat Journal. 9 Jun 2023:1455613231180031

[66] Singh Gendeh H, Singh GB. Updates on laryngo-pharyngeal reflux (LPR) and its management. In: Updates on Laryngology. London, UK: IntechOpen; 2023. DOI: 10.5772/intechopen.109733

[67] Ayyaswamy A, Saravanam PK, Latha S, Sundaram S. Laryngeal lymphoma in a child—Case report and review of literature. Iranian Journal of Otorhinolaryngology. 2022;**34**(6):337-341

[68] Dougherty T, Aitken G, Harrell RM, Edwards C, Guerrero SV, Bimston. Paraganglioma of the recurrent laryngeal nerve. AACE Clinical Case Reports. 2024;**10**:24-26

[69] OuYang Z, Lou Z. Management of adult laryngeal hemangioma with low-temperature plasma radiofrequency coblation ear. Nose and Throat Journal. 3 Jul 2023:1455613231185018

[70] Bouatay R, Bouaziz N, Abdallah H, Ben Hammouda S, Koubaa J. Isolated laryngeal tuberculosis: A diagnostic dilemma. International Journal of Surgery Case Reports. 2024;**116**:e109376

[71] Hamdan AL, Chaar JA, Rahal JA. Laryngeal manifestations of bullous pemphigoid: Case report and review of the literature. Ear, Nose and Throat Journal. 6 Feb 2024:1455613241230252

[72] Akı ES, Çorakçı O, Canpolat S. Multiple dermoid cysts in the epiglottis presenting with dysphonia and dysphagia: A rare case. Turkish Archives of Otorhinolaryngology. 2022;**60**(3):173-176

[73] Tritter AG, Spiller PT, Brown ML, Weinberger PM, Nathan CO. Pilot study: Pneumatic compression garment therapy for postradiotherapy laryngopharyngeal edema. Ear, Nose and Throat Journal. 2022;**101**(1):54-58

[74] Biswas S, Saran M. Blunt trauma to the neck presenting as dysphonia and dysphagia in a healthy young woman; a rare case of traumatic laryngocele. Bulletin of Emergency and Trauma. 2020;**8**(2):129-131

[75] Renard L, Lemaignen A, Desoubeaux BD. Case report: Progressive dysphonia and dysphagia due to laryngeal leishmaniasis. The American

Journal of Tropical Medicine and Hygiene. 2021;**105**(2):458-460

[76] Kamarudin N, Abdul Rahim N, Azman M, et al. Subchordal cyst containing non-degraded hyaluronic acid: A rare complication of injection laryngoplasty. Cureus. 2022;**14**(8):e27801

[77] Nganzeu C, Esce A, Abu-Ghanem S, Meiklejohn DA, Sims HS. Laryngeal trauma. Otolaryngologic Clinics of North America. 2023;**56**(6):1039-1053. DOI: 10.1016/j.otc.2023.06.001. Epub 2023 Jul 11

[78] Maharaj S, Ahmed S, Pillay P. Deep neck space infections: A case series and review of the literature. Clinical Medicine Insights: Ear, Nose and Throat. 2019;**12**:1179550619871274. DOI: 10.1177/1179550619871274

[79] Pesis M, Bar-Droma E, Ilgiyaev A, Givol N. Deep neck infections, life threatening infections of dental origin: Presentation and management of selected cases. The Israel Medical Association Journal. 2019;**21**(12):806-811

[80] Woodun H, Woodun H, Sethi N, Simons A. Idiopathic hypopharyngeal perforation presenting as supraglottitis and parapharyngeal abscess: Case report and literature review. Journal of Surgical Case Reports. Jan 2022;**2022**(1):rjab569. DOI: 10.1093/jscr/rjab569

[81] Kovalev V. A severe case of Ludwig's angina with a complicated clinical course. Cureus. 2020;**12**(4):e7695

[82] Mendes SC. Life-threatening complications of Ludwig's angina: A series of cases in a developed country. BML Case Reports. 2021;**14**(4):e240429

[83] Mariniello G, Corvino S, Teodonno G, Pagano S, Maiuri F. Postoperative Lemierre's syndrome: A previously unreported complication of transoral surgery. Illustrative Case. Journal of Neurosurgery Case Lessons. 2021;**1**(17):CASE20118

[84] Bates J, LaPorte S, Abraham A, et al. Spontaneous cervical haematoma caused by extracapsular haemorrhage from a parathyroid carcinoma presenting with acute onset neck swelling and dysphonia. BML Case Reports. 2021;**14**:e239150

[85] Vierendeels C, Peeters X, Bosschaert P. Retropharyngeal hematoma under rivaroxaban: A rare entity to know for its risk of airway obstruction. Journal of the Belgian Society of Radiology. 2021;**105**(1):15, 1-4

[86] Ashraf A, Bannon M, Smith C, Kaushik P, Marak C. Upper airway hematoma: An unusual presentation of acute upper airway obstruction. Respiratory Medicine Case Reports. 2022;**36**:101612

[87] Arshad W, Maqbool S, Kiany JA, Raza A, Farooq U, Ali Q, et al. A rare case of retropharyngeal liposarcoma: A rare location of a rare diagnosis. Journal of Surgical Case Reports. 2023;**3**:1-3

[88] Strüder D, Ebert J, Kalle F, Schraven SP, Eichhorst L, Mlynski R, et al. Head and neck cancer: A study on the complex relationship between QoL and swallowing function. Current Oncology. 2023;**30**:10336-10350

[89] Mirestean CC, Simionescu CE, Iancu RI, Stan MC, Iancu DPT, Badulescu F. Head and neck low grade chondrosarcoma—A rare entity. Diagnostics. 2023;**13**:3026

[90] Salameh B, Ghareeb A, Badran H, Salameh H, Hajali W, Alassaf A. Rhabdomyoma in the base of the tongue:

A case report. International Journal of Surgery Case Reports. 2022;**95**:107239

[91] Barzegar M, Akhavan-Tafti Y, Soltani HR, Goodarzi M. A large sublingual dermoid cyst causing dysphagia and dysphonia: A case review study. Case Reports in Dentistry. 28 Jul 2023;**2023**:7776558

[92] Mousa H, Aljassem R. A case report of uncommon giant epidermal inclusion cyst found in the thyroid gland. Annals of Medicine and Surgery. 2024;**86**:2214-2221

[93] Martinez-Paredes JF, Alfakir R, Kasperbauer J, Rutt A. Zenker diverticulum: Does size correlate with preoperative symptoms? International Archives of Otorhinolaryngology. 2022;**26**(3):e334-e338

[94] Kumar A, Singhal T, Krishna SM, Narayan ML. Dual thyroid ectopia: A pictorial case series and review of literature. World Journal of Nuclear Medicine. 2020;**19**:336-340

[95] Thomas C, Bhamra N, Darr A, Amlani A, Murphy J. Simultaneous dysphagia and stridor: An unreported presentation of hypocalcaemia. Journal of Surgical Case Reports. 2020;**9**:1-2

[96] Gadkaree SK, Fuller JC, Sadow DDG, Jeremy D, Richmon JD. Necrotizing sialometaplasia of the hypopharynx. Ear, Nose, and Throat Journal. 2019;**98**(9):NP138–NP141

[97] Miles A, McRae J, Clunie G, Gillivan-Murphy P, Inamoto Y, Kalf H, et al. An international commentary on dysphagia and dysphonia during the COVID-19 pandemic. Dysphagia. 2022;**37**:1349-1374

[98] Regan J, Walshe M, Lavan S, et al. Post-extubation dysphagia and dysphonia amongst adults with COVID-19 in the Republic of Ireland: A prospective multi-site observational cohort study. Clinical Otolaryngology. 2021;**46**:1290-1299

[99] Miles A, Brodsky M. Current opinion of presentation of dysphagia and dysphonia in patients with coronavirus disease 2019. Current Opinion in Otolaryngology and Head and Neck Surgery. 2022;**30**:393-399

[100] Song JG, Cho WH, Ji SM, Park JH, Kim SK. Laryngeal granulomas in patients after two-jaw surgery—Four cases report. Anesthesia and Pain Medicine (Seoul). 2019;**14**(4):489-493. DOI: 10.17085/apm.2019.14.4.489

[101] Kikura M, Suzuki Y, Itagaki T, Sato T, Nishino J. Vocal cord paralysis associated with tracheal intubation: Incidence, risk analysis, and classification of severity. Masui. 2015;**64**(1):57-59. Japanese

[102] Pan DR, Jiang N. Outcomes of intubation-induced vocal fold motion impairment. Journal of Voice. 2020;**34**(2):250-258. DOI: 10.1016/j.jvoice.2018.09.015. Epub 2018 Oct 9

[103] Llad G et al. Vagus nerve dysfunction in the post COVID-19 condition: A pilot cross-sectional study. Clinical Microbiology and Infection. 2024;**30**:515e52

Chapter 2

# Esophageal Motility Disorders and Dysphagia: Understanding Causes and Consequences

*Irfan Corovic, Mladen Maksic, Dusan Radojevic, Samir Vucelj, Sabir Sagdati, Isidora Stanisavljevic, Tijana Veljkovic, Bojana Simovic Markovic, Ivan Jovanovic, Bojan Stojanovic, Dusan Popovic, Djordje Kralj and Marina Jovanovic*

## Abstract

Esophageal motility disorders are common conditions that impede the normal movement of food and liquids from the esophagus to the stomach, frequently manifesting as dysphagia, chest pain, and regurgitation. These disorders arise from a variety of etiological factors and can greatly diminish patients' quality of life. If left untreated, esophageal motility disorders may lead to severe complications, including malnutrition, weight loss, and aspiration pneumonia. This chapter offers an in-depth examination of the etiology and pathogenesis of both primary and secondary EMDs. It thoroughly investigates the clinical manifestations and diagnostic methods, highlighting the critical role of differential diagnosis in the accurate identification of these conditions. Additionally, the chapter reviews current treatment options, including pharmacological interventions, endoscopic procedures, and surgical techniques, and discusses the potential of novel therapies and future research directions. Through a detailed analysis of these aspects, the chapter aims to provide a comprehensive understanding of esophageal motility disorders and to guide effective clinical management and innovative therapeutic approaches.

**Keywords:** esophageal motility disorders, esophagus, dysphagia, achalasia, distal esophageal spasm, jackhammer esophagus, gastroesophageal reflux disease, high-resolution manometry, endoscopy

## 1. Introduction

Esophageal motility disorders (EMDs) encompass a range of conditions that disrupt the normal passage of food and liquids from the esophagus to the stomach. Commonly marked by dysphagia (difficulty swallowing), chest pain, and regurgitation of food, these disorders are prevalent worldwide [1]. Dysphagia can result in malnutrition, weight loss, and dehydration due to swallowing difficulties. Additionally, the regurgitation of undigested food increases the risk of aspiration, potentially causing pneumonia and other respiratory issues. Furthermore, the psychological burden of living with a chronic swallowing disorder can contribute to anxiety and depression, further diminishing the quality of life [2]. The association of EMDs with complications such as esophageal cancer is well-established [3]. Using the Chicago Classification version (CCV) 4.0, EMDs are categorized as follows: achalasia, esophagogastric junction (EGJ) outflow obstruction, distal esophageal spasm (previously diffuse esophageal spasm), hypercontractile (jackhammer) esophagus, absent contractility, and ineffective esophageal motility (IEM) [4]. Given their prevalence, impact on quality of life, and potential for serious complications, this chapter aims to investigate the pathogenesis, clinical presentation, diagnosis, and treatment of primary and secondary EMDs leading to dysphagia, with particular emphasis on achalasia, distal esophageal spasm (DES), and jackhammer esophagus.

## 2. Etiology

EMDs can be broadly classified into primary and secondary types. Primary disorders are idiopathic, whereas secondary disorders are mostly associated with systemic diseases [5]. During swallowing, involuntary esophageal motility is coordinated by extrinsic nerves. Normally inactive during fasting, the esophagus undergoes specific changes during voluntary swallowing: the upper esophageal sphincter (UES) and lower esophageal sphincter (LES) relax to allow food entry and exit, respectively. Once the food bolus passes through the UES, an involuntary peristaltic wave, known as the "primary peristaltic wave," swiftly propels it toward the stomach.

Initially, sensory signals travel *via* several cranial nerves to the solitary tract nucleus in the brainstem, where motor signals are coordinated. These motor signals then travel *via* vagal fibers to the cervical esophagus (through the recurrent laryngeal nerves) and the proximal esophagus (through thoracic vagal fibers) to initiate and sustain the primary peristaltic wave [6]. The specific etiology of primary EMDs remains unknown, but research indicates that a combination of genetic, lifestyle, and environmental factors can contribute to their onset [7–9]. Understanding these complex interactions is crucial for developing effective prevention and treatment strategies for these disorders. Ongoing research aims to unravel the mechanisms underlying these conditions, shedding light on new treatments and improved patient outcomes.

### 2.1 Genetic background

The genetic etiology of EMDs is a complex and evolving field. Understanding the genetic basis of these disorders could lead to improved diagnostic tools, targeted therapies, and personalized treatment approaches for affected individuals. As genetic research advances, it holds the promise of unlocking new insights into the underlying causes of these challenging and often debilitating disorders.

#### *2.1.1 Achalasia*

Achalasia is a primary EMDs characterized by the failure of the LES to relax and the absence of esophageal peristalsis [10]. Although the exact cause is unclear, familial cases and twin studies indicate a genetic component [11, 12]. Several gene mutations have been implicated. For example, certain alleles of the human leukocyte antigen (HLA) system, specifically HLA-DQ, are associated with an increased risk of achalasia, suggesting an autoimmune component potentially triggered by genetic predisposition [13, 14]. Additionally, mutations in the ALADIN gene, which is associated with triple-A syndrome (alacrima, achalasia, adrenal insufficiency, neurologic disorder), further indicate a genetic link in some achalasia cases, providing insight into potential genetic pathways involved in the disorder [15].

#### *2.1.2 DES*

DES is defined by uncoordinated esophageal contractions, which result in symptoms such as chest pain and dysphagia [5]. While the genetic underpinnings of DES are not as well-documented as those of achalasia, existing evidence indicates a hereditary component. The presence of DES in multiple family members suggests that genetic factors may play a role in its pathogenesis [16, 17].

#### *2.1.3 Jackhammer esophagus*

This rare EMD results in dysphagia, chest pain, and gastroesophageal reflux symptoms [18, 19]. Research into its genetic etiology is still in its early stages. Future studies are needed to identify specific genetic mutations or polymorphisms associated with this condition. The terms "classic jackhammer esophagus" and "spastic jackhammer esophagus" have been introduced to distinguish between the types, indicating a heterogeneous disease with varying underlying pathophysiology [20].

Understanding these genetic factors is crucial for developing effective prevention and treatment strategies for EMDs. Ongoing research aims to unravel the mechanisms underlying these conditions, potentially leading to new treatments and improved patient outcomes.

### 2.2 Environmental and lifestyle factors in EMDs

Various environmental and lifestyle factors can influence the occurrence of EMDs. Factors such as diet, alcohol consumption, tobacco use, stress, and medication use can contribute to the development and exacerbation of these disorders by affecting the esophageal muscles, nerves, and overall function [7, 21].

#### *2.2.1 Diet and eating habits*

Consuming a diet high in fats can slow gastric emptying and affect esophageal motility. This can exacerbate symptoms such as reflux, acid regurgitation, postprandial fullness, heartburn, swallowing obstruction or pain, epigastric burning sensation, chest pain, chronic laryngopharyngitis, and cough in individuals with EMDs [22]. Similarly, spicy foods can irritate the esophagus and intensify symptoms due to capsaicin stimulating nerve endings in the esophagus, potentially triggering esophageal spasms [23, 24]. Additionally, eating large meals can increase pressure in the stomach and esophagus, leading to motility issues and gastroesophageal reflux, worsening symptoms such as chest pain and regurgitation [25]. Irregular eating patterns, such as skipping meals or eating at inconsistent times, can disrupt normal esophageal function and contribute to motility disorders [25]. Therefore, maintaining a consistent meal schedule is important for promoting healthy digestion and minimizing symptoms in individuals with EMDs. Obesity is also a significant risk factor for esophageal dysfunction, as excess body weight increases intra-abdominal pressure, leading to LES dysfunction and reflux [26].

#### *2.2.2 Alcohol, tobacco, and medication use*

Excessive alcohol intake can damage the esophageal mucosa and impair motility. Alcohol can also relax the LES, contributing to reflux and EMDs [27]. Smoking has been linked to various gastrointestinal disorders, including EMDs. Nicotine can relax the LES and impair esophageal motility, increasing the risk of reflux and dysphagia [28]. Additionally, certain medications can affect esophageal motility. For example, nifedipine, a calcium channel blocker commonly used for hypertension, can relax the LES and impair esophageal contractions [29]. Opioids and anticholinergic medications can also negatively affect esophageal motility [30, 31].

#### *2.2.3 Stress and psychological factors*

Psychological stress and anxiety have been shown to impact esophageal motility, with stressors potentially leading to increased esophageal sensitivity and altered motility patterns [32]. These effects can contribute to the development or worsening of disorders such as functional heartburn and globus sensation, characterized by the feeling of a lump in the throat. The relationship between stress and esophageal motility is complex and not fully understood. However, it is believed that stress-induced alterations in nerve signaling and hormonal responses may play a role in these effects [33].

### 2.3 Secondary EMDs

Secondary EMDs arise from various underlying conditions that affect the normal functioning of the esophagus. These disorders can manifest due to a wide range of etiologies, including collagen vascular diseases, diabetes, Chagas' disease, amyloidosis, multiple sclerosis (MS), idiopathic pseudo-obstruction, or the aging process [34]. They can affect esophageal motility through mechanisms such as nerve damage, muscle weakness, inflammation, and structural changes. Understanding the diverse causes of secondary EMDs is crucial for accurate diagnosis and effective management. Neurological diseases like Parkinson's disease, MS, and stroke can disrupt the neural pathways controlling esophageal peristalsis and sphincter function, impacting swallowing [35–37]. Systemic autoimmune conditions like systemic sclerosis (scleroderma) and systemic lupus erythematosus (SLE) can lead to fibrosis and thickening of esophageal tissues, resulting in impaired motility [38, 39]. Structural abnormalities such as hiatal hernia, esophageal strictures, and tumors (benign or malignant) can mechanically obstruct the esophagus, causing dysmotility and difficulty swallowing [40–42]. As outlined in the introduction, this section will explore the fundamental mechanisms by which secondary disorders contribute to esophageal motility dysfunction, with particular emphasis on gastroesophageal reflux disease (GERD) due to its high prevalence.

#### *2.3.1 Neurological diseases*

Neurological diseases represent a significant category of conditions leading to secondary EMDs. These disorders arise from disruptions in the neural control mechanisms responsible for coordinating esophageal peristalsis and sphincter function. Recognizing the impact of neurological diseases on esophageal motility is crucial for implementing appropriate diagnostic and therapeutic strategies to improve swallowing function and quality of life for affected individuals. Parkinson's disease is characterized by the degeneration of dopaminergic neurons in the substantia nigra, resulting in dopamine deficiency affecting the basal ganglia, which are crucial for coordinating smooth muscle movements, including those in the esophagus [35, 43]. Patients with Parkinson's disease often experience dysphagia due to impaired peristalsis and reduced LES relaxation, leading to difficulty swallowing solids and liquids [35]. MS is an inflammatory disease affecting the central nervous system, causing demyelination of nerve fibers [44]. Lesions along the neural pathways controlling esophageal function disrupt the signal transmission necessary for coordinated peristalsis, resulting in dysphagia, regurgitation, and chest pain [36]. Stroke can damage brain areas that are responsible for swallowing reflexes and esophageal muscle coordination. Depending on the stroke's location and extent, patients may experience dysphagia ranging from mild difficulty swallowing to a complete inability to swallow, along with impaired esophageal motility [37]. Amyotrophic lateral sclerosis (ALS) is a progressive neurodegenerative disease characterized by significant loss of motor neurons in the spinal cord, brainstem, and motor cortex [45]. As the disease progresses, patients may develop dysphagia due to the weakening of the muscles involved in swallowing, including those in the esophagus, leading to impaired peristalsis and reduced LES tone [46].

#### *2.3.2 Systemic autoimmune conditions*

Systemic autoimmune conditions significantly contribute to secondary EMDs by inducing structural changes and inflammation within the esophagus. These conditions result from the immune system's aberrant response, targeting various tissues and organs throughout the body, including the esophagus. This leads to impaired peristalsis, reduced LES function, and symptoms such as dysphagia and GERD. Scleroderma is a chronic autoimmune disease characterized by excessive collagen production and fibrosis in multiple organs, including the skin and internal organs. The systemic form of scleroderma, CREST syndrome (calcinosis, Raynaud phenomenon, esophageal dysmotility, sclerosis, and telangiectasia), affects both the smooth muscle and connective tissue layers, resulting in a stiffened, less compliant esophagus [47, 48]. The LES may become hypertensive or fail to relax properly, contributing to GERD. Dysphagia in scleroderma often results from both mechanical obstruction due to fibrosis and impaired peristalsis. Genetic studies have identified several susceptibility loci for scleroderma, including HLA genes, particularly HLA-DR and HLA-DQ. Polymorphisms in the interferon regulatory factor 5 (IRF5) and signal transducer and activator of transcription 4 (STAT4) genes have also been linked to an increased risk of developing scleroderma [49–51]. SLE is an autoimmune disease characterized by the deposition of immune complexes in healthy tissues, leading to the accumulation of immune cells and tissue damage. Esophageal involvement in SLE is less common but can occur due to immune complex deposition and inflammation in the esophageal mucosa. This inflammation can disrupt normal esophageal motility, leading to symptoms such as dysphagia and odynophagia. Additionally, SLE patients may experience GERD symptoms due to esophageal dysmotility and impaired LES function [39, 52].

#### *2.3.3 Structural abnormalities*

Structural abnormalities of the esophagus can result from congenital malformations, acquired conditions, or mechanical obstructions [53]. These disorders, which include hiatal hernias, esophageal strictures, and tumors, impair the normal passage of food and liquids through the esophagus, leading to symptoms such as dysphagia, odynophagia, chest pain, and food impaction. Hiatal hernia occurs when the gastroesophageal junction and a portion of the stomach protrude through the diaphragmatic hiatus into the chest cavity. There are two main types: sliding and paraesophageal [54]. Sliding hiatal hernias, where the gastroesophageal junction moves up into the chest alongside the stomach, are more common. This displacement can compromise the function of the LES, allowing gastric acid and contents to reflux into the esophagus. Chronic GERD associated with hiatal hernia can lead to esophagitis and subsequent fibrosis, contributing to impaired esophageal peristalsis and dysmotility [55]. Esophageal strictures are characterized by the narrowing of the esophageal lumen due to scar tissue formation. They can develop secondary to conditions that cause chronic inflammation or injury to the esophageal mucosa [56]. For instance, chronic GERD leads to inflammation and ulceration of the esophageal lining, which can progress to fibrotic scarring and stricture formation. Other causes include the ingestion of caustic substances, such as lye or acids, and radiation therapy for cancers in the chest region, which can lead to fibrosis and strictures [57, 58]. Esophageal strictures restrict the normal peristaltic movement of the esophagus, causing dysphagia, odynophagia, and the potential for food impaction. Esophageal tumors can be benign or malignant and can obstruct the esophageal lumen, affecting normal swallowing function. Benign tumors like leiomyomas arise from smooth muscle cells within the esophageal wall and typically present as well-circumscribed masses that can cause partial obstruction [59]. Malignant tumors, including adenocarcinoma and squamous cell carcinoma, often arise from the mucosal lining and can infiltrate the surrounding tissues, leading to significant luminal obstruction [60]. Esophageal cancer is associated with symptoms such as progressive dysphagia, unintentional weight loss, chest pain, and sometimes coughing or hoarseness due to tracheal compression. The presence of tumors in the esophagus disrupts normal peristalsis and can lead to severe dysmotility as the disease progresses [3].

### *2.3.4 Gastroesophageal reflux disease (GERD)*

Chronic acid reflux, also known as GERD, can have serious consequences for the esophagus [61]. Repeated exposure of the esophagus to stomach acid can lead to inflammation, known as esophagitis [62]. This inflammation can cause irritation and damage to the esophageal lining, resulting in symptoms such as heartburn, chest pain, and difficulty swallowing. Over time, chronic inflammation can lead to the formation of scar tissue in the esophagus, known as esophageal fibrosis, which can cause esophageal stricture and subsequent difficulty swallowing and food impaction. In addition to inflammation and scarring, persistent exposure to stomach acid can weaken the muscles that control the movement of food down the esophagus, resulting in dysmotility. This condition prevents the esophagus from contracting properly to move food into the stomach [63]. Furthermore, acid reflux can irritate the nerves in the esophagus, leading to conditions such as esophageal spasms. These spasms can cause chest pain and difficulty swallowing, further complicating the motility of the esophagus.

### *2.3.5 Metabolic diseases*

Metabolic diseases can significantly impact esophageal motility. For instance, diabetes mellitus is a major contributor to esophageal dysmotility. Diabetic neuropathy can impair the nerves that control esophageal peristalsis and the LES, leading to conditions such as gastroparesis and diabetic esophagus, which manifest as dysphagia, heartburn, and regurgitation [64]. Obesity, a key feature of metabolic syndrome, is associated with a wide array of EMDs [65]. Additionally, hypothyroidism can influence esophageal motility by decreasing the duration and percentage of relaxation [66].

#### *2.3.6 Infectious diseases*

Infectious diseases can significantly contribute to the development of EMDs. A prominent example is Chagas disease, caused by the protozoan parasite *Trypanosoma cruzi*, which is endemic in parts of Latin America. In Chagas disease, esophageal dysfunction results from damage to the esophageal myenteric plexus. This leads to the loss of esophageal peristalsis, partial or absent relaxation of the LES, and the development of megaesophagus [67]. Additionally, esophageal candidiasis, often seen in immunocompromised patients such as those with HIV/AIDS, can cause inflammation, esophageal strictures, and secondary motility issues [68].

## 3. Pathophysiology

The most studied and well-known motility disorder of the esophagus is achalasia. Other motility disorders have not been as well studied, in part due to the lack of a clear consensus in nomenclature and diagnostic criteria, which have changed over the years. Available data suggest that these disorders have their own distinctive pathophysiological pathways and may overlap with other esophageal disorders.

### 3.1 Achalasia

The mechanism behind primary achalasia has been somewhat elucidated. It is now known that achalasia is definitively caused by the loss of inhibitory neurons and the interstitial cells of Cajal (ICC) in the Auerbach's (myenteric) plexus of the distal esophagus. These cells produce nitric oxide (NO) and vasoactive intestinal peptide (VIP), which are responsible for smooth muscle relaxation. Therefore, the loss of these neurotransmitters results in the hallmark of achalasia: impaired LES relaxation [69]. The process responsible for the destruction of neurons is selective, preserving excitatory neurons and their peptides [70].

#### *3.1.1 Neuronal damage*

Achalasia does not affect only the esophagus; certain regions of the central nervous system also undergo degeneration. Patients with achalasia have degenerated nerve cells in the dorsal motor nucleus (DMN) of the vagus nerve [71]. Animal studies have shown that bilateral DMN damage can result in achalasia-like dilatation of the esophagus [72]. Additionally, vagal nerve fibers have been found to be degenerated in patients with achalasia [73]. There is a possibility that the degeneration of the vagus nucleus and vagal nerve fibers is secondary to the loss of signal input from the esophagus [74]. The most significant damage occurs in the muscle layer of the esophagus, beginning in the Auerbach's plexus. Histopathological examinations have shown the infiltration of activated cytotoxic T lymphocytes and the activation of the complement system within the myenteric ganglia, along with increased levels of IL-1β, IFNγ, TNF-α, and IL-2, especially in the early stages of the disease [75]. Thus, the primary pathological mechanism leading to myenteric ganglia loss is believed to be chronic ganglionitis [76]. This histopathological finding of ganglionitis with preserved intrinsic neurons and minimal fibrosis is linked to type III achalasia (also called "vigorous" or spastic achalasia) and is considered an early stage of achalasia. Prolonged inflammation leads to "classic" or type II achalasia through a decrease in the number of inhibitory neurons, as well as hypertrophy and neuronal fibrosis [77]. Further loss of neurons (eventually complete loss) and severe fibrosis correspond to type I achalasia. Therefore, some authors consider that the three types of achalasia represent a clinicopathological continuum [78].

#### *3.1.2 Changes in the esophagus muscle layer*

The smooth muscle of the esophagus, the muscularis propria, is irregularly and inconsistently hypertrophied in the early stages of the disease [79]. The classic dilation of the esophagus (sigmoid-like dilation and megaesophagus) proximal to the cardia occurs in the later stages of the disease. The esophagus dilates approximately 6 mm per year, while the esophagogastric junction reduces its lumen diameter by about 1 mm each year. Megaesophagus is rare and usually seen in elderly patients with longstanding disease [80]. Esophagus emptying has been studied in patients with achalasia, revealing that while the esophagus in type III achalasia patients is relatively easily emptied during most swallows, types I and II show impaired esophagus emptying. Type I achalasia shows no emptying, while food transit in type II achalasia is possible thanks to the contraction of the longitudinal muscle layer in the distal esophagus [81].

#### *3.1.3 Changes in the esophagus mucosa*

Although not primarily affected by the disease, the esophageal mucosa exhibits certain pathological alterations in achalasia, especially in patients with longstanding disease. Changes in the mucosa include diffuse squamous cellular hyperplasia, high-grade squamous dysplasia, and esophageal squamous cell carcinoma. Additionally, the esophageal mucosa of achalasia patients shows an increase in T lymphocytes. These changes are likely secondary to chronic inflammation caused by food stasis [82–84]. This state of chronic, continuous inflammation leads to an increased risk of esophageal squamous cell cancer, which may be elevated up to 140 times compared to the general population [85].

### 3.2 DES

The mechanism behind DES is poorly understood. Some authors believe it is a disorder similar to achalasia and that in some cases, it can progress to achalasia [86]. Full-thickness muscularis propria biopsies have shown atrophy and fibrosis of this layer, as well as a reduction in ICCs, a feature shared with achalasia [87]. Isolated case reports have found that DES symptoms can improve after corticosteroid or antiepileptic therapy, highlighting the general lack of understanding of this disease [88, 89]. The main characteristic of this disorder is the simultaneous contraction of multiple segments of the esophagus, primarily its distal portion. Some experimental studies have shown that the lack of NO neurotransmitter can cause DES-like simultaneous contractions of the esophagus, while reintroduction of NO reverses it. It is known that patients taking opioids experience this syndrome more frequently and that opioid-induced DES is reversible upon their withdrawal [86]. Psychiatric disease (possibly through increased opioid use), along with GERD, has also been associated with DES [90]. Although the multiple possible etiologies present a challenge in understanding the exact pathophysiological mechanism that induces the spastic contractions, they also suggest the potential for personalized therapy in each case.

### 3.3 Jackhammer esophagus

Jackhammer esophagus is diagnosed by high-resolution manometry (HRM) with normal median integrated relaxation pressure and ≥ 20% hypercontractile swallows (>8000 mmHgscm). This condition appears to be distinct from achalasia. While the diagnosis has been clarified thanks to HRM, the pathological substrate of jackhammer esophagus remains enigmatic [4]. The disorder primarily affects the distal portion of the esophagus. Although the muscle layer of the distal esophagus is hypertrophied in jackhammer esophagus, the contractions are accompanied by a lack of synchrony between the longitudinal and circular layers of the smooth muscle [19]. Recent studies have shown eosinophilic infiltration in the mucosa, submucosa, and muscle layer of the esophagus in patients with EMDs [91]. Eosinophil infiltration of the mucosa with >15 eosinophils per high power field, after excluding other more common diseases, is diagnostic of eosinophilic esophagitis (EoE). EoE is likely a separate clinical and pathological entity, with dysmotility mainly due to reduced esophageal compliance, probably secondary to fibrosis of the esophagus [92]. In some cases, jackhammer esophagus is associated with GERD, and it appears that those patients could benefit from proton pump inhibitor (PPI) therapy [93]. In the idiopathic jackhammer esophagus, the primary driving factor is likely eosinophil infiltration of the esophageal muscle layer, sometimes referred to as eosinophilic esophageal myositis (**Table 1**) [94, 95].

| EMDs | Genetics | Pathophysiology | Manometric Characteristics CCV 4.0 [4] |
|---|---|---|---|
| Achalasia | • Familial cases<br>• Twin studies<br>• HLA-DQ<br>• ALADIN gene | • Impaired LES relaxation<br>• Loss of inhibitory neurons and ICC; impaired NO and VIP production<br>• Irregular and inconsistent hypertrophy of the smooth muscle in the muscularis propria | • Integrated relaxation pressure elevated<br>• 100% absent peristalsis |
| DES | • Familial cases | • Simultaneous contraction of multiple segments of the esophagus<br>• Reduction of ICC<br>• Atrophy and fibrosis of muscularis propria | • Integrated relaxation pressure normal<br>• ≥ 20% swallows with premature contractions |
| Jackhammer esophagus | • Unknown | • Lack of synchrony between the longitudinal and circular layers of the smooth muscle<br>• Eosinophil infiltration of the esophageal muscle layer | • Integrated relaxation pressure normal<br>• ≥ 20% swallows with hypercontractile contractions |

**Table 1.**
*Differences in genetics, pathogenesis, and manometric characteristics between achalasia, DES, and jackhammer esophagus.*

## 4. Symptoms

The symptomatology indicating diseases of the esophagus is becoming an increasingly common problem that patients present to doctors. It is considered that every fifth person has experienced symptoms that would suggest a disorder in esophageal function at least once, regardless of gender and age [96]. The most common symptoms indicating a possible esophageal disorder include dysphagia, odynophagia, chest pain, heartburn, regurgitation, globus sensation, hiccups, and belching. It is also important to consider the presence of extraesophageal manifestations indicating esophageal dysfunction, such as wheezing, cough, throat pain, and hoarseness, after excluding primary diseases that lead to them [97].

### 4.1 Dysphagia

The leading symptom of EMDs is dysphagia. Around 15% of patients experience a sensation of difficulty swallowing, and its frequency increases with age. Dysphagia is of Greek origin and consists of two parts: "dis" (difficulty) and "phagia" (eating), representing a disorder in the passage of food from the mouth to the stomach. The sensation of difficulty swallowing may be associated with numerous neuromuscular and structural disorders, not only of the esophagus in the case of esophageal dysphagia but also of oropharyngeal diseases in the case of oropharyngeal dysphagia. The presence of this sensation has been confirmed in patients with psychiatric disorders, based on abnormal sensory perception at the level of the esophagus [98]. The swallowing process itself represents a complex neuromuscular action that affects oropharyngeal movements and esophageal peristaltic movements with the aim of transporting liquids and food to the stomach, lasting on average about 10 seconds. Any deviation from the correct act manifests in some of the symptoms of esophageal disorders, most commonly dysphagia [99].

Oropharyngeal dysphagia is defined as the inability to transport food from the oral cavity to the esophagus. The most common causes leading to the development of oropharyngeal dysphagia of neuromuscular origin are Parkinson's disease, ALS, MS, and polymyositis, while structural disorders are dominated by cancers, infections of the pharynx and throat, thyroid enlargement, and Zenker's diverticulum. In this type of dysphagia, symptoms occur immediately after swallowing food, indicating potential localization. Food impaction and difficulty swallowing saliva often occur, leading to manual evacuation of the bolus, vomiting, and increased saliva production. Potential causes that can lead to similar complaints are associated with atrophy of the masticatory muscles, inadequate chewing of food, lack of teeth, swallowing large food bites, and inadequate functioning of salivary glands [100].

The second type of dysphagia is esophageal dysphagia, which can also occur due to structural disorders such as cancers, diverticula, benign tumors, EoE, peptic changes, Schatzki's ring, and foreign bodies, as well as neuromuscular causes such as achalasia, DES, jackhammer esophagus, and hypertensive esophageal sphincter [101].

Valuable help in assessing the cause is obtained based on whether the patient has difficulty swallowing food or liquids, whether dysphagia is progressive or intermittent, whether heartburn occurs, and whether there is weight loss [101]. Patients experiencing a sensation of dysphagia during swallowing liquid and solid food, as well as after swallowing liquids, indicate a neuromuscular problem. In patients who have dysphagia only when swallowing solid food, without problems swallowing mushy food or liquids, it is usually due to mechanical obstruction. When it comes to the impaction of a foreign body, it is most often accompanied by regurgitation and hypersalivation that passes after removing the foreign body. In patients who have liquid dysphagia, these complaints occur only during the consumption of liquids [102]. In patients with malignancy, there is a sudden onset of dysphagia symptoms, accompanied by weight loss and anorexia, as well as the appearance of heartburn with progressive worsening of symptoms. Dysphagia may also occur on the ground of previous esophagitis as well as on the ground of caustic damage to the esophagus in patients with esophagitis caused by drugs, when in addition to difficulty swallowing, there is also painful swallowing, a feeling of burning behind the sternum. In younger people who have previously had food bolus impaction, it is necessary to exclude the development of EoE. Any occurrence of dysphagia requires an adequate diagnostic approach to investigate it [103].

### 4.2 Chest pain

A major differential diagnostic challenge in medicine is chest pain. It can occur in patients with cardiovascular diseases, pulmonary system diseases, vascular diseases, and musculoskeletal disorders or may originate from the gastrointestinal tract [104]. It is considered that in 57% of patients who had chest pain and who underwent coronary angiography and did not have findings on coronary blood vessels, the pain was of esophageal origin [105]. Chest pain of esophageal origin can simulate pain of cardiac origin due to its retrosternal localization as well as due to the sharing of innervation pathways with the heart. Esophageal pain may have a lateral localization or spread to the neck, chin, or back, but less commonly, most often in the form of burning behind the sternum or smoldering. It occurs most often after a meal, can worsen with a meal, and can occur during the night. After taking PPIs or antacids, pain can be suppressed [104]. There are several theories that explain the appearance of esophageal pain of origin. So far, the most acceptable theory is associated with the action of hydrochloric acid on chemoreceptors in the esophagus, whose activation changes the electric charge of the membrane of smooth muscle cells and leads to spontaneous and repeated contractions of the muscles of the esophagus that cause pain. The above theory is followed by during the high-tone muscle tone, slow blood flow through the muscles of the esophagus, which leads to ischemia of the said organ and worsens the pain. In addition to the thermoreceptors, it is also important to consider the effect of the mechanoreceptors that are activated in the dilation of the esophagus, and there is no lesser importance. The cooling of the solutions comes to an end, activating the thermoreceptors, which manifests as dilation, and the esophagus comes to the activation of the mechanoreceptors, causing pain [106].

### 4.3 Regurgitation

Another important manifestation of the esophagus is the appearance of regurgitation. It is defined as the backward flow of food, stomach acid, and bile content into the mouth. It is necessary to make a distinction between regurgitation and vomiting, where the contents of the stomach are found in the mouth but there is no previous retching or activation of the abdominal muscles. Special importance is given to the difference between regurgitation and rumination, where the role of the short-term and periodic re-orientation of food in the oral cavity is to eat. Regurgitation occurs most often at night and in patients who have been bending forward for a long time [107].

### 4.4 Impact on nutrition and quality of life

The diversity of symptoms in patients with esophageal dysmotility is significant. The onset of one or more symptoms leads to discomfort, frustration, and a reduction in daily activities. In addition to these manifestations, there are psychological changes such as anxiety, depression, and social isolation among these patients, further compromising their quality of life. A multidisciplinary approach to these patients is essential, starting with dietary habits. Firstly, it is necessary to chew food adequately during meals to prevent possible impaction and the sensation of difficulty swallowing, as well as consuming moderate amounts of fluids to facilitate easier passage of food boluses. Patients are advised to have more frequent meals throughout the day, with smaller quantities, which aids in easier emptying and reduces the activation of mechanoreceptors in the esophagus [108]. It is crucial to break daily habits such as alcohol consumption, which weakens the tight junctions between esophageal cells, allowing acid passage and activating chemoreceptors, as well as weakening the LES. In addition to alcohol, patients are advised to quit smoking and avoid sweets, chocolates, fatty foods, and excessively hot or cold beverages. Limited consumption of citrus juices and spicy foods is also recommended to avoid heartburn. Patients should avoid running and performing isometric exercises or lifting heavy weights [109]. Emotional instability in the form of frequent stress, worry, and discomfort also worsens existing symptoms by lowering visceral sensitivity. The use of certain medications has been noted to exacerbate symptoms, including calcium channel blockers, theophylline, aspirin, non-steroidal anti-inflammatory drugs (NSAIDs), and bisphosphonates. In addition to the above, patients with esophageal dysmotility are advised against late meals and sleeping on the right side due to possible worsening of existing symptoms [110].

### 4.5 Association with other gastrointestinal symptoms

In addition to the previously mentioned symptoms of esophageal dysmotility, odynophagia, globus sensation, hiccups, and extraesophageal manifestations of esophageal dysfunction should be noted. Odynophagia, or painful swallowing, is a symptom associated with various conditions. The pain is typically retrosternal and is experienced while swallowing food or sometimes even saliva. It can result from inflammation of the esophageal mucosa or deeper structures and may occur due to caustic injuries, viral and fungal infections, or after radiation therapy to this area. Odynophagia can also be caused by improper use of tetracyclines. In severe cases of GERD, swallowing may become difficult and painful [111]. Globus sensation, or globus pharyngeus, is experienced by at least half of the population during their lifetime. It is believed to be primarily a psychological disorder leading to the sensation of a lump in the throat, difficulty swallowing, or throat tightening, without any abnormality in the tone of the upper esophageal sphincter or any other pathological changes within the esophageal lumen [112]. Hiccups represent a systemic manifestation of various conditions, not limited to gastrointestinal diseases such as achalasia, peptic ulcer, and GERD. They can also occur in patients with chest or abdominal trauma, or those with renal insufficiency. Despite being a multisystem manifestation, most patients with hiccups are initially evaluated by gastroenterologists, who may prescribe medications such as metoclopramide, baclofen, or gabapentin. In extreme cases where hiccups are frequent and uncontrollable with medications, and other causes are ruled out, surgical ablation of the phrenic nerve may be necessary [113]. Patients with asthma, chronic cough, laryngitis, or pulmonary fibrosis are sometimes referred to gastroenterologists for further evaluation. Studies have shown that 35–80% of asthma patients also have GERD. The pathogenesis is bidirectional; therapy given to asthma patients often leads to GERD because bronchodilators relax the LES. Conversely, patients with the established reflux disease may develop asthma symptoms, particularly at night, including coughing, wheezing, hoarseness, and inflammation of the arytenoids. This is attributed to micro-aspiration of gastric contents and vagus-mediated neural reflexes [114].

## 5. Diagnosis

### 5.1 Clinical assessment

EMDs encompass a range of conditions that disrupt the normal function of the esophagus, hindering the passage of food from the mouth to the stomach. Clinical assessment of patients with these disorders requires a thorough medical history, detailed physical examination, and specific diagnostic tests. Gathering information about symptoms such as dysphagia, retrosternal pain, regurgitation, and possible weight loss is crucial. These symptoms may progress gradually over several months or years. Patients often report difficulty swallowing solid foods, while liquids pass more easily. Symptoms such as heartburn, the sensation of food sticking in the esophagus, and related issues should also be noted. Typically, physical examination does not reveal significant abnormalities but is essential for ruling out other potential causes of symptoms. Collecting a detailed medical history and family history can provide insights into genetic predispositions or inherited risk factors. Risk factors such as smoking, alcohol consumption, and previous gastrointestinal diseases should also be considered. Diagnostic procedures include upper gastrointestinal endoscopy, which allows visualization of the esophageal mucosa and exclusion of mechanical obstructions such as strictures or tumors. Esophageal manometry is used to assess functional aspects of motility, identifying abnormalities in peristalsis and LES tone, which may indicate disorders like achalasia. Radiological tests, such as barium swallow, can depict esophageal dilation, delayed emptying, and other characteristic changes indicating motility disorders. In certain cases, pH monitoring may be necessary to assess acid reflux, which can contribute to symptoms and complications [115].

### 5.2 High-resolution manometry

Manometry of the esophagus is a crucial diagnostic method for identifying esophageal motility disorders. This procedure allows for detailed analysis of the functional aspects of the esophagus, which is essential for the precise diagnosis of various forms of dysmotility. Disorders such as achalasia, DES, and hypomotility can significantly impair patients' quality of life, causing symptoms like dysphagia, chest pain behind the sternum, and regurgitation. Esophageal manometry is performed using a catheter equipped with pressure sensors, which is inserted through the nose or mouth into the stomach. During the procedure, the patient swallows small amounts of water, allowing for the measurement of pressures and peristaltic waves along the esophagus. Modern manometry utilizes HRM, providing a more detailed and precise pressure map within the esophagus compared to traditional methods. Manometry is essential for the differential diagnosis of various esophageal motility disorders. In the case of achalasia, manometry reveals the absence of esophageal peristalsis and elevated pressure of the LES that fails to relax properly during swallowing. In DES, manometry shows simultaneous, high-pressure contractions that disrupt normal food transport. Hypomotility of the esophagus is characterized by reduced amplitude of peristaltic waves or their complete absence. The results of manometry enable a personalized approach to treatment [116].

### 5.3 Barium swallow studies

Swallowing barium is a non-invasive radiological method that plays a crucial role in assessing patients with esophageal motility disorders. This procedure allows for detailed visualization of the anatomical structure and functional state of the esophagus, which is essential for making an accurate diagnosis and planning appropriate treatment. During this procedure, the patient consumes a barium suspension that coats the esophageal mucosa, enabling detailed imaging of the esophagus using fluoroscopy. As the barium passes through the esophagus, radiographs are taken to capture a series of images showing peristaltic waves, the shape of the esophagus, and any abnormalities present. Swallowing barium is particularly useful for detecting structural and functional abnormalities that may contribute to esophageal motility disorders. This method can identify strictures, diverticula, tumors, or hernias that

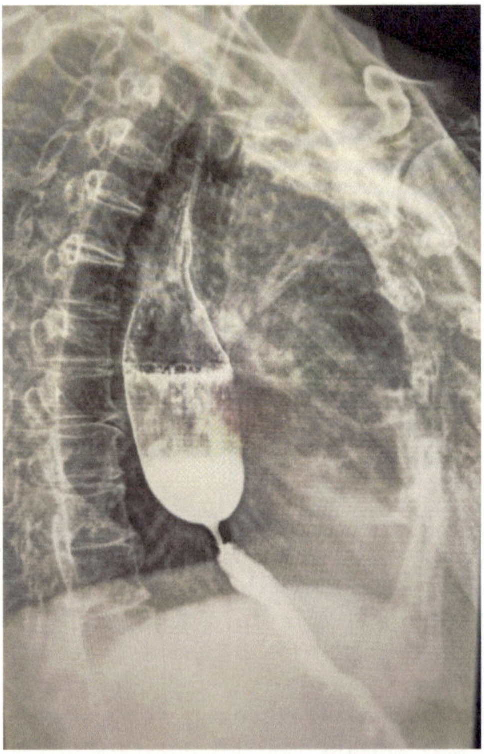

**Figure 1.**
*A dilated esophagus with a retained column of barium and a "bird's beak" appearance indicates achalasia.*

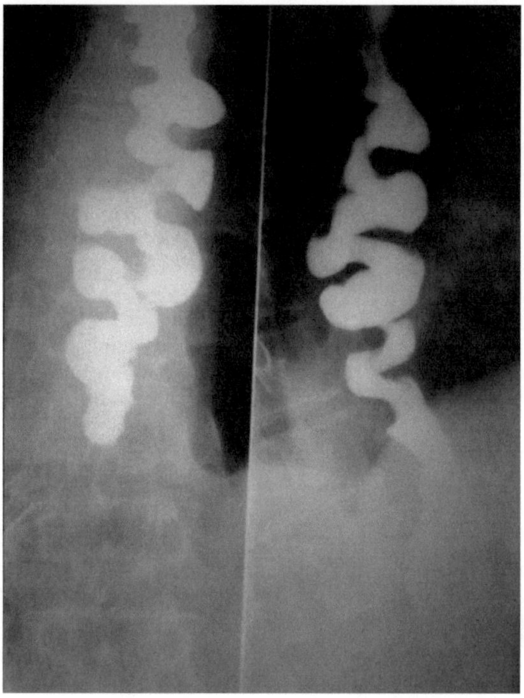

**Figure 2.**
*The esophagus exhibits a corkscrew appearance caused by DES. Attribution to: © Nevit Dilmen, https://commons.wikimedia.org/wiki/File:Radiology_0012_Nevit.jpg, "Radiology 0012 Nevit," https://creativecommons.org/licenses/by-sa/3.0/legalcode.*

may obstruct normal food passage. Additionally, swallowing barium can reveal delayed emptying of the esophagus, dyskinesia, and non-rhythmic contractions, which are characteristic of various types of esophageal motility disorders [117]. The results of barium swallow provide valuable information for differential diagnosis and further evaluation of patients with symptoms such as dysphagia, chest pain, and regurgitation. Combining this method with other diagnostic procedures such as manometry and endoscopy allows for a comprehensive understanding of the pathophysiology of esophageal motility disorders. For example, in patients suspected of achalasia, barium swallow may reveal characteristic findings such as esophageal dilation and a "bird's beak" narrowing at the junction of the esophagus and stomach (see **Figure 1**). In DES, images may show segmental contractions that disrupt the normal passage of barium (see **Figure 2**). This data is crucial for planning therapy, whether it involves endoscopic interventions, pharmacological treatment, or surgical procedures [118].

### 5.4 Endoscopy

Upper gastrointestinal endoscopy is a crucial diagnostic tool for evaluating patients with esophageal motility disorders. This procedure allows for direct visualization of the interior of the esophagus using a flexible endoscopic device, providing a detailed examination of the mucosa and identification of potential structural or functional abnormalities. Equipped with a high-quality camera, the endoscope enables precise visualization of the mucosal condition, assessing its color, integrity, and any pathological changes that may affect esophageal motility [119]. Endoscopy is essential for identifying various pathological conditions that can impact esophageal function. This procedure can detect benign or malignant tumors, strictures, Barrett's esophagus, and other anatomical variations that may be causes or contributors to symptoms of esophageal motility disorders. In clinical practice, endoscopy is used to comprehensively evaluate the esophageal mucosa to accurately diagnose and plan further therapeutic approaches. Based on endoscopic findings, additional diagnostic steps such as biopsy or therapeutic interventions like dilation of strictures or ablation of pathological changes may be undertaken [120]. Integrating endoscopy with other diagnostic methods such as esophageal manometry and barium swallow allows for a comprehensive analysis of esophageal motility. This multidisciplinary approach is crucial for understanding the pathophysiology of disorders and tailoring individualized therapy, significantly contributing to treatment efficacy and patients' quality of life.

### 5.5 Differential diagnosis

Differential diagnosis of esophageal motility disorders encompasses a wide range of conditions. Dysphagia is a significant finding. It is essential to differentiate between oropharyngeal dysphagia (difficulty swallowing in the mouth and throat) and esophageal dysphagia (difficulty swallowing in the esophagus). Diagnostic approaches include upper endoscopy, HRM, barium swallow, and others (see **Figure 3**). Malignancy should be primarily ruled out, followed by investigation into other causes of dysphagia such as EMDs, scleroderma, peptic stricture, esophageal ring, dysphagia lusoria, and thyroid enlargement [121]. In addition to dysphagia,

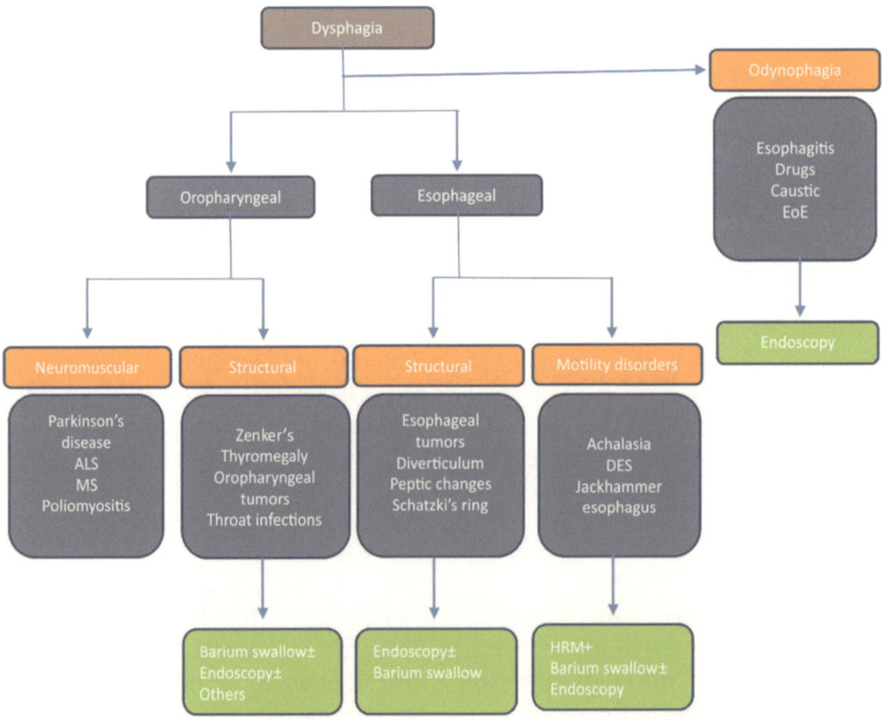


**Figure 3.**
*Differential diagnosis of dysphagia with diagnostic workup.*

chest pain, often associated with difficulty swallowing, commonly prompts patients to seek cardiology evaluation. Chest pain can also indicate pneumonia, pleuritis, pneumothorax, aortic dissection, musculoskeletal chest pain with radiation to the arms, and neck in cervical spine disorders. It is crucial to exclude pericarditis, pericardial tamponade, and thromboembolism [122]. Accurate diagnosis and management of these disorders require a multidisciplinary approach involving gastroenterology, cardiology, pulmonology, and other relevant specialties to ensure appropriate treatment tailored to each patient's condition.

## 6. Treatment

### 6.1 Pharmacologic treatment

Pharmacologic treatment for achalasia is generally considered the least effective option and is typically used only as a temporary measure before more effective interventions or for patients who do not respond to botulinum toxin injections and are not suitable for myotomy [123]. The primary medications used are calcium channel blockers and nitrates. Calcium channel blockers work by inhibiting calcium uptake in cells, which is necessary for the contraction of the LES, thereby promoting relaxation. However, these drugs often lead to tolerance, reducing their long-term effectiveness [124]. Nifedipine has shown some long-term benefits and even physiological normalization in a small subset of patients [125]. Nitrate therapy aims to counteract the decrease in NO, reducing LES tone and pressure. Sublingual isosorbide dinitrate effectively decreases basal LES pressure and improves esophageal emptying, but significant side effects such as hypotension, headaches, and peripheral edema limit its use [123, 125]. Other less commonly used treatments include anticholinergics, beta-adrenergic agonists, theophylline, and phosphodiesterase inhibitors. These inhibitors work by preventing the breakdown of cyclic GMP, which mediates nitric oxide-induced relaxation, thereby reducing LES tone [1, 125]. While experimental data are promising, further clinical studies are needed to confirm their efficacy in treating achalasia [125]. All the aforementioned smooth muscle relaxants might be used in patients with spastic esophageal disorders (DES and jackhammer esophagus) and non-cardiac chest pain as the primary symptom. Moreover, neuromodulators can be considered for this indication, such as tricyclic antidepressants, serotonin-norepinephrine reuptake inhibitors, and selective serotonin reuptake inhibitors. Additionally, PPIs are indicated in these disorders whenever there is increased gastric acid secretion and symptoms of GERD, such as regurgitation and heartburn [123].

### 6.2 Endoscopic treatment

#### *6.2.1 Botulinum toxin*

Botulinum toxin, a strong inhibitor of acetylcholine release from nerve endings, was introduced as a treatment for achalasia in 1995. It counteracts the unopposed contraction of the LES mediated by cholinergic nerves, thus reducing LES pressure [126]. Botulinum toxin is endoscopically injected at the squamocolumnar junction, extending up to 1 cm proximally. This minimally invasive treatment has a low rate of side effects and complications but is less effective than other non-pharmacological treatments. The success rate drops from 82% after 1 month to 48% after 1 year and is particularly less effective in patients younger than 50 years [127]. Consequently, ACG guideline recommends botulinum toxin injection as first-line therapy for achalasia patients who are unfit for definitive therapies. While botulinum toxin can initially provide effective results, with only slightly lower effectiveness compared to myotomy, its benefits quickly diminish over time. This makes it a suboptimal intervention for patients with a reasonable life expectancy who are suitable candidates for endoscopic or surgical interventions [1]. For spastic disorders, botulinum toxin injections have demonstrated significant improvement and a reduction in chest pain. However, the sample sizes in these studies are small, and the effects appear to be short term. More research is needed in this area to confirm these findings [128].

#### *6.2.2 Pneumatic dilation*

Pneumatic dilation (PD) is a highly effective treatment for achalasia, especially when standard dilators fail to achieve symptom relief by disrupting the muscularis propria. Patients undergoing PD must also be candidates for surgery due to the potential risk of esophageal perforation, which occurs in about 1.9% of cases. The most frequently used dilators are non-radiopaque graded polyethylene balloons (Rigiflex), available in sizes of 3.0, 3.5, and 4.0 cm, typically used in a sequential manner. The procedure is carried out under sedation, with or without fluoroscopy, and requires significant operator expertise. During the procedure, the balloon is precisely positioned across the LES and inflated to a pressure of 10–15 psi for 15–60 seconds to achieve maximum dilation. After the procedure, patients are closely monitored for signs of perforation, with imaging tests conducted if perforation is suspected. If no complications are detected, patients can be discharged with antiemetics and instructed to seek immediate medical attention if they experience severe chest pain or fever, as delayed perforation can occur [1]. PD offers an excellent success rate of 91% after a 5-year follow-up, with 25% of PD patients requiring redilation during this period [129].

#### *6.2.3 Peroral endoscopic myotomy*

The hybrid technique of peroral endoscopic myotomy (POEM) was developed in Japan, combining endoscopic approaches with natural orifice transluminal endoscopic surgery principles to perform a myotomy. The procedure involves creating a submucosal plane with an endoscope to access and cut the circular muscle fibers over at least 6 cm into the esophagus and 2 cm below the squamocolumnar junction [1]. The International POEM survey, conducted across 16 expert centers and reporting 841 completed procedures, signifies a groundbreaking advancement in the treatment of achalasia, demonstrating a high overall clinical response rate of 98% [130]. POEM also demonstrates high long-term effectiveness, achieving over 90% clinical success at the 5-year follow-up, but with a higher incidence of GERD compared to PD [131, 132]. POEM has been employed for other EMDs, such as diffuse esophageal spasm, though with less success than with achalasia [133].

### 6.3 Surgery

#### *6.3.1 Heller myotomy*

Heller myotomy, first performed approximately a century ago, was considered the gold standard for achalasia before the emergence of POEM. Initially performed through a thoracotomy, this procedure involves dividing the muscle fibers of the LES without disrupting the mucosa. While thoracoscopic myotomy has been used successfully, laparoscopic myotomy is now the preferred method due to its lower morbidity and faster recovery [1, 133]. Laparoscopic Heller myotomy (LHM) offers significant symptom relief, with approximately 90% of patients experiencing improvement. The most frequent complication associated with this procedure is GERD. However, when fundoplication is added to the laparoscopic myotomy, the incidence of postoperative GERD significantly decreases from 31.5 to 8.8% [134]. A meta-analysis of nine studies on LHM (583 patients) indicated that LHM is effective, but its success rate varies by achalasia subtype. Patients with types I and II achalasia experienced higher success rates post-LHM at 81 and 92%, respectively, compared to 71% for type III patients [135]. Overall, graded PD, LHM, and POEM are all first-line treatment options for type I or type II achalasia, offering similar efficacy. POEM and LHM are more invasive than PD, with POEM having higher rates of post-myotomy GERD compared to PD and LHM with fundoplication. For type III achalasia, POEM and LHM are recommended over PD. For patients not suitable for any of these definitive treatments, endoscopic botulinum toxin injection and smooth muscle relaxants are recommended [1]. LHM has shown effectiveness in treating "diffuse esophageal spasm." Studies using the criteria of the new classification for DES and jackhammer esophagus, along with surgical treatment of these conditions, are still not available [136].

#### *6.3.2 Esophagectomy*

Patients with achalasia often manage symptoms like dysphagia and regurgitation through dietary and lifestyle changes, making it challenging to accurately assess treatment outcomes. Both patients and physicians may initially underestimate the severity of the condition or the effects of interventions. As achalasia progresses, it can lead to severe complications such as significant esophageal dilation (megaesophagus) or tortuosity (sigmoid esophagus), increasing the risk of aspiration, aspiration pneumonia, and malnutrition. For these patients, treatments such as PD, surgical myotomy, or POEM may be less effective. Ultimately, up to 5% of achalasia patients may require esophagectomy, which can be safely performed by experienced surgeons in appropriately selected cases [1, 137, 138]. Esophagectomy can be performed *via* open transthoracic, thoracoscopic, or transhiatal routes. The surgical approach depends on the anastomosis location and the choice of esophageal replacement conduit (stomach, colon, or small bowel), with resection options ranging from limited to the EGJ to near-total esophagectomy [137].

## 7. Conclusion

While significant progress has been made in the diagnosis and treatment of EMDs, ongoing research, and a multidisciplinary approach will be crucial for enhancing patient outcomes and developing new, more effective therapies. Conducting long-term follow-up studies on the efficacy and safety of different treatment options will provide more robust data to guide clinical practice.

## Conflict of interest

The authors declare no conflict of interest.

## Author details

Irfan Corovic[1,2*], Mladen Maksic[3,4], Dusan Radojevic[3,4], Samir Vucelj[2], Sabir Sagdati[2], Isidora Stanisavljevic[1], Tijana Veljkovic[5,6], Bojana Simovic Markovic[1], Ivan Jovanovic[1], Bojan Stojanovic[1,7], Dusan Popovic[8,9], Djordje Kralj[10] and Marina Jovanovic[3,4]

1 Faculty of Medical Sciences, Center for Molecular Medicine and Stem Cell Research, University of Kragujevac, Kragujevac, Serbia

2 Department of Internal Medicine, General Hospital of Novi Pazar, Novi Pazar, Serbia

3 Faculty of Medical Sciences, Department of Internal Medicine, University of Kragujevac, Kragujevac, Serbia

4 Clinic for Internal Medicine, Department for Gastroenterology and Hepatology, University Clinical Center Kragujevac, Kragujevac, Serbia

5 Faculty of Medical Sciences, Department of Pediatrics, University of Kragujevac, Kragujevac, Serbia

6 Clinic for Pediatrics, Department of Gastroenterology and Hepatology, University Clinical Center Kragujevac, Kragujevac, Serbia

7 Faculty of Medical Sciences, Department of Surgery, University of Kragujevac, Kragujevac, Serbia

8 Clinic for Internal Medicine, Department for Gastroenterology and Hepatology, Dr Dragisa Misovic-Dedinje University Clinical Hospital Center, Belgrade, Serbia

9 Faculty of Medicine, Department of Internal Medicine, University of Belgrade, Belgrade, Serbia

10 Clinic for Internal Medicine, Department for Gastroenterology and Hepatology, University Clinical Hospital Center Zvezdara, Belgrade, Serbia

*Address all correspondence to: ira.corovic@gmail.com

## References

[1] Vaezi MF, Pandolfino JE, Yadlapati RH, Greer KB, Kavitt RT. ACG clinical guidelines: Diagnosis and management of achalasia. The American Journal of Gastroenterology. 2020;**115**:1393-1411. DOI: 10.14309/ajg.0000000000000731

[2] Bendsen BB, Jensen D, Westmark S, Krarup AL, Riis J, Melgaard D. The quality of life in citizens with oropharyngeal dysphagia-A cross-sectional study. Journal of Clinical Medicine. 2022;**11**:4212. DOI: 10.3390/jcm11144212

[3] Tustumi F, de Sousa JHB, Dornelas NM, Rosa GM, Steinman M, Bianchi ET. The mechanisms for the association of cancer and esophageal dysmotility disorders. Medical Sciences (Basel, Switzerland). 2021;**9**:32. DOI: 10.3390/medsci9020032

[4] Yadlapati R, Pandolfino JE, Fox MR, Bredenoord AJ, Kahrilas PJ. What is new in Chicago classification version 4.0? Neurogastroenterology and Motility. 2021;**33**:e14053. DOI: 10.1111/nmo.14053

[5] Herbella FA, Raz DJ, Nipomnick I, Patti MG. Primary versus secondary esophageal motility disorders: Diagnosis and implications for treatment. Journal of Laparoendoscopic & Advanced Surgical Techniques. Part A. 2009;**19**(2):195-198. DOI: 10.1089/lap.2008.0317

[6] Zenilman ME. Origin and control of gastrointestinal motility. The Surgical Clinics of North America. 1993;**73**:1081-1099. DOI: 10.1016/s0039-6109(16)46181-5

[7] Engel LS, Chow WH, Vaughan TL, Gammon MD, Risch HA, Stanford JL, et al. Population attributable risks of esophageal and gastric cancers. Journal of the National Cancer Institute. 2003;**95**:1404-1413. DOI: 10.1093/jnci/djg047

[8] Zou M, Liang Q, Zhang W, Zhu Y, Xu Y. Causal association between dietary factors and esophageal diseases: A Mendelian randomization study. PLoS One. 2023;**18**:e0292113. DOI: 10.1371/journal.pone.0292113

[9] Zheng Z, Nordenstedt H, Pedersen NL, Lagergren J, Ye W. Lifestyle factors and risk for symptomatic gastroesophageal reflux in monozygotic twins. Gastroenterology. 2007;**132**:87-95. DOI: 10.1053/j.gastro.2006.11.019

[10] Zilberstein B, de Cleva R, Gabriel AG, Neto SG, Gama-Rodrigues JJ. Congenital achalasia: Facts and fantasies. Diseases of the Esophagus. 2005;**18**:335-337. DOI: 10.1111/j.1442-2050.2005.00513.x

[11] Zimmerman FH, Rosensweig NS. Achalasia in a father and son. The American Journal of Gastroenterology. 1984;**79**:506-508

[12] Stein DT, Knauer CM. Achalasia in monozygotic twins. Digestive Diseases and Sciences. 1982;**27**:636-640. DOI: 10.1007/BF01297220

[13] Wong RK, Maydonovitch CL, Metz SJ, Baker JR Jr. Significant DQw1 association in achalasia. Digestive Diseases and Sciences. 1989;**34**:349-352. DOI: 10.1007/BF01536254

[14] Ruiz-de-León A, Mendoza J, Sevilla-Mantilla C, Fernández AM, Pérez-de-la-Serna J, Gónzalez VA, et al. Myenteric antiplexus antibodies

and class II HLA in achalasia. Digestive Diseases and Sciences. 2002;**47**:15-19. DOI: 10.1023/a:1013242831900

[15] Vezzoli V, Duminuco P, Pogliaghi G, Saccone M, Cangiano B, Rosatelli MC, et al. Two novel truncating variants of the AAAS gene causative of the triple a syndrome. Journal of Endocrinological Investigation. 2020;**43**:973-982. DOI: 10.1007/s40618-020-01180-1

[16] O'Brien CJ, Smart HL. Familial coexistence of achalasia and non-achalasic oesophageal dysmotility: Evidence for a common pathogenesis. Gut. 1992;**33**:1421-1423. DOI: 10.1136/gut.33.10.1421

[17] Kaye MD, Demeules JE. Achalasia and diffuse oesophageal spasm in siblings. Gut. 1979;**20**:811-814. DOI: 10.1136/gut.20.9.811

[18] Sirinawasatien A, Sakulthongthawin P. Manometrically jackhammer esophagus with fluoroscopically/endoscopically distal esophageal spasm: A case report. BMC Gastroenterology. 2021;**21**:222. DOI: 10.1186/s12876-021-01808-3

[19] Roman S, Pandolfino JE, Chen J, Boris L, Luger D, Kahrilas PJ. Phenotypes and clinical context of hypercontractility in high-resolution esophageal pressure topography (EPT). The American Journal of Gastroenterology. 2012;**107**:37-45. DOI: 10.1038/ajg.2011.313

[20] Hong YS, Min YW, Rhee PL. Two distinct types of hypercontractile esophagus: Classic and spastic jackhammer. Gut Liver. 2016;**10**(5):859-863. DOI: 10.5009/gnl15388

[21] Zhong C, Liu K, Wang K, Liu H, Su H, Wu J, et al. Developing a diagnostic understanding of GERD phenotypes through the analysis of levels of mucosal injury, immune activation, and psychological comorbidity. Diseases of the Esophagus. 2018;**31**:doy039. DOI: 10.1093/dote/doy039

[22] Yuan L, Tang D, Peng J, Qu N, Yue C, Wang F. Study on lifestyle in patients with gastroesophageal reflux disease. Zhong Nan Da Xue Xue Bao. Yi Xue Ban. 2017;**42**:558-564. Chinese. DOI: 10.11817/j.issn.1672-7347.2017.05.013

[23] Yi CH, Lei WY, Hung JS, Liu TT, Orr WC, Chen CL. Sleep disturbance and enhanced esophageal capsaicin sensitivity in patients with gastroesophageal reflux disease. Journal of Gastroenterology and Hepatology. 2016;**31**:1940-1945. DOI: 10.1111/jgh.13428

[24] Yu M, Chang C, Undem BJ, Yu S. Capsaicin-sensitive vagal afferent nerve-mediated interoceptive signals in the esophagus. Molecules. 2021;**26**:3929. DOI: 10.3390/molecules26133929

[25] Wu KL, Rayner CK, Chuah SK, Chiu YC, Chiu KW, Hu TH, et al. Effect of liquid meals with different volumes on gastroesophageal reflux disease. Journal of Gastroenterology and Hepatology. 2014;**29**:469-473. DOI: 10.1111/jgh.12457

[26] Zacchi P, Mearin F, Humbert P, Formiguera X, Malagelada JR. Effect of obesity on gastroesophageal resistance to flow in man. Digestive Diseases and Sciences. 1991;**36**:1473-1480. DOI: 10.1007/BF01296818

[27] Yazir Y, Tugay M, Utkan Z, Utkan T. Effects of chronic ethanol consumption on rat upper gastrointestinal system: Functional and histologic findings. Alcohol. 2012;**46**:649-655. DOI: 10.1016/j.alcohol.2012.06.003

[28] Rattan S, Goyal RK. Effect of nicotine on the lower esophageal

sphincter. Studies on the mechanism of action. Gastroenterology. 1975;**69**:154-159

[29] Yoshida K, Furuta K, Adachi K, Ohara S, Morita T, Tanimura T, et al. Effects of anti-hypertensive drugs on esophageal body contraction. World Journal of Gastroenterology. 2010;**16**:987-991. DOI: 10.3748/wjg.v16.i8.987

[30] Xue P, Canakis A, Lee DU, Kadiyala J, Fan GH, Kim RE. Active narcotic use and post-peroral endoscopic myotomy outcomes in esophageal motility disorders. Gastrointestinal Endoscopy. 2024;**99**:490-498.e10. DOI: 10.1016/j.gie.2023.10.046

[31] Dow TG, Brock-Utne JG, Rubin J, Welman S, Dimopoulos GE, Moshal MG. The effect of atropine on the lower esophageal sphincter in late pregnancy. Obstetrics and Gynecology. 1978;**51**:426-430. DOI: 10.1097/00006250-197804000-00009

[32] Zamani M, Alizadeh-Tabari S, Chan WW, Talley NJ. Association between anxiety/depression and gastroesophageal reflux: A systematic review and meta-analysis. The American Journal of Gastroenterology. 2023;**118**:2133-2143. DOI: 10.14309/ajg.0000000000002411

[33] Zerbib F, Rommel N, Pandolfino J, Gyawali CP. ESNM/ANMS review. Diagnosis and management of globus sensation: A clinical challenge. Neurogastroenterology and Motility. 2020;**32**:e13850. DOI: 10.1111/nmo.13850

[34] Richter JE. Oesophageal motility disorders. Lancet. 2001;**358**:823-828. DOI: 10.1016/S0140-6736(01)05973-6

[35] Taira K, Fujiwara K, Fukuhara T, Koyama S, Morisaki T, Takeuchi H. Evaluation of the pharynx and upper esophageal sphincter motility using high-resolution pharyngeal manometry for Parkinson's disease. Clinical Neurology and Neurosurgery. 2021;**201**:106447. DOI: 10.1016/j.clineuro.2020.106447

[36] Daly DD, Code CF, Andersen HA. Disturbances of swallowing and esophageal motility in patients with multiple sclerosis. Neurology. 1962;**12**:250-256. DOI: 10.1212/wnl.12.4.250

[37] Silva AC, Fabio SR, Dantas RO. A scintigraphic study of oral, pharyngeal, and esophageal transit in patients with stroke. Dysphagia. 2008;**23**:165-171. DOI: 10.1007/s00455-007-9117-0

[38] Zaninotto G, Peserico A, Costantini M, Salvador L, Rondinone R, Roveran A, et al. Oesophageal motility and lower oesophageal sphincter competence in progressive systemic sclerosis and localized scleroderma. Scandinavian Journal of Gastroenterology. 1989;**24**:95-102. DOI: 10.3109/00365528909092245

[39] Tatelman M, Keech MK. Esophageal motility in systemic lupus erythematosus, rheumatoid arthritis, and scleroderma. Radiology. 1966;**86**:1041-1046. DOI: 10.1148/86.6.1041

[40] Sohda M, Kato H, Sakai M, Suzuki S, Tanaka N, Sakai M, et al. Combination of hiatal hernia with nonspecific esophageal motility disorder (NEMD) successfully treated with thoracic and abdominal surgery: Report of a case. International Surgery. 2010;**95**:309-314

[41] Zimmer T, Tschiedrich M, Ritz JP, Cornely D, Liehr RM, Wolf KJ, et al. Intramurale pseudodivertikulose des osophagus [Intramural pseudodiverticulosis of the esophagus].

Zeitschrift für Gastroenterologie. 1997;**35**:939-944

[42] Ziaja D, Stasiów B, Sznapka M, Domalik J, Kuczmik W, Ziaja K, et al. Adaptation of endovascular technique of self-expandable metal esophageal stent implantation in palliative treatment of malignant dysphagia in the course of esophageal and bronchial cancers: A one-center study. Advances in Clinical and Experimental Medicine. 2020;**29**:1363-1366. DOI: 10.17219/acem/111810

[43] Zweig RM, Disbrow EA, Javalkar V. Cognitive and psychiatric disturbances in parkinsonian syndromes. Neurologic Clinics. 2016;**34**:235-246. DOI: 10.1016/j.ncl.2015.08.010

[44] Zavalishin IA. Sovremennye predstavleniia Ob étiologii rasseiannogo skleroza [Current theories on the etiology of multiple sclerosis]. Zhurnal Nevropatologii i Psikhiatrii Imeni S.S. Korsakova. 1990;**90**:3-8

[45] Zona C, Pieri M, Carunchio I. Voltage-dependent sodium channels in spinal cord motor neurons display rapid recovery from fast inactivation in a mouse model of amyotrophic lateral sclerosis. Journal of Neurophysiology. 2006;**96**:3314-3322. DOI: 10.1152/jn.00566.2006

[46] Umemoto G, Furuya H, Tsuboi Y, Fujioka S, Arahata H, Sugahara M, et al. Characteristics of tongue and pharyngeal pressure in patients with neuromuscular diseases. Degenerative Neurological and Neuromuscular Disease. 2017;**7**:71-78. DOI: 10.2147/DNND.S132745

[47] Wollheim FA. Classification of systemic sclerosis. Visions and reality. Rheumatology (Oxford, England). 2005;**44**:1212-1216. DOI: 10.1093/rheumatology/keh671

[48] Zuber-Jerger I, Müller A, Kullmann F, Gelbmann CM, Endlicher E, Müller-Ladner U, et al. Gastrointestinal manifestation of systemic sclerosis–thickening of the upper gastrointestinal wall detected by endoscopic ultrasound is a valid sign. Rheumatology (Oxford, England). 2010;**49**:368-372. DOI: 10.1093/rheumatology/kep381

[49] Xu Y, Mo N, Jiang Z, Lu S, Fu S, Wei X, et al. Human leukocyte antigen (HLA)-DRB1 allele polymorphisms and systemic sclerosis. Modern Rheumatology. 2019;**29**:984-991. DOI: 10.1080/14397595.2018

[50] Zhou XD, Yi L, Guo XJ, Chen E, Zou HJ, Jin L, et al. Association of HLA-DQB1*0501 with scleroderma and its clinical features in Chinese population. International Journal of Immunopathology and Pharmacology. 2013;**26**:747-751. DOI: 10.1177/039463201302600318

[51] Xu Y, Wang W, Tian Y, Liu J, Yang R. Polymorphisms in STAT4 and IRF5 increase the risk of systemic sclerosis: A meta-analysis. International Journal of Dermatology. 2016;**55**:408-416. DOI: 10.1111/ijd.12839

[52] Varghese B, Haase N, Low PS. Depletion of folate-receptor-positive macrophages leads to alleviation of symptoms and prolonged survival in two murine models of systemic lupus erythematosus. Molecular Pharmaceutics. 2007;**4**:679-685. DOI: 10.1021/mp0700615

[53] Ariel I, Wells TR. Structural abnormalities of the myenteric (Auerbach's) plexus in familial dysautonomia (Riley-day syndrome) as demonstrated by flat-mount preparation of the esophagus and stomach. Pediatric Pathology. 1985;**4**:89-98. DOI: 10.3109/15513818509025906

[54] Sillcox R, Carrera R, Wright AS, Oelschlager BK, Yates RB, Tatum RP. Esophageal motility patterns in paraesophageal hernia patients compared to sliding hiatal hernia: Bigger is not better. Journal of Gastrointestinal Surgery. 2023;**27**:2039-2044. DOI: 10.1007/s11605-023-05754-1

[55] Zhu HM. Study of the influence of hiatus hernia on gastroesophageal reflux. World Journal of Gastroenterology. 1997;**3**:27-30. DOI: 10.3748/wjg.v3.i1.27

[56] Zouari M, Kamoun H, Bouthour H, Ben Abdallah R, Hlel Y, Ben Malek R, et al. Peptic oesophageal stricture in children: Management problems. African Journal of Paediatric Surgery. 2014;**11**:22-25. DOI: 10.4103/0189-6725.129206

[57] Youn BJ, Kim WS, Cheon JE, Kim WY, Shin SM, Kim IO, et al. Balloon dilatation for corrosive esophageal strictures in children: Radiologic and clinical outcomes. Korean Journal of Radiology. 2010;**11**:203-210. DOI: 10.3348/kjr.2010.11.2.203

[58] Yeoh E, Holloway RH, Russo A, Tippett M, Bermingham H, Chatterton B, et al. Effects of mediastinal irradiation on oesophageal function. Gut. 1996;**38**:166-170. DOI: 10.1136/gut.38.2.166

[59] Zucchetti F, Negro F, Bock E, Stroppa I, Triveri P. Leiomyoma of the esophagus. (A case report). Annali Italiani di Chirurgia. 1997;**68**:541-545. discussion 545-547

[60] Swain CP, Bown SG, Edwards DA, Kirkham JS, Salmon PR, Clark CG. Laser recanalization of obstructing foregut cancer. The British Journal of Surgery. 1984;**71**:112-115. DOI: 10.1002/bjs.1800710211

[61] Zürcher B. Phytotherapeutic approaches in the treatment of laryngopharyngeal reflux in the ENT practice [Phytotherapeutische Ansätze zur Behandlung des laryngopharyngealen reflux in der HNO-Praxis]. Complementary Medicine Research. 2021;**28**:446-452. German. DOI: 10.1159/000514337

[62] Fuchs KH, Breithaupt W. Benigne Erkrankungen des Ösophagus. Refluxkrankheit, diffuser Ösophagusspasmus, Achalasie [Benign esophageal disorders. Gastroesophageal reflux disease, diffuse esophageal spasm, achalasia]. Chirurg. 2011;**82**:271-279. quiz 280-281 German. DOI: 10.1007/s00104-010-2033-0

[63] Valdovinos Díaz MA, Flores C, Facha MT, Koller LJ. Manometría esofágica en la enfermedad por reflujo gastroesofágico. Incompetencia del esfínter esofágico inferior o dismotilidad esofágica? [Esophageal manometry in gastroesophageal reflux disease. Lower esophageal sphincter incompetence or esophageal dismotility?]. Revista de Gastroenterología de México. 1999;**64**(1):16-18

[64] Lin J, Liu G, Duan Z. The mechanism of esophagus dysmotility in diabetes and research progress of relating treatments. Expert Review of Gastroenterology & Hepatology. 2021;**15**:919-927. DOI: 10.1080/17474124.2021.1945921

[65] Chang P, Friedenberg F. Obesity and GERD. Gastroenterology Clinics of North America. 2014;**43**:161-173. DOI: 10.1016/j.gtc.2013.11.009

[66] İlhan M, Arabaci E, Turgut S, Karaman O, Danalioglu A, Tasan E. Esophagus motility in overt hypothyroidism. Journal of Endocrinological Investigation. 2014;**37**:639-644. DOI: 10.1007/s40618-014-0085-6

[67] Dantas RO. Management of esophageal dysphagia in chagas disease. Dysphagia. 2021;**36**:517-522. DOI: 10.1007/s00455-021-10297-1

[68] Mohamed AA, Lu XL, Mounmin FA. Diagnosis and treatment of esophageal candidiasis: Current updates. Canadian Journal of Gastroenterology & Hepatology. 2019;**2019**:3585136. DOI: 10.1155/2019/3585136

[69] Nikaki K, Sawada A, Ustaoglu A, Sifrim D. Neuronal control of esophageal peristalsis and its role in esophageal disease. Current Gastroenterology Reports. 2019;**21**:59. DOI: 10.1007/s11894-019-0728-z

[70] Villanacci V, Annese V, Cuttitta A, et al. An immunohistochemical study of the myenteric plexus in idiopathic achalasia. Journal of Clinical Gastroenterology. 2010;**44**:407-410. DOI: 10.1097/MCG.0b013e3181bc9ebf

[71] Penagini R, Cantù P, Grigolon A. Chest trauma and aetiology of achalasia. Gut. 2006;**55**:1052. DOI: 10.1136/gut.2006.094359

[72] Higgs B, Kerr FW, Ellis FH Jr. The experimental production of esophageal achalasia by electrolytic lesions in the medulla. The Journal of Thoracic and Cardiovascular Surgery. 1965;**50**:613-625

[73] Cassella RR, Ellis FH Jr, Brown AL Jr. Fine-structure changes in achalasia of the esophagus. I. Vagus Nerves. American Journal of Pathology. 1965;**46**:279-288

[74] Ates F, Vaezi MF. The pathogenesis and Management of Achalasia: Current status and future directions. Gut Liver. 2015;**9**:449-463. DOI: 10.5009/gnl14446

[75] Kilic A, Owens SR, Pennathur A, Luketich JD, Landreneau RJ, Schuchert MJ. An increased proportion of inflammatory cells express tumor necrosis factor alpha in idiopathic achalasia of the esophagus. Diseases of the Esophagus. 2009;**22**:382-385. DOI: 10.1111/j.1442-2050.2008.00922.x

[76] Clark SB, Rice TW, Tubbs RR, Richter JE, Goldblum JR. The nature of the myenteric infiltrate in achalasia: An immunohistochemical analysis. The American Journal of Surgical Pathology. 2000;**24**(8):1153-1158. DOI: 10.1097/00000478-2

[77] Goldblum JR, Rice TW, Richter JE. Histopathologic features in esophagomyotomy specimens from patients with achalasia. Gastroenterology. 1996;**111**:648-654. DOI: 10.1053/gast.1996.v111.pm8780569

[78] Sodikoff JB, Lo AA, Shetuni BB, Kahrilas PJ, Yang GY, Pandolfino JE. Histopathologic patterns among achalasia subtypes. Neurogastroenterology and Motility. 2016;**28**:139-145. DOI: 10.1111/nmo.12711

[79] Faussone-Pellegrini MS, Cortesini C. The muscle coat of the lower esophageal sphincter in patients with achalasia and hypertensive sphincter. An electron microscopic study. Journal of Submicroscopic Cytology. 1985;**17**:673-685

[80] Csendes P, Csendes A, Cortes C, Burgos AM. Evolutive radiological changes of the esophagus in patients with achalasia who did not receive treatment. Surgery Today. 2007;**37**:183-186. DOI: 10.1007/s00595-006-3365-8

[81] Kim JH. A unique esophageal motor pattern that involves longitudinal muscles is responsible for emptying in achalasia esophagus (gastroenterology 2010;**139**:102-111). Neurogastroenterology and

Motility. 2011;**17**:96-97. DOI: 10.5056/jnm.2011.17.1.96

[82] Streitz JM Jr, Ellis FH Jr, Gibb SP, Heatley GM. Achalasia and squamous cell carcinoma of the esophagus: Analysis of 241 patients. The Annals of Thoracic Surgery. 1995;**59**:1604-1609. DOI: 10.1016/0003-4975(94)00997-l

[83] Fujii T, Yamana H, Sueyoshi S, Fujita H, Tanaka Y, Kubota M, et al. Histopathological analysis of non-malignant and malignant epithelium in achalasia of the esophagus. Diseases of the Esophagus. 2000;**13**:110-116. DOI: 10.1046/j.1442-2050.2000.00088.x

[84] Pressman A, Behar J. Etiology and pathogenesis of idiopathic achalasia. Journal of Clinical Gastroenterology. 2017;**51**:195-202. DOI: 10.1097/MCG.0000000000000780

[85] Dunaway PM, Wong RK. Risk and surveillance intervals for squamous cell carcinoma in achalasia. Gastrointestinal Endoscopy Clinics of North America. 2001;**11**:425-434

[86] Gorti H, Samo S, Shahnavaz N, Qayed E. Distal esophageal spasm: Update on diagnosis and management in the era of high-resolution manometry. World Journal of Clinical Cases. 2020;**8**:1026-1032. DOI: 10.12998/wjcc.v8.i6.1026

[87] Nakajima N, Sato H, Takahashi K, Hasegawa G, Mizuno K, Hashimoto S, et al. Muscle layer histopathology and manometry pattern of primary esophageal motility disorders including achalasia. Neurogastroenterology and Motility. 2017;**29**:e12968. DOI: 10.1111/nmo.12968

[88] He YQ, Sheng JQ, Wang JH, An HJ, Wang X, Li AQ, et al. Symptomatic diffuse esophageal spasm as a major ictal manifestation of post-traumatic epilepsy: A case report. Diseases of the Esophagus. 2013;**26**:327-330. DOI: 10.1111/j.1442-2050.2012.01442.x

[89] Roman S, Kahrilas PJ. Distal esophageal spasm. Current Opinion in Gastroenterology. 2015;**31**:328-333. DOI: 10.1097/MOG.0000000000000187

[90] Zaher EA, Patel P, Atia G, Sigdel S. Distal esophageal spasm: An updated review. Cureus. 2023;**15**:e41504. DOI: 10.7759/cureus.41504

[91] Sato H, Takeuchi M, Takahashi K, et al. Nutcracker and jackhammer esophagus treatment: A three-case survey, including two novel cases of eosinophilic infiltration into the muscularis propria. Endoscopy. 2015;**47**:855-857. DOI: 10.1055/s-0034-1391985

[92] Muir A, Falk GW. Eosinophilic esophagitis: A review. Journal of the American Medical Association. 2021;**326**:1310-1318. DOI: 10.1001/jama.2021.14920

[93] Clément M, Zhu WJ, Neshkova E, Bouin M. Jackhammer esophagus: From manometric diagnosis to clinical presentation. Canadian Journal of Gastroenterology & Hepatology. 2019;**2019**:5036160. Published 2019 Mar 3. DOI: 10.1155/2019/5036160

[94] Sato H, Nakajima N, Takahashi K, Hasegawa G, Mizuno KI, Hashimoto S, et al. Proposed criteria to differentiate heterogeneous eosinophilic gastrointestinal disorders of the esophagus, including eosinophilic esophageal myositis. World Journal of Gastroenterology. 2017;**23**:2414-2423. DOI: 10.3748/wjg.v23.i13.2414

[95] Sato H, Takeuchi M, Takahashi K. Eosinophilic infiltration of the

muscularis propria in a patient with jackhammer esophagus treated with per-oral endoscopic myotomy. Clinical Gastroenterology and Hepatology. 2015;**13**:e33-e34. DOI: 10.1016/j.cgh.2014.11.005

[96] Zuercher P, Moret CS, Dziewas R, Schefold JC. Dysphagia in the intensive care unit: Epidemiology, mechanisms, and clinical management. Critical Care. 2019;**23**:103. DOI: 10.1186/s13054-019-2400-2

[97] Johnston BT. Oesophageal dysphagia: A stepwise approach to diagnosis and management. The Lancet Gastroenterology & Hepatology. 2017;**2**:604-609. DOI: 10.1016/S2468-1253(17)30001-8

[98] Nigam GB, Vasant DH, Dhar A. Curriculum review: Investigation and management of dysphagia. Frontline Gastroenterology. 2021;**13**:254-261. DOI: 10.1136/flgastro-2021-101917

[99] Eslick GD, Talley NJ. Dysphagia: Epidemiology, risk factors and impact on quality of life–A population-based study. Alimentary Pharmacology & Therapeutics. 2008;**27**:971-979. DOI: 10.1111/j.1365-2036.2008.03664.x

[100] Rommel N, Hamdy S. Oropharyngeal dysphagia: Manifestations and diagnosis. Nature Reviews. Gastroenterology & Hepatology. 2016;**13**:49-59. DOI: 10.1038/nrgastro.2015.199

[101] Thiyagalingam S, Kulinski AE, Thorsteinsdottir B, Shindelar KL, Takahashi PY. Dysphagia in older adults. Mayo Clinic Proceedings. 2021;**96**:488-497. DOI: 10.1016/j.mayocp.2020.08.001

[102] Bhattacharyya N. The prevalence of dysphagia among adults in the United States. Otolaryngology and Head and Neck Surgery. 2014;**151**:765-769. DOI: 10.1177/0194599814549156

[103] Drossman DA, Li Z, Andruzzi E, Temple RD, Talley NJ, Thompson WG, et al. U.S. householder survey of functional gastrointestinal disorders. Prevalence, sociodemography, and health impact. Digestive Diseases and Sciences. 1993;**38**:1569-1580. DOI: 10.1007/BF01303162

[104] Nasr I, Attaluri A, Hashmi S, Gregersen H, Rao SS. Investigation of esophageal sensation and biomechanical properties in functional chest pain. Neurogastroenterology and Motility. 2010;**22**:520-526, e116. DOI: 10.1111/j.1365-2982.2009.01451.x

[105] Schofield PM, Brooks NH, Colgan S, Bennett DH, Whorwell PJ, Bray CL, et al. Left ventricular function and oesophageal function in patients with angina pectoris and normal coronary angiograms. British Heart Journal. 1987;**58**:218-224. DOI: 10.1136/hrt.58.3.218

[106] Katz PO, Castell DO. Approach to the patient with unexplained chest pain. The American Journal of Gastroenterology. 2000;**95**:S4-S8. DOI: 10.1016/s0002-9270(00)01072-8

[107] Chahal PS, Rao SS. Functional chest pain: Nociception and visceral hyperalgesia. Journal of Clinical Gastroenterology. 2005;**39**:S204-S209. discussion S210. DOI: 10.1097/01.mcg.0000156108.20871.bb

[108] Kaltenbach T, Crockett S, Gerson LB. Are lifestyle measures effective in patients with gastroesophageal reflux disease? Archives of Internal Medicine. 2006;**166**:965-971. DOI: 10.1001/archinte.166.9.965

[109] Sethi S, Richter JE. Diet and gastroesophageal reflux disease.

Current Opinion in Gastroenterology. 2017;**33**:107-111. DOI: 10.1097/MOG.0000000000000337

[110] Djärv T. Physical activity, obesity and gastroesophageal reflux disease in the general population. World Journal of Gastroenterology. 2012;**18**:3710-3714. DOI: 10.3748/wjg.v18.i28.3710

[111] Slee GR, Wagner SM, McCullough FS. Odynophagia in patients with malignant disorders. Cancer. 1985;**55**:2877-2879. DOI: 10.1002/1097-0142(19850615)55:12

[112] Harar RP, Kumar S, Saeed MA, Gatland DJ. Management of globus pharyngeus: Review of 699 cases. The Journal of Laryngology and Otology. 2004;**118**:522-527. DOI: 10.1258/0022215041615092

[113] Pechlivanis I, Seiz M, Barth M, Schmieder K. A healthy man with intractable hiccups. Journal of Clinical Neuroscience. 2010;**17**:781-783. DOI: 10.1016/j.jocn.2009.08.022

[114] Rey E, Elola-Olaso CM, Rodríguez-Artalejo F, Locke GR 3rd, Díaz-Rubio M. Prevalence of atypical symptoms and their association with typical symptoms of gastroesophageal reflux in Spain. European Journal of Gastroenterology & Hepatology. 2006;**18**:969-975. DOI: 10.1097/01.meg.0000230081.53298.03

[115] Gambescia RA, Rogers AI. Gastroenterology. Dysphagia: Diagnosis by history. Postgraduate Medicine. 1976;**59**:211-216. DOI: 10.1080/00325481.1976.11714311

[116] Van Daele DJ. Esophageal manometry, pH testing, endoscopy, and videofluoroscopy in patients with globus sensation. The Laryngoscope. 2020;**130**:2120-2125. DOI: 10.1002/lary.28289

[117] Ishii T, Akaishi T, Abe M, Takayama S, Koseki K, Kamei T, et al. Importance of barium swallow test and chest CT scan for correct diagnosis of achalasia in the primary care setting. The Tohoku Journal of Experimental Medicine. 2019;**247**:41-49. DOI: 10.1620/tjem.247.41

[118] O'Neill OM, Johnston BT, Coleman HG. Achalasia: A review of clinical diagnosis, epidemiology, treatment and outcomes. World Journal of Gastroenterology. 2013;**19**(35):5806-5812. DOI: 10.3748/wjg.v19.i35.5806

[119] ASGE Standards of Practice Committee, Early DS, Ben-Menachem T, Decker GA, Evans JA, Fanelli RD, et al. Appropriate use of GI endoscopy. Gastrointestinal Endoscopy. 2012;**75**:1127-1131. DOI: 10.1016/j.gie.2012.01.011

[120] Zhang L, Zou DW. Endoscopy in the diagnosis and management of esophageal motility disorders. Zhonghua Wei Chang Wai Ke Za Zhi. 2012;**15**:656-658

[121] Chilukuri P, Odufalu F, Hachem C. Dysphagia. Missouri Medicine. 2018;**115**:206-210

[122] Lenfant C. Chest pain of cardiac and noncardiac origin. Metabolism. 2010;**59**(Suppl. 1):S41-S46. DOI: 10.1016/j.metabol.2010.07.014

[123] Patel DA, Yadlapati R, Vaezi MF. Esophageal motility disorders: Current approach to diagnostics and therapeutics. Gastroenterology. 2022;**162**:1617-1634. DOI: 10.1053/j.gastro.2021.12.289

[124] Short TP, Thomas E. An overview of the role of calcium antagonists in the treatment of achalasia and diffuse oesophageal spasm. Drugs. 1992;**43**:177-184. DOI:10.2165/00003495-199243020-00004

[125] Dughera L, Chiaverina M, Cacciotella L, Cisarò F. Management

of achalasia. Clinical and Experimental Gastroenterology. 2011;**4**:33-41. DOI: 10.2147/CEG.S11593

[126] Pasricha PJ, Ravich WJ, Hendrix TR, Sostre S, Jones B, Kalloo AN. Intrasphincteric botulinum toxin for the treatment of achalasia. The New England Journal of Medicine. 1995;**332**:774-778. DOI: 10.1056/NEJM199503233321203

[127] Shim CS. Endoscopic botulinum toxin injection: Benefit and limitation. Gastrointestinal Intervention. 2014;**3**:19-23. DOI: 10.1016/j.gii.2014.03.001

[128] Sterling JL, Schey R, Malik Z. The role of botulinum toxin injections for Esophageal motility disorders. Current Treatment Options in Gastroenterology. 2018;**16**:528-540. DOI: 10.1007/s11938-018-0212-0

[129] Moonen A, Annese V, Belmans A, Bredenoord AJ, Bruley des Varannes S, Costantini M, et al. Long-term results of the European achalasia trial: A multicentre randomised controlled trial comparing pneumatic dilation versus laparoscopic Heller myotomy. Gut. 2016;**65**:732-739. DOI: 10.1136/gutjnl-2015-310602

[130] Stavropoulos SN, Modayil RJ, Friedel D, Savides T. The international per Oral endoscopic Myotomy survey (IPOEMS): A snapshot of the global POEM experience. Surgical Endoscopy. 2013;**27**:3322-3338. DOI: 10.1007/s00464-013-2913-8

[131] Modayil RJ, Zhang X, Rothberg B, Kollarus M, Galibov I, Peller H, et al. Peroral endoscopic myotomy: 10-year outcomes from a large, single-center U.S. series with high follow-up completion and comprehensive analysis of long-term efficacy, safety, objective GERD, and endoscopic functional luminal assessment. Gastrointestinal Endoscopy. 2021;**94**:930-942. DOI: 10.1016/j.gie.2021.05.014

[132] Ponds FA, Fockens P, Lei A, Neuhaus H, Beyna T, Kandler J, et al. Effect of peroral endoscopic myotomy vs pneumatic dilation on symptom severity and treatment outcomes among treatment-naive patients with achalasia: A randomized clinical trial. Journal of the American Medical Association. 2019;**322**:134-144. DOI: 10.1001/jama.2019.8859

[133] Cappell MS, Stavropoulos SN, Friedel D. Updated systematic review of achalasia, with a focus on POEM therapy. Digestive Diseases and Sciences. 2020;**65**:38-65. DOI: 10.1007/s10620-019-05784-3

[134] Campos GM, Vittinghoff E, Rabl C, Takata M, Gadenstätter M, Lin F, et al. Endoscopic and surgical treatments for achalasia: A systematic review and meta-analysis. Annals of Surgery. 2009;**249**:45-57. DOI: 10.1097/SLA.0b013e31818e43ab

[135] Andolfi C, Fisichella PM. Meta-analysis of clinical outcome after treatment for achalasia based on manometric subtypes. The British Journal of Surgery. 2019;**106**:332-341. DOI: 10.1002/bjs.11049

[136] Schlottmann F, Patti MG. Primary Esophageal motility disorders: Beyond achalasia. International Journal of Molecular Sciences. 2017;**18**:1399. DOI: 10.3390/ijms18071399

[137] Watson TJ. Esophagectomy for end-stage achalasia. World Journal of Surgery. 2015;**39**:1634-1641. DOI: 10.1007/s00268-015-3012-x

[138] Aiolfi A, Asti E, Bonitta G, Bonavina L. Esophagectomy for end-stage achalasia: Systematic review and Meta-analysis. World Journal of Surgery. 2018;**42**:1469-1476. DOI: 10.1007/s00268-017-4298-7

Chapter 3

# Dysphagia: Esophageal Motility Disorders and Advancement in Management

*Emmanuel Ocheli*

## Abstract

Motility disorder of the esophagus is a functional cause of dysphagia classified into primary and secondary motility disorders. While secondary causes of motility disturbances of the esophagus arise from some systemic conditions and their management including diagnostic and therapeutic approach which is outlined in standard medical textbooks. Primary motility disorders are either oropharngeal and esophageal motility disorders. Esophageal motility disorders, largely amenable to some surgical intervention include such conditions as achalasia, diffuse esophageal spasm (DES) and hypertensive lower esophageal sphincter. Dysphagia, chestpain, regurgitation and weight loss constitute the predominant symptomatology of motility disorders of the esophagus. There are few physical findings on examination. The main diagnostic tools in properly diagnosing this group of conditions include contrast esophagogram and high-resolution impedance manometry, which have revolutionized management decisions and expectations in terms of prognosis. Surgical treatment is more effective and longer-lasting than medical therapies. Laparoscopic esophagomyotomy, in addition to partial fundoplication, has proven to be more efficacious than other techniques. However, the recent introduction of peroral endoscopic myotomy is the new optimism in the treatment of this age-long disorder. Early, appropriate, and standardized management protocol can lead to resolution of symptoms and improvement in outlook.

**Keywords:** dysphagia, barium swallow, manometry, Heller's myotomy, fundoplication

## 1. Introduction

Dysphagia is defined as difficulty in swallowing or transferring bolus or ingested materials from the mouth to the stomach. In consonance with the phases of deglutition, dysphagia is classified, therefore, as oropharyngeal and esophageal. Oropharyngeal dysphagia arises from functional abnormalities in the swallowing mechanisms in the mouth or pharynx – occurring mostly as a result of infection, neurologic, metabolic, myopathic disease. Physiologically, dysphagia occurring in the early phase of the swallowing process is most likely due to oropharyngeal dysphagia.

Other distinguishing symptoms include drooling, coughing, inability to chew, nasal regurgitation of solids and liquids [1, 2].

### 1.1 Brief anatomy of the esophagus

The esophagus is a conduit from the throat to the stomach. It is a muscular contracting tube starting from the pharynx, running caudally to exit through the diaphragmatic crura, ending in the stomach below the diaphragm as shown in **Figure 1**. The esophagus begins immediately inferior to the cricoid cartilage located anteriorly, at the level of the sixth cervical spinous process, lower border of the sixth cervical vertebral body and transverse processes. The cricopharyngeus muscle, which forms a collar around the esophagus acts as the superior esophageal sphincter [1, 3, 4].

In its upper aspect, the esophagus lies in the midline for 3–5 cm in front of the trachea, then deviates to the left down to the region of bronchial bifurcation, only to return to the midline in its middle third. The esophagus then deviates again to the left, angulating antero-inferiorly adjacent to the thoracic aorta passing through the diaphragmatic crura and terminating in the stomach at 2–3 cm below the diaphragm. There are three natural constrictions in the esophagus. The first of these constrictions is at the level of the cricopharyngeus muscles which forms the superior sphincter (cricoid cartilage). The second is at the level of bronchial bifurcation and the aortic arch crossing; while the third is at the gastroesophageal junction narrowed by the muscular tension effect of the diaphragmatic opening and crural condensation. All three constrictions may be visible on contrast barium/gastrografin swallow and can be appreciated during upper gastrointestinal (GI) endoscopic examinations. The importance of these natural narrowing is significant in cases of swallowed foreign

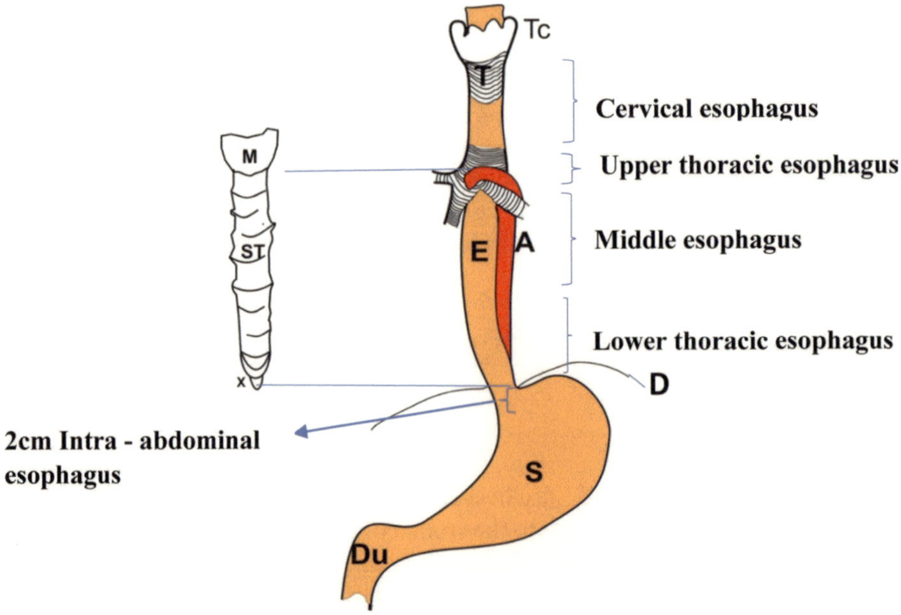


**Figure 1.**
*Schematic diagram of anatomy of the esophagus (Tc – Thyroid cartilage; T – Trachea; E-Esophagus; A – Aorta; D – Diaphragm; S – Stomach; Du – Duodenum; M – Manubrium; ST – Sternum; X-Xiphoid). The horizontal lines from the sternum to the esophagus corresponds to the regions of the esophagus symptomatically. Source: Author's original work.*

bodies acting as points of impaction and are susceptible to greater extent of injury in times of ingestion of caustic substances. The esophagus is divided into three portions, the cervical, thoracic and gastric parts (as seen in **Figure 1**). The cervical portion begins at level of the cricoid cartilage to the thoracic inlet marked by the lower border of the second vertebral body. While the thoracic portion extends from the thoracic inlet to the level of diaphragmatic hiatus; and, the gastric portion remains intraabdominal and constitutes a part of the lower esophageal sphincter. The length of the cervical portion is about 5 cm, the thoracic is 20 cm and the gastric is about 2 cm. In the groove between the trachea and the esophagus in the upper third lies the recurrent laryngeal nerve on the right and left sides.

Circumferentially from the inner to outer section, the lumen of the esophagus consists of stratified epithelium and few columnar epithelia at the gastroesophageal junction (GEJ). This is surrounded by the lamina propria, the intramural musculature consisting of an inner circular which is striated in the upper third gradually turning into smooth muscle in its middle third and wholly smooth muscle in the lower third; and, outer longitudinal smooth muscles in its entire length.

Blood supply to the esophagus derives from several sources. The cervical portion is supplied by the right and left inferior thyroidal arteries, the thoracic esophagus receives its blood supply from the bronchial arteries and direct arterial branches from the aorta on both sides while the lower third is supplied by the ascending esophageal branch of the left gastric artery and the inferior phrenic arteries. Within the wall of the esophagus, the arteries form two plexuses – muscular and submucosal plexuses. These longitudinal arterial plexuses make mobilization of the esophagus less hazardous without compromise to the vascular supply. The venous system also forms an arcade of venous plexuses which coalesce to drain into the inferior thyroidal veins in the neck, into the azygos, hemiazygos and bronchial veins in the thorax; and, in the abdomen empty into the coronary veins. At the GEJ, the esophageal and gastric plexuses are continuous forming a portosystemic anastomosis, the significance of which becomes important in patients with portal hypertension due to liver cirrhosis.

The nervous supply to the esophagus arises from diverse origins. The vagus nerve (cranial nerve X) and its recurrent laryngeal nerve branches predominantly innervates the pharynx and the cervical esophagus with little contributions from the IX cranial or glossopharyngeal nerve. The affectation of these nerves not only interferes with the function of the vocal cords but also affects swallowing due to interference with cricopharyngeal sphincter function and cervical esophageal motility. Sensory pathways are by afferent non-synaptic sensory nerve fibers integrated into the first to fourth thoracic spinal segments consisting of both sympathetic and parasympathetic vagal pathways; the same segments receiving fibers from the heart are integrated, giving rise to similarity of symptoms in diseases of both organs. This partially explains the reason coronary artery disease is an important differential diagnosis of benign esophageal diseases.

The lymphatic drainage of the esophagus has an extensive submucosal plexus and runs longitudinal in the submucosa before penetrating radially to join the lymphatic channels in the adventitia. Hence, cancer cell metastasis can occur early and to a considerable distance from the primary lesion without recognition. Drainage of lymph in the upper two thirds of the esophagus is superiorly; and, in the lower third is inferiorly toward the gastric and coeliac plexuses/lymph nodes. Thus, efferent lymphatics channels in the cervical esophagus drain into the deep cervical and paratracheal lymph nodes, while those from the upper and middle thoracic regions of the esophagus flow into the paratracheal lymph nodes [1, 3, 4].

## 1.2 Physiology of swallowing

Swallowing or deglutition is a coordinated physiological function that moves a bolus from the mouth through the esophagus into the stomach. It consists of both voluntary and involuntary phases – depending on the phases: oropharyngeal and esophageal phases. It starts with the voluntary actions on a bolus of food material in the mouth and involves mastication, as long as the senses or the individual determines, rolling reasonably-sized bolus, positioning, elevation of the tongue, which pushes the food posteriorly into the back of the throat or pharynx. Propulsion of the bolus into the pharynx beyond the upper esophageal sphincter triggers the involuntary phase of deglutition. This results in the generation of primary and secondary peristaltic waves initially from the peritonsillar cells – primary esophageal pacemakers. These peristaltic waves generate a contractile esophageal activity behind the bolus which is propelled forward; and, by reflex mechanism of neural loop connecting to the swallowing center in the lower medulla and pons. There is concomitant relaxation in front of the advancing bolus including the lower esophageal sphincter (LES), thus aiding the forward movement through the esophagus and into the stomach. Any remaining food in the esophagus generates secondary peristalsis both from the primary centers and the body of the esophagus. These secondary waves are mediated principally by vagus nerves via the myenteric plexuses [4, 5].

The process involved in a single swallowing effort is repetitive when food is chewed and swallowed in bits and pieces. A bolus is propelled through the esophagus by peristalsis. Two types of peristaltic waves are generated: primary and secondary [4, 5]. The primary peristalsis is a continuation of waves that propel food in the pharyngeal phase of swallowing into the esophagus. The pharyngeal phase is somewhat more complex and involves combined coordination with the respiratory pathway. A bolus entering the retropharynx stimulates contraction of the glossopalatine muscles which retracts medially leaving a slit in the midline, allowing morsels (bits/pieces of bitten foods) to pass through; elevation of the larynx and epiglottis with closure of the vocal cords. This allows the bolus to drop into the upper esophagus without entering the trachea. The pharyngeal phase takes a few seconds during which the respiration is on hold; and, this break is inconsequentially unrecognizable. Sometimes, this coordination is integrated with when talking during eating. Secondary peristalsis is generated to clear the esophagus of any residual contents. They arise both from intrinsic 'pacemakers' in the body of the esophagus and through vagal reflex arc and glossopharyngeal efferent nerve fibers. Each esophageal phase takes about 8–10 seconds or less, in an erect posture, aided by gravity.

Generally, dysphagia is a symptom arising from myriads of etiological factors; however, this chapter sets out to dwell more on esophageal dysphagia resulting from primary intrinsic esophageal wall motility disorders, as shown in **Table 1**. Patients who classically present with perceived dysphagia to liquids, less to solids (referred to as paradoxical dysphagia), regurgitation, night cough, and insidious weight loss over months or years may be indications of esophageal motility disorders. Notably, symptoms of esophageal dysphagia are principally in the chest or abdomen [1, 2, 4, 6]. It may present as chest pain, localized to the area affected – retrosternal or epigastric burning sensation which radiates mimicking coronary artery disease (CAD); regurgitation, perceptible level of arrest of bolus. In general, precise perception of location of obstructive lesion during swallowing is often described by patients [1, 2] in 75% of cases. Other symptoms include dysphagia to solids, progressing to liquids when there is mechanical esophageal obstruction, is relieved by regurgitation or a change in diet to semi-solids or liquids. Associated weight loss, anorexia, and low-grade fever, in

| |
|---|
| a. PRIMARY ESOPHAGEAL MOTILITY DISORDERS |
| • Achalasia, 'Vigorous' Achalasia. |
| • Diffuse esophageal spasm. |
| • Nutcracker esophagus. |
| • Hypertensive lower esophageal segment. |
| b. SECONDARY ESOPHAGEAL MOTILITY DISORDERS |
| • Endocrine and metabolic disorders (Diabetes mellitus, Myxedema). |
| • Connective tissue diseases, systemic sclerosis, systemic lupus erythematosus, Scleroderma, Amyloidosis, etc. |
| • Alcoholism. |
| • Neuromuscular diseases – parkinsonism, muscle dystrophies, etc. |
| • Crohn's disease. |

**Table 1.**
*Summary etiology of esophageal motility disorders.*

addition to obstructive symptoms, suggest cancer of the upper gastrointestinal (GI) tract.

## 2. Clinical features

### 2.1 Primary motility disorders: Consists of these four classes

a. Achalasia

b. Diffuse esophageal spasm

c. Hypertensive lower esophageal sphincter

d. Nutcracker esophagus

#### *2.1.1 Achalasia*

##### *2.1.1.1 Epidermiology*

Achalasia is a rare primary motility disorder of the esophagus. The incidence is 1–6: 100,000 in the United States of America [4, 6, 7, 8]. Males and females are affected, and it is common between the ages of 20–60 years.

##### *2.1.1.2 Pathology*

The cause of achalasia in majority of cases is unknown. However, evidence is accumulating in support of autoimmune-derived ganglionitis arising from viral infections in genetically susceptible individuals [2]. The basic lesion is the absence of ganglion cells in the Auerbach's (Myenteric) plexus in the body of the esophagus. This results in a pathophysiological dysfunction, resulting in ineffective peristalsis in the body of the esophagus, with persistent contraction or non-relaxation of the lower esophageal segment (LES) and a functional esophageal obstruction. While the cause is unknown, secondary causes have been known to occur with similar nature in Chagas disease, DM and malignant infiltration of the LES (pseudoachalasia). Chaga's disease is caused by flagellated protozoa, trypanosoma cruzi, endemic in Central and South America, where it is prevalent as the commonest etiological factor of achalasia and has the same pathological resemblance with achalasia [1, 2]. Infection by the trypanosome involves the destruction of the esophageal myenteric plexus frequently associated with neurological disturbances in other extra-esophageal sites, giving rise to accompanying ureteral (megaureter), duodenal (megaduodenum), colonic dilatation (megacolon) and myocarditis [2]. The pathogenesis in these extra-esophageal sites may have similar underlying mechanisms worthy of further research.

Sustained pressure in the LES, functional obstruction often causes gradual dilatation of the esophagus greater than 4 cm in diameter in an adult. Progressive dilatation can increase to great dimensions resembling the sigmoid colon, referred to as sigmoid or megaesophagus. Achalasia is regarded as a precancerous condition as there is an increased risk of esophageal malignancy from chronic mucosal irritation by toxic degradation retention products in the esophageal lumen [1, 2].

#### *2.1.1.3 Clinical features*

The history is one of insidious, indistinct progressive onset of dysphagia initially to solids. As the disease progresses, the dysphagia is to solids and liquids in 70–97% of cases [7, 8]. However, in late stages, it is perceived that the dysphagia is more to liquids, especially hot liquids, than solids (paradoxical dysphagia); regurgitation of foul-smelling undigested foods previously eaten several days ago occurs in 75% of patients [5, 6] thus constituting major characteristic symptomatology of achalasia. Other presentations include weight loss in 60% (as sufferers may adduce to some loss of weight noticed as a result of loose clothing, increasing waist belt holes), retrosternal chest pain present among 40% (which must be excluded from angina), heartburn, halitosis and sometimes, sensation of fluid lapping in the chest in long-standing cases. Features of aspiration is accompanied by night coughs, choking episodes, voice change, wheezing and recurrent pneumonia [1, 4–9].

Among the different scores to assess the severity and frequency of symptoms of achalasia is the Eckardt score (**Table 2**). The symptom-grading system was adopted to determine the presence of specific stage of the disease and efficacy of treatment modalities. Weighted points (0–3) are assigned for four major symptoms, viz.: dysphagia, regurgitation, chest pain and weight loss. A total score ranging from 0

| **Notations** | | SCORE | | |
|---|---|---|---|---|
| Symptoms | 0 | 1 | 2 | 3 |
| Weight loss (Kg) | None | < 5 | 5–10 | >10 |
| Dysphagia | None | Occasional | Daily | Each meal |
| Retrosternal chestpain | | | | |
| Regurgitation | | | | |

**Table 2.**
*Eckardt score for symptomatic Evaluation of Achalasia. Source: Author's original conception.*

to 12, categorized as stage 0 (0–1); stage I (2–3); stage II (4–6) and a score of 6–12 corresponds to stage III.

Symptoms alone does not conclusively diagnose achalasia, as other esophageal conditions overlap in their various manifestations. The Eckardt score and its staging do not correlate with degree of esophageal dilatation, manometric findings or response to treatment. Complete application of full diagnostic investigative tools assists in decision-making in relation to the choice of treatment early in the course of management of patients. Physical examination is largely unremarkable with mild dehydration in some instances. Rales may be presents in regions of the lung zones when pneumonic process complicates the condition.

#### *2.1.1.4 Diagnostic workup*

##### *2.1.1.4.1 Chest radiograph*

The very first investigative tool employed in the diagnosis of achalasia is routine chest radiograph, mostly deriving from the evaluation of a patient with persistent night cough, wheezy respiration and recurrent pneumonia. The chest X-ray (CXR) features in early stages, as shown in **Figure 2**, is essentially normal; however, there could be mediastinal widening in late stages. Additionally, suggestive features are absent gastric gas bubble sign and a right-sided posterior mediastinal shadow indicating the outline of the fluid-filled esophagus [1, 4].

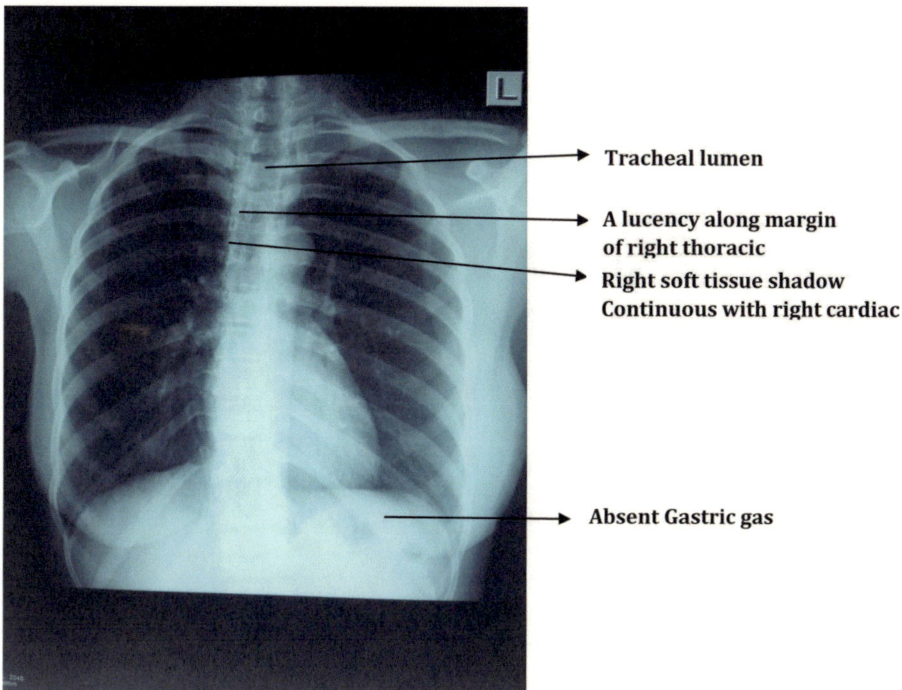


**Figure 2.**
*Suggestive CXR appearance of achalasia in a 39—old female patient presenting with an Echardt score grade I after a 5-year history of dysphagia. Source: Author' archives.*

#### *2.1.1.4.2 Barium (contrast) study*

Barium swallow fully outlines the esophageal configuration. As shown in **Figure 3**, it is characterized by dilatation of the body of the esophagus with the classic pencil-tip, bird-beak or rat-tail appearance resulting from distal esophageal narrowing tapering gradually toward the stomach [1, 4, 6]. The dilated body may show mottling within the esophageal lumen due to retained food particles undergoing putrefaction. A full column, double-contrast or cine-radiology may be necessary to further confirm the underlying pathology [1, 4, 10]. In advanced disease, due to massive distension, the esophagus is grossly dilated and tortuous, resembling the sigmoid colon referred to as sigmoid esophagus (**Figure 4**).

#### *2.1.1.4.3 Upper GI endoscopy*

Upper GI endoscopy is usually undertaken to exclude peptic ulcer disease or obstructive esophageal diseases such as stricture, web and malignancy – either developing in situ; or, as pseudoachalasia [1, 4, 5, 8, 10]. It further strengthens the diagnosis by visualization of putrid fluid filling and lapping in the esophagus real-time and suctioning of same to see the terminal constricted segment, which may or may not be passable, as shown in **Figure 5a-c**. The finding of an empty stomach further strengthens the near absence of passage of esophageal contents into the distal gastric space. While the description of the procedure for conducting upper GI endoscopy is beyond the scope of this discuss, it simply allows the use of telescopic flexible fibre-optic instrument to visualize the entire esophageal lumen including obtaining biopsy specimens for histological analyses.

#### *2.1.1.4.4 Esophageal manometry*

Esophageal manometry is the gold standard for the definitive diagnosis of motility disorders of the esophagus, notably achalasia. This is a specialized investigation consisting of a catheter system connected along its length to pressure sensors that

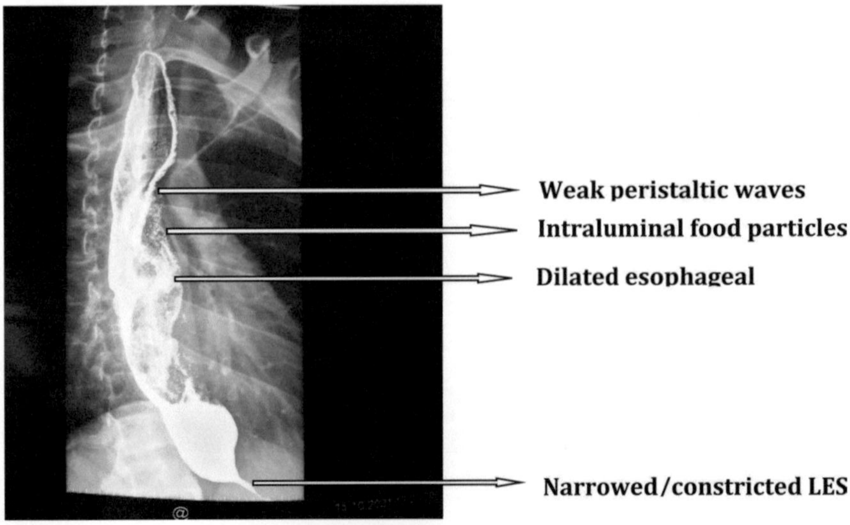


**Figure 3.**
*Barium swallow of a patient with suspected achalasia. Source: Author's archives.*

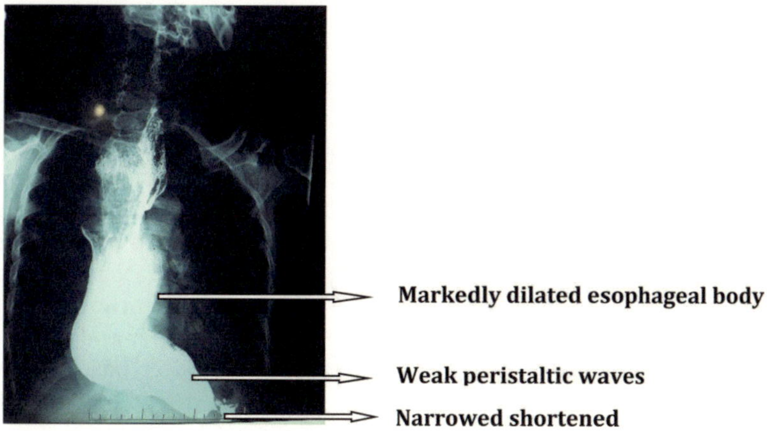


**Figure 4.**
*Sigmoid or megaesophagus. Source: Author's archives.*

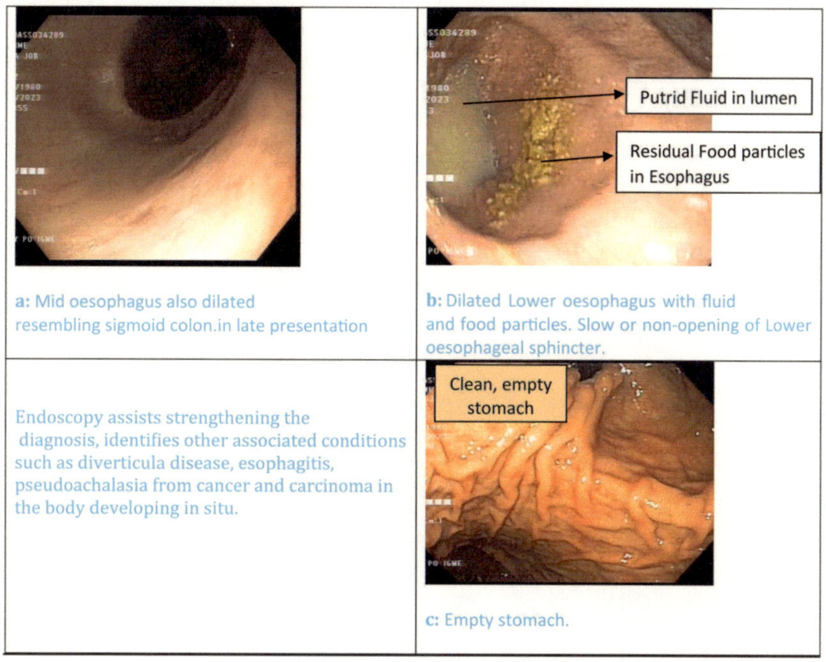


**Figure 5.**
*Endoscopic findings in achalasia. Source: Author's archives.*

measure the 'segmental' pressure along different zones of the esophagus down to the cardia of the stomach [4–8, 11, 12]. In diagnosing achalasia, four distinct manometric features stand out:

- Hypertensive LES, with intraesophageal pressure greater than 8–12 mmHg which is 92% sensitive.

- Failure of the LES to relax on swallowing.

- Absent peristalsis in the body of the esophagus.
- Elevated LES baseline pressure.

Ray Clouse, in 1991 [13], pioneered the innovative advancement in conventional esophageal manometry by adding 36 miniaturized pressure-measuring sensors recording multiple longitudinal and circumferential sites into the modern-day high-resolution manometry (HRM), creating a color-coded mapping of esophageal and sphincter pressure pattern (**Figure 6**). These catheter systems are embedded with miniaturized sensors aligned to cover every centimeter along the entire length of the esophagus. Data so acquired from the upper and lower esophageal sphincters, esophageal body, LES is analyzed by computer-based software. The test is easy to perform, the time of testing is shortened, and interpretation is simplified, and it has been configured into the Chicago Classification. This has increased the sensitivity in measuring pressure gradients along the esophagus, predicting bolus propagation, and aids the diagnosis of various localized motor abnormalities [4, 7].

The advent of technologically-enabled HRM not only increased the diagnostic accuracy but also has assisted in the identification of other variants of the disease from the quality of data acquisition [4, 7, 8, 10]. Parameters such as Integrated Relaxation Pressure (IRP) and analysis of esophageal body are available. The IRP accurately defines the LES relaxation by corresponding to the mean pressure of 4 s in a 10 s gap of greatest post-deglution relaxation as a bolus enters into the initial phase of swallowing. Analysis of the esophageal body based on aperistalsis, pressurization of the esophageal body and/or presence of spastic ineffectual esophageal contractions. In all three classes or variants of the Chicago Classification, there

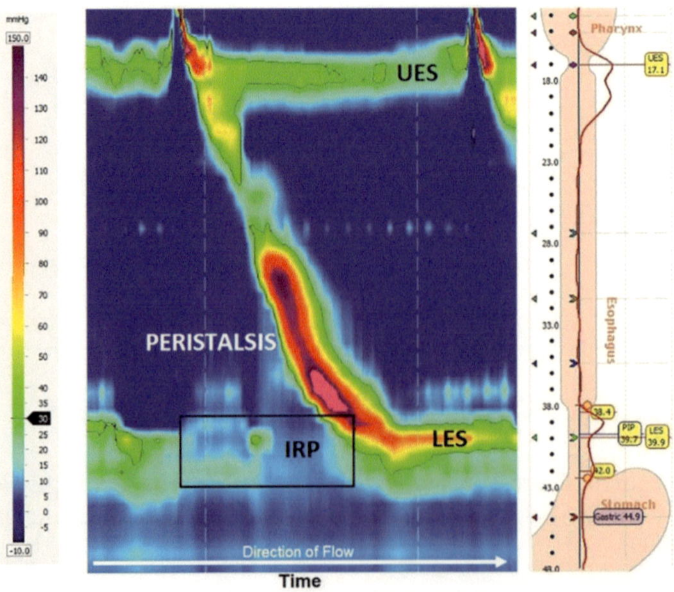


**Figure 6.**
*High-resolution esophageal manometry with pressure tracing. Source: Mari et al. [8]. Available from: https://www.researchgate.net/publication/330674046_Open_Access_Rambam_Maimonides_Medical_Journal_Achalasia_Insights_into_Diagnostic_and_Therapeutic_Advances_for_an_Ancient_Disease. CC-BY 4.0.*

is incomplete relaxation of the LES. The main criterion that has led to emergence of Chicago Classification or Criteria is based on the analysis of esophageal body (shown in **Table 3**).

The advent of the Chicago Classification (CC) has aided the recognition of subtypes of motility disorders of the esophagus. The Chicago Classification based on various parameters, is able to identify the different subtypes or classes [7, 8, 10]. Three distinguished classes have been designated Class I, II and III (**Figure 7a–c**), which bear a direct relationship with response to treatment. Type I – has a 56% positive response; Type II – 96% and Type III has only 29% response rate. Studies tend to suggest that Class I and II are amenable, to a higher degree, to dilatation and surgical myotomy; and, Class III is best managed by peroral endoscopic myotomy (POEM). These decisions are best taken in the initial approach to tackling the disease. Treatment outcomes with different classes have been recognized when different management protocols are used, whether medical or surgical [7, 9, 14].

The introduction of the concept, research into and development of esophageal impedance has revolutionized the determination of esophageal function and gastroesophageal reflux. Further improvement in combining HRM with impedance measurement has improved its predictive value in terms of choice of appropriate therapeutic management, specific diagnosis, results and assessment of treatment; and, prognostication of outcome [4, 7, 9]. The development and application of intraluminal electrical impedance catheters, the sensitivity of which is validated by cine-radiology, reinforces the diagnosis of motility disorders of the gastrointestinal system and type of reflux including acid, nonacid and gaseous materials. Intraluminal impedance (ratio of voltage to current) is inversely proportional to the electrical conductivity in the hollow organ. Gas has low electrical conductivity and high impedance, so does increased luminal diameter. Contraction with narrowing of the lumen has the opposite effect. While saliva and food in the esophagus are of high conductivity and reduced impedance levels. Thus, bolus transport along the esophagus is well-defined by impedance waveform characteristics hence allowing esophageal function and gastroesophageal reflux to be simultaneously integrated confirming actual esophageal dysfunction in an individual [4, 7].

#### *2.1.1.5 Treatment*

Treatment could be medical or surgical. Achalasia is a disease of unknown etiology and characterized by irreversible nerve damage of nervous plexuses, and treatment can only be directed at reducing the symptoms., as the restoration of the nerves is currently considered unattainable.

| Type | Lower esophageal sphincter | Esophageal body |
|---|---|---|
| I | Incomplete Relaxation (with increased pressure in LES) | Aperistalsis and absence of esophageal pressurization |
| II | | Aperistalsis and pan-esophageal pressurization in at least 20% of swallows |
| III | | Premature (spastic) contractions with distal contractility integral (DCI) >450 mmHg-s-cm with ≥20% of swallows |

**Table 3.**
*Specific criteria for manometric Chicago classification in achalasia. Source: Author's original conception.*

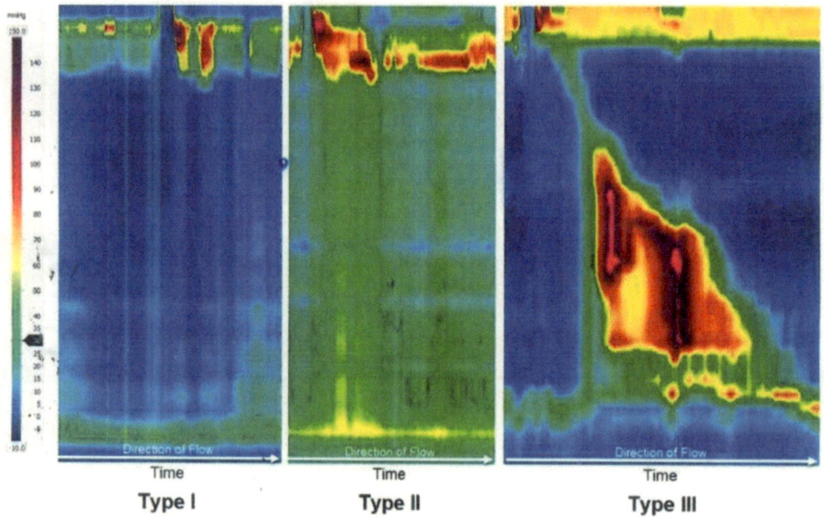


| a: Class 1 cc | b: Class II cc | c: Class III cc |
|---|---|---|
| Is characterized by the total absence of peristalsis for all swallows. | Peristalsis is replaced by pan-esophageal pressurizations. | Is characterized by the presence of premature spastic contraction. |

**Figure 7.**
*Chicago classification (cc) achalasia subtypes. Source: Mari et al. [8]. Available from: https://www.researchgate.net/publication/330674046_Open_Access_Rambam_Maimonides_Medical_Journal_Achalasia_Insights_into_Diagnostic_and_Therapeutic_Advances_for_an_Ancient_Disease. CC-BY 4.0.*

Medical management – Efficacy of medical treatment is inconsistent, unreliable and offers only short-term relief. It is best applied to early, mild, or when surgery is not feasible. Medical treatment is carried out with drug administration using calcium channel blockers and nitrates [15, 16]. These drugs are generally smooth muscle relaxants, but evidence-based proof of their efficacy is questionable. Nitrates are ubiquitous and widely used vasodilator drugs in cardiovascular diseases. These groups of drugs act in dual inter-related pathways to produce relaxation of smooth muscles of the body, including vascular, cardiac and smooth muscles of the esophagus. The mechanism of action involves the release of nitrous oxide (NO), a known powerful, smooth muscle relaxant and also activates guanylate cyclase. The activated guanylate cyclase converts AMP to cyclic 3′,5′-amino monophosphate (cAMP) in gastrointestinal (GI) smooth muscles to produce protein kinase. The protein kinase produced by the interaction of guanylate cyclase with nitric acid cause a dephosphorylated process in the GI smooth muscles, leading to inhibition of normal contractility. Thus, nitrous acid is an inhibitory non-adrenergic, non-cholinergic neurotransmitter mediated by cAMP. Nitroglycerin has been known to have been used in the treatment of achalasia for over 50 years [9, 15, 17].

Calcium channel blockers interfere with calcium ion ($Ca^{2+}$) influx into the cell across the cell membrane through the slow $Ca^{2+}$ channels. The mechanism may involve reduced contractility of smooth muscles in most luminal GI structures, vascular, cardiac and specialized nerve cells; thus, hypothetically leading to pan-relaxation in these structures. Calcium channel blockers reduce the amplitude of contractions [9, 15, 17]. The exact mechanism, whether by reduction in the initiation or force of contractions, is definitely known. Its use in esophageal motility in early, mild cases are questionable, but better symptom relief has been recorded in spastic, painful esophageal disorders such as nutcracker esophagus in which it has been observed to reduce amplitude of contractions and reducing associated chest pain. Calcium channel blockers and nitrates may reduce pain associated with esophageal spasms.

However, a more invasive medical management is the use of Botulinum toxin A injection (Botox injection). Botulinum toxin binds irreversibly to nerve endings, reducing the release of acetylcholine (ACH), the neurotransmitter necessary to transmit impulses [9, 15] at synapses. This effectively reduces the force of contraction of all muscle types including smooth muscles. Botulinum toxin is usually injected endoscopically into the wall of the esophagus proximal to the LES, ostensibly to paralyze smooth muscles of the immediate surrounding of the LES, thus relaxing the uninhibited LES characteristic of achalasia.

Botox, introduced by Pasricha et al. in 1993, involves the injection of 100 units of constituted Botox, divided into aliquots into the four quadrants of the LES. It offers 80% initial transient success, reducing to 60% recurrence in 1 year and 80% in 2 years [9]. The second drawback is that it causes inflammation resulting in submucosal fibrosis in the distal esophagus, peri-esophagitis jeopardizing subsequent myotomy as a result of adhesions in the layers of the esophagus. Thus, the planes of dissections are rendered difficult. It is not deemed a popular method of treatment, especially when myotomy is an option. However, reports suggest some improvement in symptoms of patients with spastic disorders. The resolution of symptoms with Botox is temporary and response decreases with repeated injections. Repetitive injection is necessary every 10 (11) months [1, 4, 5]. It finds its use mainly in unfit patients.

Pneumatic balloon dilatation (PBD) is the most effective nonsurgical therapy undertaken under fluoroscopic control in which high-pressure 30–35 mm diameter balloons are applied serially to the LES [9]. Documented results range from 60 to 90% initial success rate [1]. Initial results showed 70% symptom relief over 6 months after a mean of two sessions, decreasing to 36% over 20 years. Subsequent dilatations following a recurrence of symptoms are much less effective. Pneumatic balloon dilatation is even poorer with Chicago Class III [7, 9]. Recurrence is common in 5 years. Predictors of recurrence include young age less than 40 years, symptom duration of less than 5 years and post-dilatation LES pressure greater than 10 mmHg. Esophageal bleeding, rupture and perforation at 2–5% rate sometimes complicate this procedure [1]. These interventions provide short-term relief with subsequent recurrence within 6 months and are less effective than surgical modes of management. The high rate of 3–6% of esophageal perforation in the use of balloon dilatation has been a major limiting factor in the general adoption of this procedure [7].

#### *2.1.1.5.1 Surgical management*

As sequelae of the prolonged, insidious course of the disease, inanition, the physiological effects of anemia, dehydration, electrolyte, nutritional derangement, contact esophagitis and precursor to cancer, proper preoperative evaluation is necessary. This is more important in ensuring the correction of such abnormalities and optimization of the patient toward safe anesthesia and eventual satisfactory surgical outcomes. The preoperative investigations, apart from those special tests aiding diagnosis, are intended to fully elucidate patients' status and fitness for any surgical intervention or therapy. They include hematocrit (Hct), hemoglobin level (Hb), Serum electrolyte, urea and creatinine levels, urinalysis, fasting blood glucose (FBG), liver function tests (LFT), prothrombin/bleeding time, electrocardiogram (especially in elderly patients), chest X-ray (CXR) and endoscopy and respiratory function tests.

The goal of surgical treatment in achalasia is twofold – reduction of LES pressure and prevention of reflux:

Reduction of les pressure: A modified Heller's procedure was developed to reduce the tension in the contracted lower esophageal segment. Simply stated, it involves anterior longitudinal myotomy through the entire length of the contracted zone of the lower esophageal segment, extending 2 cm proximally and distally into the cardia of the stomach. Heller's esophagocardiomyotomy can be accomplished by open operation through thoracotomy (thoracic approach) or laparotomy (abdominal approach) (**Figure 8**) or by minimal access surgery (VATS – Left thoracoscopic myotomy or laparoscopic or endoscopic) [1, 4, 6, 9, 16]. Whichever procedure is chosen, it is recommended that the procedure be combined with an anti-reflux procedure. The thoracic (thoracotomy or thoracoscopic) procedures are better accompanied by the Belsey-type anti-reflux repairs as fundoplication from this approach is impossible. Conversely, the abdominal (laparotomy or laparoscopic) approach in undertaking Heller's myotomy is best combined with an anti-reflux procedure, preferably partial fundoplication (Dor's, Toupet or Guarner's) [1, 4, 6].

*2.1.1.5.2 Anti-reflux procedures*

The partial fundoplication (partial wrap-around) usually undertaken include Dor's procedure which is an anterior 180° fundal wrap-around or Toupet – a posterior 270° fundoplication [**Figure 9**].

*2.1.1.5.3 Minimal access surgery techniques*

Currently, Minimal access surgical techniques have overtaken open operations and have become the gold standard in advanced countries, driven by technological advancements in high-resolution optical instruments, thus facilitating pin-hole surgery, the need for cosmesis, less pain, less tissue destruction and shorter

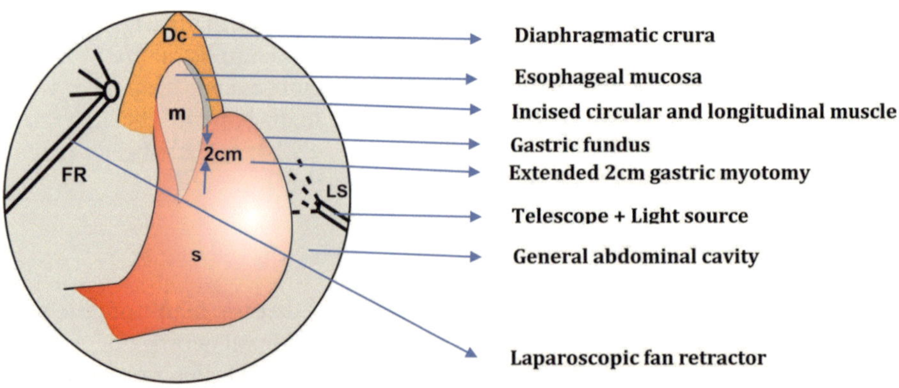


**Figure 8.**
*Schematic diagram of modified Hellers myotomy (abdominal/laparoscopic approach): Dc – Diaphragmatic crura; m – Putting mucosa; S – Stomach; LS – Light source; FR – Fan retractor. Source: Author's original work.*

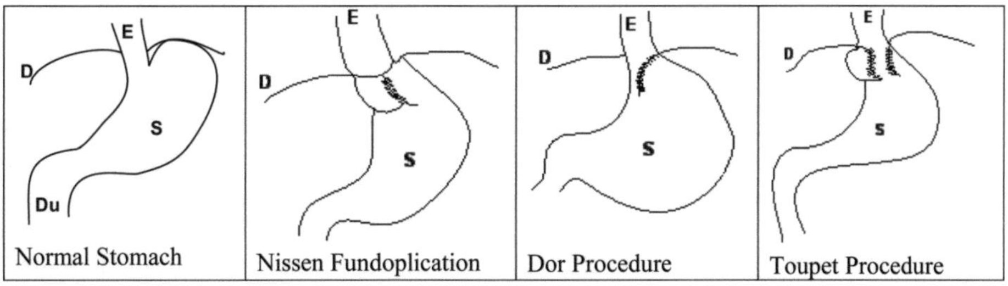


**Figure 9.**
*Schematic diagrams of anti-reflux techniques (E – Esophagus; S – Stomach; Du – Duodenum; D – Diaphragm). Source: Author's original conception.*

hospital stay [1, 5, 17]. Among the minimal access surgery (MAS) techniques, Laparoscopic is preferred to thoracoscopic approach, thus gaining currency with an outcome, complication rate and recurrence that are acceptably lower than other procedures. Thoracoscopic left Heller myotomy has been abandoned, and in its place, laparoscopic Hellers' myotomy and partial fundoplication [13, 18] have become the gold standard. The results are excellent and comparable in terms of outcome to open procedures, with the added advantages of less post-operative pain and faster recovery. Dysphagia is eliminated in over 90% of patients [4, 5, 7]. In the late stages of the disease associated with sigmoid or megaesophagus, esophagectomy and esophageal replacement surgeries have been recommended [4, 5]. Alternatively, some thoracic surgeons carry out myotomy, which may be either as a primary procedure or as a reoperation. Efficacy of symptom relief ranges from 85 to 93% success rate [4, 5, 7]. Post-operative gastroesophageal reflux is between 0 and 2% [5] and operative mortality is about 2%. However, persistent dysphagia may be treated initially with pneumatic dilatation or POEM.

*2.1.1.5.3.1 Complications*

1. Pneumothorax.

2. Wound infection and esophageal leak – 10 to 15% (5).

3. Perforation – 0 to14% (5).

4. Residual dysphagia if the myotomy is not extended down to the cardia of the stomach.

5. Abnormal gastroesophageal reflux if the myotomy is extended too far into gastric wall. It may be asymptomatic or characterized by heartburn, necessitating follow-up post-operative evaluation. Medical treatment is advocated in the elderly while laparoscopic partial fundoplication in younger persons has an expected better outcome.

*2.1.1.5.4 Right thoracoscopic myotomy*

Right thoracoscopic myotomy is recommended for DES; nutcracker esophagus in which the pathology extends to the entire length of the thoracic esophagus, sparing the LES whose function is normal. The myotomy extends from the diaphragm to the thoracic inlet. However, easier and simpler than left thoracoscopic myotomy, the complications of perforation or residual dysphagia are obviated as the gastroesophageal junction is largely intact and undisturbed with the hazardous dissection into the gastric extension avoided [1, 4]. The most fearsome complication with this procedure is delayed esophageal leak. However, long-term follow-up shows excellent results with DES. The results with nutcracker esophagus have a more uncertain and unpredictable outcome with surgery and medical management. Persistent chest pain remains a major complaint by patients. For any viable options, medical therapy is still being undertaken by a number of practitioners.

*2.1.1.5.5 Endoscopic method of esophageal myotomy*

The term, peroral endoscopic myotomy (POEM) has been added to the dictum of esophageal surgical procedures recently. This novel intervention via upper GI endoscopic route between 2010 and 2014 to carry out esophagomyotomy is a milestone in the treatment of achalasia. The immense collaboration and innovations between giants in industrial medical manufacturers and practitioners in the field of endoscopy and minimal access procedures have had a positive effect in this regard. The experience over the period has provided impetus to these developments and expanded the scope of conditions to which this procedure is applicable. This endoscopy-enabled myotomy starts by making a short 1 cm longitudinal incision 1–2 cm proximal to the constricted lower esophageal zone, after saline mixed with indigo-carmine dye is injected into the submucosal space, to create the dissection plane [6, 16]. The endoscopy tip is covered in an appropriate dissection hood which is passed through the incision with identification of the circular fibers. The myotomy commences using a hooked triangle-tip knife to lift up the circular muscle bundle perpendicular to the orientation of the muscle fibers, as shown in **Figure 10**. This progresses deliberately and slowly; it should be extended distally to 2–3 cm of the stomach. The gastric end is the most challenging aspect of the dissection due to the thin muscular layer in the region of lower esophageal sphincter.

POEM has found applicability in the various types of esophageal motility disorders, including spastic disorders and sigmoid esophagus. This is made possible by the possibility of short, medium, and extended myotomies. However, its use in sigmoid esophagus, though possible, has certain challenges due to abnormal angulations in the body of the esophagus distorting the LES and the shortened thin gastroesophageal junction (GEJ), which increases the risk of mucosal perforation or counter-mucosal injury. For advanced cases of sigmoid esophagus, the simultaneous use of two endoscopes – a second thin gastroscopes in the esophageal lumen to guide the distal 2–3 cm myotomy toward the stomach [15, 19].

Symptom remission with POEM has been considered comparable to laparoscopic Heller myotomy with partial fundoplication from a number of non-randomized studies. In fact, one study found POEM and laparoscopic Hellers' myotomy to be equally effective [17]. Some of these studies show [15, 19, 20] an initial improvement of symptoms in 89–97% of patients, with a change of Eckardt score of 7 to 1, reducing to 82% after 12 months, with a lesser Eckardt score in left Heller myotomy and balloon dilatation. The use of POEM in recurrences from previous interventions such as in Botox injections, and balloon dilatations, shows it is safe and effective [12]. POEM is 94% effective in cases of non-spastic achalasia and 90% in Chicago Class III [9, 17]. Randomized clinical trials (RCT) are necessary to prove its efficacy and safety profile in a conclusive way compared to other methods.

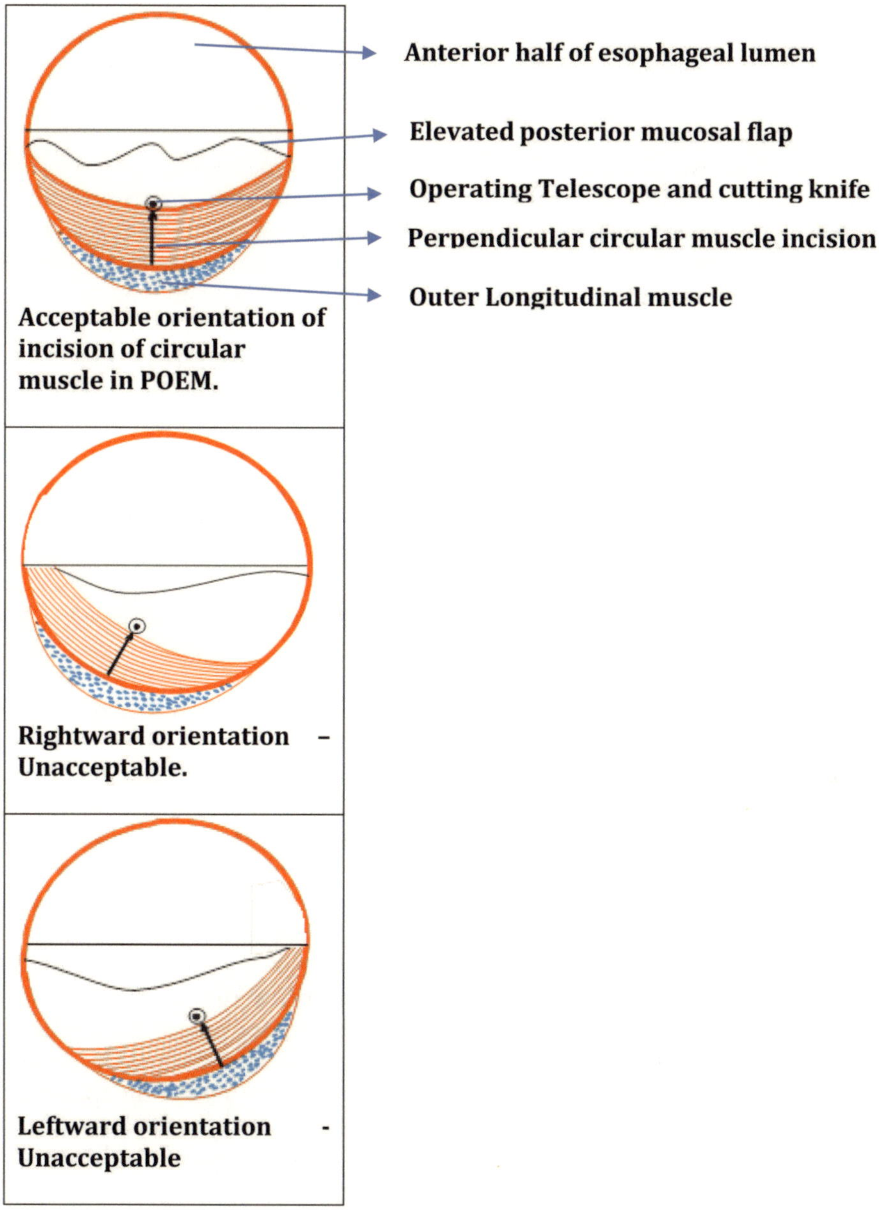


**Figure 10.**
*Schematic diagram showing the direction of circular muscle incision perpendicular to the direction of the muscle fibers in POEM. Source: Author's original conception.*

An important complication with most myotomies is the occurrence of gastroesophageal reflux, theoretically attributed to the extension of the myotomy into the stomach, rendering the lower esophageal sphincter mechanism incompetent. Reports of reflux in studies mixed with some studies showing comparable incidence [16, 17]. This has technically made an addition of anti-reflux procedures complementary. POEM as an option leads to a higher rate of abnormal esophageal acid exposure without a concomitant increase in the rate of gastroesophageal reflux symptoms when marched against laparoscopic Hellers' myotomy [17]. In the only RCT comparing POEM with other interventions, gastric reflux was found to occur at a rate higher than other surgical myotomies such as laparoscopic Hellers' myotomy with reflux symptoms in 20–37% [15]. Majority of reflux symptoms after POEM is treated by proton pump inhibitors [9, 16].

The procedure, which belongs to the minimal access procedures, is yet to be fully adopted and current ongoing evaluations indicate great promise of its future. So far, documented outcome studies appear comparable to laparoscopic Heller's myotomy; and, may in fact, provide a permanent solution for esophageal achalasia management. Recently, peroral endoscopic myotomy has shown remarkable promise in the hands of practitioners experienced in the procedure. It is still limited to a few centers and surgeons. However, the learning curve in its application has been shortening since its introduction to the armamentarium of surgical options [16, 21]. The results are adjudged to be satisfactory and even superior to other methodologies, though cautious evaluation is ongoing [5]. The detailed description of the procedure is beyond the scope of this book. Observed complications with POEM include bleeding, perforation/laceration of the esophagus, subcutaneous emphysema and post-operative pneumonia.

##### *2.1.1.5.6 Indications for reoperation for esophageal achalasia*

Laparoscopic Heller's myotomy is effective in relieving dysphagia in greater than 90% of patients [1]. Causes of failure are sometimes unknown but commonly characterized by persistent or recurrent dysphagia after a variable period of remission following the initial operation and include (i). Technical procedural reasons are either too short a myotomy distally or proximally. (ii). A constricting fundoplication at the LES. (iii) Transmural fibrosis leads to constricting scarring and strictures, especially in patients previously treated by Botox injections in who peri-esophageal fibrosis is common and myotomy is more difficult and less reliable in alleviating symptoms [9].

If the initial management of achalasia fails, a full evaluation is essential and should be undertaken before a decision is made on further treatment option(s). The diagnostic bundle for re-evaluation encompasses upper GI series, upper GI endoscopy, esophageal manometry, and PH-impedance monitoring to identify residual reflux [4, 7, 9]. Treatment failure consists of two options, depending on the previous therapy, which are either laparoscopic Hellers' myotomy plus a Dor fundoplication or POEM [9, 15, 19] has been advocated. In exceptional circumstances, balloon dilatation is carried out. Reintervention is based on the results of re-evaluation studies carried out on the patient and the subsisting information gathered therefrom. In the event of persisting or reoccurrence of symptoms, reoperation may be difficult; technically challenging, risk-prone and esophageal perforation is common. While small perforations can be repaired, large ones may necessitate esophagectomy. All options must be discussed with the patient before consent is given.

### *2.1.2 Diffuse esophageal spasm-DES (corkscrew esophagus)*

The etiology is unknown, and the pathophysiology is poorly understood. Spastic esophageal disorders are characterized by the impairment of inhibitory innervation in the distal esophagus leading to both premature, rapidly propagated, or simultaneous contractions and incomplete LES relaxation. The stimulatory motor fibers to the distal esophagus are from neurons mediated via the midbrain by efferent excitatory vagal (cholinergic) nerve endings or inhibitory nitrous oxide from myenteric plexuses. However, an inconstant neuropathic abnormality with degeneration of vagal branches to the esophageal body has been described [3, 11]. The distal latency (DL) measured by HRM at the onset of the swallowing to the onset distal esophageal peristalsis was found to be shorter in patients with simultaneous contractions than in those with normal peristalsis in spastic disorders [11]. Diffuse esophageal spasm (DES) is defined by repetitive high-pressure smooth muscle contractions that occur and are associated with normal esophageal pressures in the entire length of the esophagus with normal pressure in the LES. The esophageal musculature is hypertrophic, a consequence of repetitive high-pressure contractions. It remains a much rarer condition than achalasia.

Clinically, dysphasia secondary to DES is non-progressive to both liquids and solids. It is sometimes associated with chest pain which is nonspecific and responds to nitrates (nitroglycerin); and, odynophagia. An important differential diagnosis of DES is coronary artery disease [1, 3], from which it must be differentiated.

#### *2.1.2.1 Investigation*

Barium esophagogram may show the classic corkscrew appearance in the distal two-thirds of the esophagus.

Esophageal manometric studies display a pattern of repetitive, simultaneous, uncoordinated high-pressure contractions with, at least 30% waveforms in 10 swallows [3], often of high amplitude or prolonged duration. Unlike in classical achalasia, peristaltic waves are present and strong and may span the entire length of the esophageal body, but they are usually confined to the lower two-thirds of the organ. Another clear feature is the presence of apparent normal physiology and swallowing response [3]. It is a mixture of abnormal strong esophageal peristaltic contractility interspersed with normal peristalsis. That is, periodic occurrence of simultaneous high-amplitude contractions with periodic normal peristalsis – a distinguishing point of DES from nutcracker esophagus [3, 11]. Electrocardiography and two-dimensional echocardiography are included in the investigations to exclude ischemic heart disease (**Figure 11**).

#### *2.1.2.2 Treatment*

Exclusion of coronary artery disease is paramount, with which it shares similar symptoms. Thereafter, reassurance and resuscitation of patient is accomplished. Treatment is both Medical and Surgical.

Medical management involves the use of drugs (Nitrates and calcium channel blockers), botulinum toxin injection and pneumatic dilatation, a procedure much less effective since DES affects the entire esophagus (see details in the subtopic on Achalasia Management). Classical Heller's myotomy is attended by poor success as the disease involves almost the whole length of the esophagus. Surgically, extended esophagomyotomy, either by open or right thoracoscopic myotomy plus anti-reflux operations in combination, improves symptoms in 50–86% of cases [1]. Available studies from the experiences of diverse surgeon practitioners in this field suggest that POEM, a procedure where extended esophageal myotomy is achievable [12, 15], could bring some relief to the effects of this disease.

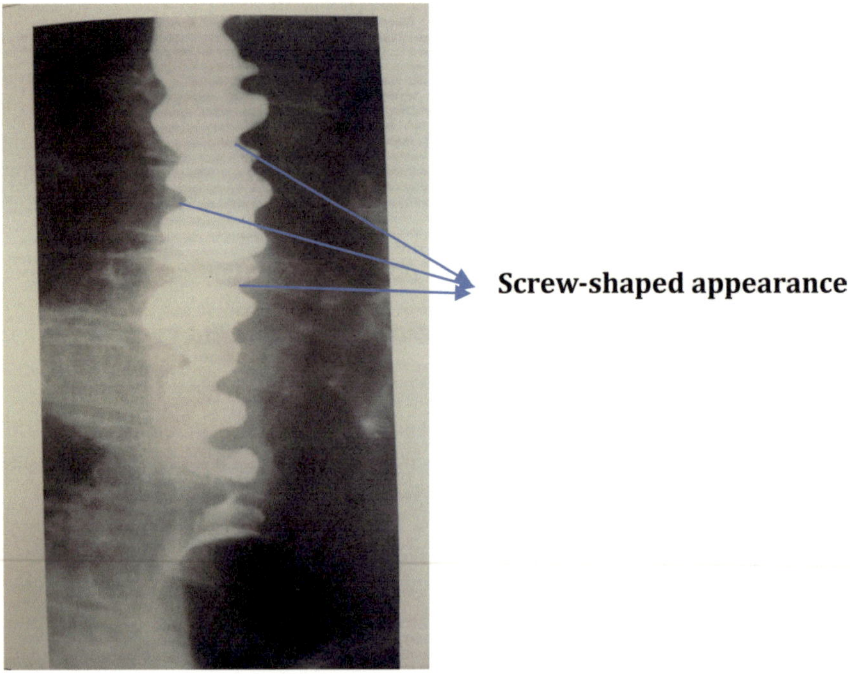


**Figure 11.**
*Barium swallow of DES (corkscrew esophagus). Source: From the author's archives.*

*2.1.3 Nutcracker esophagus*

The etiology of the nutcracker esophagus is unknown, with females more affected than males. As with most spastic motility disorders, the basic defect is neuronal inhibition in the distal esophageal body (Refer to DES). High-resolution manometry in spastic achalasia displays impaired LES relaxation (IRP ≥15 mm Hg) associated with at least 20% premature contractions [11] or Distal Contractile Integral (DCI), measurement of the contractile vigor, greater than 8000 mm Hg s cm in at least one swallow. It probably remains a primary motility disorder of the esophagus which has been poorly studied. Chest pain rather than dysphagia is the principal symptom arising from gastroesophageal reflux disease (GERD) and not due to the contractile dysfunction of the esophageal body. Barium swallow shows rapid esophageal emptying, appearing characteristically normal. Manometry shows peristalsis with markedly elevated intraesophageal pressures above 180 mmHg (**Figure 12**) [1, 3, 5].

*2.1.3.1 Treatment*

Medical management is unpredictable and ineffective but still remains an option. The outcome of surgical procedures employed in classical achalasia for spastic motility disorder is poor [11]. However, extended esophagomyotomy done as in DES is adjudged a better option [1, 5]. Today, the introduction of POEM which facilitates these extensive myotomies has brought renewed optimism [9, 11] in the treatment of this condition.

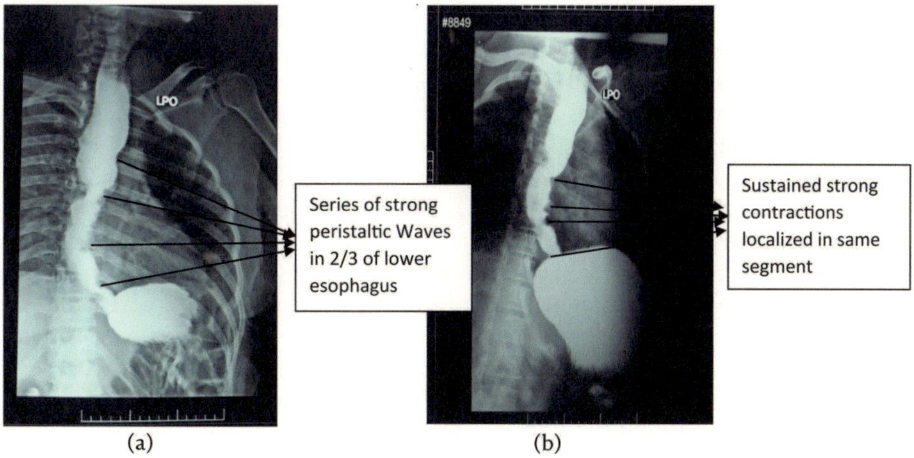


**Figure 12.**
*(a) Nut-cracker esophagus – A 46-year-old woman showing a 15s barium swallow. (b) The same patient 60 min post-deglutition (from author's archives).*

### *2.1.4 Hypertensive lower esophageal spasm*

Its origin is unknown. Clinically, it is characterized by dysphagia to solids and liquids and classically, manometric studies generally record mean intraesophageal pressures greater than 45 mmHg in mid-respiration [1, 5]. The current Chicago Classification aggregates this condition as a subtype of Class III [7, 11]. It may occur in isolation or in association with other motility disorders.

Treatment is mainly medical by drug therapy and balloon dilatation which has shown some promise in relieving persistent dysphagia [1, 11].

## 3. Summary

Esophageal motility disorders classified as primary and secondary disorders consist of both medical and surgical causes. While majority of the secondary causes arise from medical etiologies whose investigations and therapies are nonsurgical. Primary motility disorders usually are of unknown etiologies, are physiologically functional disturbances of neuromuscular origin and mechanism. They consist of variants of conditions including achalasia, diffuse esophageal spasm, nutcracker esophagus and hypertensive lower esophageal segment. The classical primary motility disorder, or achalasia pathologically is found to have degenerative nerve endings in the myenteric (Auerbach's) plexus leading to derangement of normal physiological function of the esophagus. The net effect is failure of the lower esophageal segment to relax during swallowing, absent or reduced peristalsis in the body of the esophagus, causing stasis of swallowed bolus in the lumen and subsequent gradual esophageal dilatation. Achalasia is regarded as a premalignant condition.

The prevalent symptoms of achalasia are dysphagia, regurgitation, chest pain and weight loss with few physical findings on examination. The mechanisms at play in spastic motility disorders – DES, nutcracker esophagus and hypertensive lower esophageal segment are poorly understood and their symptoms include dysphagia and chest pain essentially.

The diagnosis is usually suspected from the symptomatology; and not invariably, by the symptom or Eckardt score. However, definitive diagnosis of primary motility disorders is made using High-Resolution Manometry (HRM), by which the disease is categorized into classes I, II and III based on the esophageal body analysis referred to as Chicago Criteria or Classification. This classification plays significant role in decision-making as regards initial selection of appropriate therapy and in prognostication.

Treatment of primary motility disorders is essentially for relief of symptoms. Medical and surgical modalities have been employed with varying successes. Medical therapies include use of drugs such as calcium channel blockers, nitrates, Botox injection and pneumatic balloon dilatation. Surgical management is either by open operative techniques, minimal access (thoracoscopic or laparoscopic) or peroral endoscopic myotomy (POEM). While the combined laparoscopic Heller myotomy and partial fundoplication is the gold standard of therapeutic interventions, recent introduction of POEM is gaining prominence and fast threatening to become the new gold standard, possibly applicable to all variants or classes of the disease. While the results of POEM and laparoscopic Heller myotomy plus partial fundoplication are comparable, the higher incidence of post-intervention reflux in POEM is an issue. Hence, the search for an ideal procedure for this age-old disorder continues.

## 4. Future work

Consequent to the possible variability of the pathological microcellular interactions, defects, the ultimate functional state of the esophagus and effectiveness of the swallowing mechanism; a one-fit-all therapy is not to be expected. Phosphodiesterase-5 inhibitors (e.g., sildenafil), a sex-enhancing drug, block the degradation of nitrous oxide (NO) – a powerful smooth muscle relaxant resulting in more prolonged smooth muscle relaxation represent a new therapeutic option. This drug reduces both contractile amplitude and propagation velocity in patients with motility disorders. Symptom relief and evidence of improved manometric parameters in patients with spastic motility disorders have been recorded. Hence, a new therapeutic perspective has been made available. Endoscopically, deployment of special stents to the constricted lower esophageal segment is currently being undertaken in some centers. At the molecular level, scientists are tinkering with stem cell culture and re-implantation into the esophagus to restore damaged neurons in the tissues, research that is ongoing. Efficacy of such undertaking is yet inconclusive. The scientific world will continue the search for an optimal treatment option providing prolonged elimination of symptom, with minimal or no complication. Currently, the author is working on an innovative method of conserving massive sigmoid esophagus instead of esophagectomy.

## 5. Conclusion

Primary motility disorders, an age-old dysfunction of the esophagus remain an enigma, presenting as a spectrum of functional disturbances of esophageal physiology. It ranges from the classical achalasia to the spastic anomalies, which were hitherto confounding, both in diagnosis and management. However, over several decades, advancements in technology and the diligence of researchers have thrown some light on and opened new horizons in the management of this poorly understood condition, whose etiology remains obscure.

The development and introduction of high-resolution impedance manometry (HRIM) is an illuminating milestone in both the definitive diagnosis, identification of subtypes and formulation of appropriate treatment strategies. Therapeutic protocol for motility disorders, as a consequence, has undergone significant modifications for the best possible outcome. Incidentally, there are still some gaps to attend.

## Author details

Emmanuel Ocheli
Cardiothoracic and Vascular Surgery Unit, University of Port Harcourt Teaching Hospital, Port Harcourt, Nigeria

*Address all correspondence to: ocheliemmanuel@gmail.com

## References

[1] Souba WW, Fink MP, Jurkovich GJ, Kaiser LR, Pearce WH, Pemberton JH, et al. ACS Surgery: Principles and Practice. New York: WebMD; 2006

[2] Kumar V, Abbas AK, Fausto N, editors. Robbins and Cotran: Pathologic Basis of Disease. 7th ed. (International Edition) ed. Philadelphia: Elsevier Publishing Company; 2005

[3] Ellis H, Mahadevan V. Clinical Anatomy: Applied Anatomy for Students and Junior Doctors. 14th ed. New Jersey: Wiley-Blackwell; 2018

[4] Brunicardi FC, Anderson DK, Billiar TR, Dunn DL, Hunter JG, Mattews JB, et al., editors. Schwartz's Principles of Surgery. 9th ed. New York: The McGraw Hill Companies; 2010

[5] Guyton AC, Hall JE. Textbook of Medical Physiology. 10th ed. New York: W.B. Saunders Company; 2000

[6] Franco KL, Thourani VH. Cardiothoracic Surgery Review. Philadelphia: Lippincott Williams and Wilkins; 2012

[7] Kahrilas PJ, Bredenoord AJ, Fox M, Gyawali CP, Roman S, Smout AJPM, et al. Advances in achalasia management. Nature Reviews: Gastroenterology & Hepatology. 2017;**14**:677

[8] Mari A, Patel K, Mahamid M, Khoury T, Pesce M. Achalasia: Insights into diagnostic and therapeutic advances for an ancient disease. Rambam Maimonides Medical Journal. 2019;**10**(1):e0008. Review. DOI: 10.5041/RMMJ.10361

[9] Swanström LL. Achalasia: Treatment, current status and future advances. The Korean Journal of Internal Medicine. 2019;**34**(6):1173-1180. DOI: 10.3904/kjim.2018.43

[10] Laurino-Neto RM, Herbella F, Schlottmann F, Patti M. Evaluation of esophageal achalasia: From symptoms to the Chicago classification. ABCD. Arquivos Brasileiros de Cirurgia Digestiva. 2018;**31**(2):e1376. DOI: 10.1590/0102-672020180001e1376

[11] Roman S, Kahrilas PJ. Management of spastic disorders of the esophagus. Gastroenterology Clinics of North America. 2013;**42**(1):27-43. DOI: 10.1016/j.gtc.2012.11.002

[12] Clouse RE, Staiano A, Alrakawi A, Haroian L. Application of topographical methods to clinical esophageal manometry. The American Journal of Gastroenterology. 2000;**95**(10):2720-2730. DOI: 10.1111/j.1572-0241.2000.03178.x

[13] Wen Z, Gardener E, Wang Y. Nitrates for achalasia. Cochrane Database of Systematic Reviews. 2004;(1):1-11. DOI: 10.1002/14651858.CD002299

[14] Malas A. Esophageal spasm - Calcium channel blocker and nitrates. Gastroenterology. Medscape eMedicine publication. 2019

[15] Von Renteln D, Fuchs KH, Fockens P, Bauerfeind P, Vassiliou MC, Werner YB, et al. Peroral endoscopic myotomy for the treatment of achalasia: An international prospective multicenter study. Gastroenterology. 2013;**145**(2):309-311. e1-3. DOI: 10.1053/j.gastro.2013.04.057

[16] Bechara R, Onimaru M, Ikeda H, Inoue H. Per-oral endoscopic myotomy, 1000 cases later: Pearls, pitfalls, and

practical considerations. Gastrointestinal Endoscopy. 2016;**84**(2):330-338. DOI: 10.1016/j.gie.2016.03.1469

[17] Sharata AM, Dunst CM, Pescarus R, Shlomovitz E, Wille AJ, Reavis KM. Peroral endoscopic myotomy (POEM) for esophageal primary motility disorders: Analysis of 100 consecutive patients. Journal of Gastrointestinal Surgery. 2015;**19**(1):161-170. DOI: 10.1007/s11605-014-2610-5

[18] Richards WO, Torquati A, Holzman MD, Khaitan L, Byrne D, Lutfi R, et al. Heller myotomy versus Heller myotomy with Dor fundoplication for achalasia: A prospective randomized double-blind clinical trial. Annals of Surgery. 2004;**240**(3):405-412. DOI: 10.1097/01.sla.0000136940.32255.51

[19] Zhang Y, Wang H, Chen X, Liu L, Wang H, Liu B, et al. Per-Oral endoscopic myotomy versus laparoscopic Heller myotomy for achalasia: A meta-analysis of nonrandomized comparative studies. Medicine (Baltimore). 2016;**95**(6):e2736. DOI: 10.1097/MD.0000000000002736

[20] Boeckxstaens GE, Zaninotto G, Richter JE. Achalasia. Lancet. 2014;**383**:83-93. DOI: 10.1016/S0140-6736(13)60651-0

[21] Hungness ES, Sternbach JM, Teitelbaum EN, Kahrilas PJ, Pandolfino JE, Soper NJ. Per-oral endoscopic myotomy (POEM) after the learning curve: Durable long-term results with a low complication rate. Annals of Surgery. 2016;**264**(3):508-517. DOI: 10.1097/SLA.0000000000001870

Chapter 4

# Perspective Chapter: Aging with Dysphagia

*Nur Simsek Yurt*

## Abstract

Swallowing problems, or dysphagia, are a common geriatric syndrome that becomes more prevalent with age. Various studies have identified age-related effects on swallowing, impacting both the oral and pharyngeal stages. Patients and their families may often view swallowing difficulties as a normal aspect of aging and, therefore, might not report them unless specifically investigated by a physician. Dysphagia is linked to significant negative outcomes, including weight loss, dehydration, pneumonia, reduced life expectancy, decreased quality of life, and increased caregiver burden. This study examines the changes in swallowing associated with normal aging and explores common causes of dysphagia in elderly patients.

**Keywords:** swallowing, dysphagia, aging, elderly, management

## 1. Introduction

Swallowing is a complex biomechanical process that involves both motor and sensory functions. It is known that swallowing function declines with age. Presbyphagia, which denotes the alterations in the swallowing process due to aging, is linked to various health issues and presents in multiple forms [1]. Among the disorders caused by diseases accompanying aging, perhaps the clinical condition that has the greatest impact on quality of life is dysphagia [2]. Dysphagia is a clinical symptom defined as difficulty in the safe transport of oral contents from the oral cavity to the esophagus or irregular swallowing [3]. Oropharyngeal dysphagia has been identified as a 'geriatric syndrome,' as it is a common clinical condition in old age and is associated with multiple comorbidities and poor patient outcomes [4]. As individuals age, multiple factors independently impact their ability to eat, drink, and swallow. These factors encompass the heightened use of medications and polypharmacy, reduced appetite, and greater susceptibility to frailty. Additionally, the likelihood of encountering clinical conditions that may lead to dysphagia also rises. These include neurodegenerative diseases such as dementia, stroke, progressive neurological conditions, respiratory diseases, and cancers [5]. With the increase in the elderly population worldwide, it is crucial to recognize the impact of aging on normal swallowing and thus prevent its effects on nutrition, hydration, pulmonary function, activities of daily living, long-term healthcare issues, and overall swallowing safety [6, 7]. Older individuals require protection and prevention by identifying and eliminating any iatrogenic risk factors that may cause or worsen dysphagia [5].

## 2. Changes in swallowing function in the elderly

Understanding normal swallowing is essential to identify swallowing disorders in older people. Swallowing is a complex process that involves six cranial nerves—specifically the trigeminal (V), facial (VII), glossopharyngeal (IX), vagus (X), accessory (XI), and hypoglossal (XII)—several muscle groups, and brain inputs, all of which require precise coordination [8]. The normal swallowing process is divided into four phases (**Table 1**):

- In the oral preparation phase, food is chewed in the mouth and mixed with saliva to form a bolus (a ball of food ready for swallowing).
- In the oral phase, the bolus is pushed to the back of the oral cavity with the tongue, and the swallowing reflex is initiated. These two phases are under voluntary control.
- In the pharyngeal phase, when the bolus reaches the pharynx, the involuntary swallowing reflex is activated. The soft palate rises, the larynx moves up and forwards, and the epiglottis closes, protecting the airways and allowing the bolus to move along the pharynx.
- In the esophageal phase, the bolus enters the esophagus by opening the upper esophageal sphincter. The esophagus pushes the bolus toward the stomach with peristaltic movements. This phase is also involuntarily controlled.

All these phases work in a coordinated manner and often overlap. The pharyngeal phase occurs rapidly (about 0.7 seconds) but may be prolonged in older individuals. The passage of the bolus from the esophagus to the stomach normally takes less than 10 seconds. The airway is protected during the passage of the bolus and remains closed until the bolus has completely passed. During the laryngeal phase, the glottis (vocal cords) closes, and hyolaryngeal elevation helps to open the upper esophageal

| Oral preparatory phase | Oral phase | Pharyngeal phase | Esophageal phase |
|---|---|---|---|
| • Food is chewed in the mouth.<br>• It is mixed with saliva.<br>• A bolus ready for swallowing is formed. | • The bolus is pushed to the back of the oral cavity by the tongue.<br>• The swallowing reflex is initiated. | • The bolus reaches the pharynx.<br>• The involuntary swallowing reflex becomes active.<br>• The soft palate elevates, and the larynx moves upwards and forwards.<br>• The epiglottis closes, protecting the airway.<br>• The bolus moves downward through the pharynx. | • The bolus enters the esophagus through the opening of the upper esophageal sphincter.<br>• The esophagus propels the bolus toward the stomach through peristaltic movements. |

**Table 1.**
*The four phases of swallowing.*

sphincter. Disruption in any of these processes can affect swallowing function and lead to dysphagia. Therefore, proper functioning of all phases is critical for swallowing health [2].

Swallowing problems are classified as oral, pharyngeal, or esophageal dysphagia, according to the phase in which they occur. However, many patients experience impairments in more than one phase of swallowing. These impairments may result from motor planning, coordination, timing, or displacement of anatomical structures during swallowing and may result in airway penetration or aspiration. Penetration is when the bolus enters the laryngeal vestibule without reaching the vocal cords; aspiration is when the bolus enters the trachea and lungs. Not all patients with dysphagia will have silent aspiration. Healthy individuals respond to this with coughing, whereas patients with dysphagia experience silent aspiration and do not respond.

In swallowing assessments, these biomechanical disorders are examined to determine the treatment plan [8]. Robbins et al. extensively studied swallowing in community-dwelling older adults. The most prominent changes are a slowing of the increase in swallowing pressure, an increase in post-swallowing residue, and the presence of a permanent cricopharyngeal rod in barium studies. As these changes are often asymptomatic, they can be confusing in symptomatic patients and lead to misdiagnosis [9]. Although normal swallowing pressures are measured in the elderly, maximum isometric tongue pressures decrease with aging, indicating that the elderly use more tongue force to maintain normal pressures. Elderly patients may make multiple tongue movements to achieve sufficient pressure. This coincides with the fact that the elderly eat more slowly and rarely chew their food. It is also noted that unrelated diseases can lead to swallowing disorders because of depletion of functional reserve. These findings explain the mechanisms that transform the elderly from healthy individual to patient with dysphagia [2].

## 3. Prevalence of swallowing disorders in the elderly

Esophageal motility disorders are quite common in the elderly. Epidemiology statistics for dysphagia in healthy elderly people range from 15 to 35% [7, 10, 11]. However, these figures are affected by the definition of dysphagia used, the methods employed to determine its presence, and the methodological limitations of studies involving small sample sizes. Studies have reported that dysphagia is observed in 10-33% of elderly individuals, and it is estimated to be between 26.2 and 56.7% in hospitalized geriatric patients [12–14]. It has been reported that 40% of institutionalized older adults have a diagnosis of dysphagia [2]. A recent meta-analysis reported a prevalence of dysphagia of 35.9% among older adults in nursing homes [15]. Alzheimer's is common among elderly people living in nursing homes and causes a loss of the ability to chew and swallow non-reflexively [1].

Dysphagia is commonly observed among older adults in community settings, and it is closely associated with considerable declines in quality of life due to eating and feeding difficulties [16]. Wilkinson and Picciotto conducted a study examining the prevalence of swallowing problems among residents of a retirement village. Their findings showed that 44% of participants experienced swallowing problems that affected their daily living functions [17]. In Turkey, the prevalence of dysphagia in geriatric individuals receiving home care services was reported as 44.6% [18]. In Denmark, it was found that 50% of elderly people admitted to a geriatric unit had dysphagia symptoms [14]. Increased dysphagia symptoms were reported in 78.7% of elderly individuals receiving home care services in Japan [19].

## 4. Assessment of swallowing

When assessing for oropharyngeal dysphagia, the clinician begins with a clinical evaluation, including a comprehensive review of the patient's medical history, an interview with the patient or their caregiver/family, a cranial nerve examination, and the administration of liquids and foods of various textures and sizes. The purpose of the clinical evaluation is to ascertain whether signs of dysphagia are present, necessitating further investigation with instrumental assessments. The clinician also gathers important information regarding the patient's reported symptoms, cognitive status, meal-related fatigue, posture, positioning, environmental factors, and readiness for further assessment [8, 20].

Esophageal dysphagia is often assessed using endoscopy or a barium swallow (esophagram), frequently in collaboration with a gastroenterologist to identify and address the underlying cause. When both oropharyngeal and esophageal dysphagia are suspected, a combined videofluoroscopic swallow study with a barium swallow may be employed. Common signs of swallowing difficulties include coughing during swallowing, nasal regurgitation, a wet-sounding voice after swallowing, poor management of secretions, a weak cough, or a sensation of food being stuck or necessitating regurgitation. These issues may be particularly concerning in patients with known neurological or aerodigestive disorders, such as those who have had a stroke or those who have undergone chemoradiation for head and neck cancers. Moreover, it is crucial that the patient can actively participate in the clinical or instrumental swallowing assessment and in any subsequent recommendations, such as swallowing exercises. Therefore, performing these assessments on patients who are delirious and unable to participate may not be effective [8].

When a clinical swallow evaluation raises suspicion of oropharyngeal dysphagia, patients typically undergo an instrumental assessment to identify the precise structural or physiological aspects of the swallowing disorder [21]. These evaluations also assist in determining the safest consistency of solids and liquids that the patient can swallow. Swallowing evaluations are generally categorized into clinical assessments, typically conducted at the bedside, and instrumental assessments, which include videofluoroscopic swallowing studies (VFSS) and fiberoptic endoscopic evaluations of swallowing (FEES). During a VFSS, patients are asked to consume varying consistencies of barium contrast, as well as foods mixed or coated with barium, while the process is visualized using videofluoroscopy. When the VFSS is performed, a trained therapist visualizes the mechanics of swallowing, including the oral cavity, tongue movement, velar elevation, hyolaryngeal excursion, complete inversion of the epiglottis, and the opening of the upper esophageal sphincter [22, 23]. FEES involves inserting an endoscope through the nostrils to directly observe the naso-oropharyngeal and laryngeal structures [24]. Swallowing is then evaluated as the patient consumes foods and liquids of different textures that are tinted with food coloring. During both assessments, a therapist trained in dysphagia can observe the effectiveness of various therapeutic techniques, such as postural adjustments like the chin tuck.

Each method has its own benefits and limitations, and there is limited consensus on the best approach for different clinical scenarios. The decision on which test is most appropriate typically depends on the specific characteristics of the patient. Older adults are more prone to silent aspiration than younger adults, making clinical bedside assessments less reliable in these cases. Additional research is needed to better determine which patients will benefit most from these evaluations in terms of prognosis and treatment [23]. Clinicians must also consider the patient's ability to participate in each test. For instance, VFSS necessitates travel to the radiology suite, the ability to sit upright, and a body size that accommodates the fluoroscopy machine. In contrast, FEES requires the patient to tolerate an endoscope inserted through the nose, which carries risks such as bleeding and may increase agitation, particularly in delirious patients. The availability of mobile dysphagia diagnostic testing units is increasing, which can be advantageous in rural or long-term care settings where resources may be constrained [25]. In 2016, a systematic review comparing the accuracy of VFSS and FEES found that FEES exhibited greater sensitivity for detecting aspiration (0.88 vs. 0.77; $p = 0.03$), penetration (0.97 vs. 0.83; $p < 0.001$), and post-swallow residue (0.97 vs. 0.80; $p < 0.001$) compared to VFSS. The review also noted that sensitivity for premature spillage was comparable between the two methods (FEES: 0.69, VFSS: 0.80; $p = 0.28$), and the specificity for both procedures was similar, ranging from 0.93 to 0.98 [26].

## 5. Factors associated with swallowing disorders in the elderly

Dysphagia is not a disease in itself; instead, it is caused by various medical conditions. Many common and rare conditions associated with aging can also affect swallowing [2]. The most frequent causes of oropharyngeal dysphagia include stroke, head and neck cancer, and progressive neurological disorders such as dementia, amyotrophic lateral sclerosis, and Parkinson's disease [27]. Esophageal dysphagia, on the other hand, has various etiologies, including esophagitis, achalasia, esophageal strictures, Zenker's diverticulum, among others. A patient's medical history is valuable in evaluating these causes and guiding appropriate diagnostic workup. Esophageal dysphagia that begins with difficulty swallowing solids and later progresses to include liquids is often indicative of mechanical obstruction, such as a tumor or stricture. Conversely, when dysphagia affects both solids and liquids from the beginning, it typically points to a motor disorder like achalasia. Additionally, medical procedures (e.g., endotracheal intubation and tumor removal) and specific medications (e.g., anticholinergics) may also lead to dysphagia [8].

The aging process leads to changes in the sense of smell and taste, affecting appetite, diet selection, and oral intake. Sarcopenia affects the muscles used for swallowing, leading to reduced pressure production in the oral phase and inadequate bolus clearance [28, 29]. Changes in masticatory muscles lead to slower and less effective chewing, increasing the risk of asphyxia [30]. In addition, aging can cause low salivary flow rates and xerostomia, which are exacerbated by the effects of certain medications [31]. Many medications consumed by older adults contribute to decreased appetite, incoordination, and esophagitis. Therefore, if there are concerns about eating in older adults, the role of dysphagia and potential influence of other factors should be carefully assessed [8].

## 6. Complications associated with swallowing issues in the elderly

Dysphagia is associated with malnutrition, dehydration, respiratory infections, mortality, increased hospitalization rates, and health care costs [12, 19]. In elderly care settings, individuals are often at risk of asphyxia during eating and drinking. This not only creates challenges for healthcare professionals but also affects the quality of life of individuals and their families [32]. Dysphagia worsens nutritional status, reduces food consumption, and leads to malnutrition and weight loss. This leads to physical weakness and increased vulnerability to acute illnesses such as infections, heart disease, and dehydration [12, 18]. Melgaard et al. found a significant increase in the length of hospital stay and mortality in patients with dysphagia hospitalized in the geriatrics department compared to patients without dysphagia [14]. Banda et al. reported that oropharyngeal dysphagia is associated with pneumonia, malnutrition, and mortality [33]. According to Cabre et al., oropharyngeal dysphagia is a very common clinical sign in elderly people with pneumonia [34].

In addition to the physical consequences of dysphagia, emotional and social effects are also observed. Dysphagia negatively impacts the quality of life by contributing to depression and social isolation. Cognitive and perceptual changes, which are especially common in the elderly, constitute an important risk factor for swallowing disorders. In addition, another often overlooked but critical issue is the self-perception of health status of older adults and the sense of loss of well-being that arises due to swallowing and feeding disorders [1]. A study by Holland et al. showed that dysphagia is associated with age and depression [35].

## 7. Management of dysphagia in the elderly

Considering the aging of the population, multidisciplinary collaboration comes to the fore in dysphagia management [7]. In managing dysphagia in older adults, a combination of compensatory and rehabilitative strategies is essential, though evidence supporting their long-term efficacy is limited. Dysphagia management involves adaptive strategies and rehabilitative methods to enhance swallowing function and reduce complications such as aspiration, pneumonia, and choking [8]. Adaptive strategies aim to alleviate the symptoms and consequences of dysphagia without changing the underlying swallowing mechanics. These include oral hygiene, posture adjustments, swallowing maneuvers, modified eating strategies, and dietary changes. Oral care may help reduce pneumonia risk from aspiration in non-ventilated patients, though evidence is limited. Postural changes, like chin tuck or head turn, can modify swallowing biomechanics and decrease aspiration in individuals with swallowing disorders [36]. Adjusting food and liquid consistency is another common approach, but its effectiveness remains unclear. A recent Cochrane review found insufficient evidence on the benefits of consistency changes, with only two studies (from the same trial) showing that nectar-like and honey-like liquids reduced aspiration compared to thin liquids in patients with dementia or Parkinson's disease [37]. Overall, the evidence on adaptive methods, including consistency alterations, is limited and does not provide conclusive guidance on clinical outcomes [8].

Feeding tubes are used in patients with dysphagia either to eliminate oral intake or alongside to mitigate aspiration risks. However, feeding tubes do not improve swallowing ability and do not reduce aspiration pneumonia from contaminated oral secretions [38]. They may even increase the risk of aspiration pneumonia due to reflux

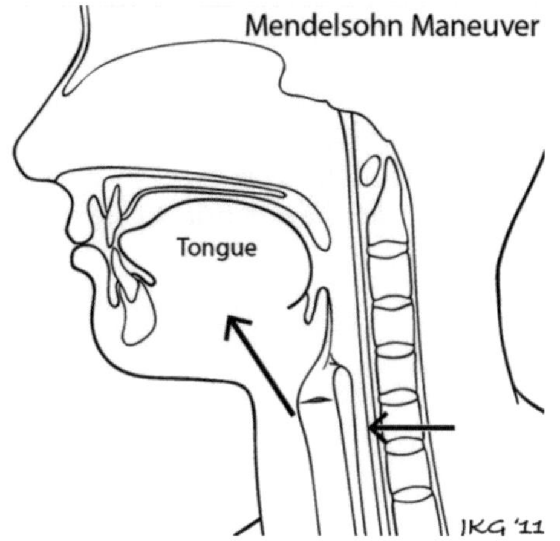


**Figure 1.**
*Illustration of the Mendelsohn maneuver's effects includes enhanced vertical and anterior laryngeal motion, as well as increased width and duration of upper esophageal sphincter opening.*

from the reduced pressure of the lower esophageal sphincter [39]. Feeding tubes are also linked to complications such as cellulitis, bacteremia, agitation, sinus infections, nasal irritation, and diarrhea [8]. A tracheostomy may be considered for patients with silent aspiration and recurrent pneumonia. It aids with tracheal toileting.

Rehabilitative interventions for dysphagia aim to improve swallowing mechanics through strength and skill training. Techniques such as effortful swallows and the Mendelsohn maneuver have shown benefits in various patient groups [40]. Studies have shown that the Mendelsohn maneuver improves swallowing function in patient populations (**Figure 1**) [41, 42]. In a group of head and neck cancer patients treated with primary radiotherapy or chemoradiotherapy, the results indicated that laryngeal movements were longer and wider with the Mendelsohn maneuver compared to initial swallows. Additionally, the use of the Mendelsohn maneuver in this study was associated with reduced frequency and occurrence of pharyngeal phase motility disorders and decreased aspiration [42]. Exercises, including progressive lingual strengthening and expiratory muscle strength training, can enhance swallowing function. However, a Cochrane review indicates that while these interventions may reduce dysphagia and hospital stays, more high-quality research is needed to confirm their effectiveness [43].

Management of dysphagia in the elderly remains a complex process that requires a multidisciplinary approach that balances compensatory strategies with rehabilitation efforts. Despite a variety of interventions, evidence supporting their long-term effectiveness is limited, highlighting the need for more rigorous research. Furthermore, potential risks associated with certain treatments, such as feeding tubes, emphasize the importance of care plans tailored to each patient's unique needs and circumstances.

## 8. Conclusion

Dysphagia in the elderly is associated with serious morbidity and potential mortality and should be addressed with a comprehensive and multidisciplinary approach. The complex nature of swallowing, increasing comorbidities, and the fact that symptoms in the elderly population are often considered a normal part of aging may lead to delays in the clinical diagnosis and treatment of dysphagia. This leads to a marked decrease in quality of life, increasing the risk of malnutrition, aspiration, and death. A good understanding of swallowing disorders in the elderly and available treatment options is critical to optimizing care for this vulnerable population. Dysphagia prevention strategies offer the potential to maximize swallowing function and support healthy aging.

## Author details

Nur Simsek Yurt
Samsun Training and Research Hospital, Clinic of Family Medicine, Samsun, Turkey

*Address all correspondence to: nursimsekyurt@gmail.com

## References

[1] Nogueira D, Reis E. Swallowing disorders in nursing home residents: How can the problem be explained? Clinical Interventions in Aging. 2013;**8**:221-227

[2] Tulunay-Ugur OE, Eibling D. Geriatric dysphagia. Clinics in Geriatric Medicine. 2018;**34**(2):183-189

[3] Olesen MD, Modlinski RM, Poulsen SH, Rosenvinge PM, Rasmussen HH, Holst M. Prevalence of signs of dysphagia and associated risk factors in geriatric patients admitted to an acute medical unit. Clinical Nutrition ESPEN. 2021;**41**:208-216

[4] Baijens LW, Clavé P, Cras P, Ekberg O, Forster A, Kolb GF, et al. European society for swallowing disorders–European Union Geriatric Medicine Society white paper: Oropharyngeal dysphagia as a geriatric syndrome. Clinical Interventions in Aging. 2016;**11**:1403-1428

[5] Wolf U, Eckert S, Walter G, Wienke A, Bartel S, Plontke SK, et al. Prevalence of oropharyngeal dysphagia in geriatric patients and real-life associations with diseases and drugs. Scientific Reports. 2021;**11**(1):21955

[6] Walshe M. Swallowing and ageing. Speech, Language and Hearing. 2019;**22**(1):2-8

[7] Liu T, Zheng J, Du J, He G. Food processing and nutrition strategies for improving the health of elderly people with dysphagia: A review of recent developments. Food. 2024;**13**(2):215

[8] Christmas C, Rogus-Pulia N. Swallowing disorders in the older population. Journal of the American Geriatrics Society. 2019;**67**(12):2643-2649

[9] Robbins JA, Levine R, Wood J, Roecker EB, Luschei E. Age effects on lingual pressure generation as a risk factor for dysphagia. The Journals of Gerontology Series A: Biological Sciences and Medical Sciences. 1995;**50**(5):M257-M262

[10] Madhavan A, LaGorio LA, Crary MA, Dahl WJ, Carnaby GD. Prevalence of and risk factors for dysphagia in the community dwelling elderly: A systematic review. The Journal of Nutrition, Health & Aging. 2016;**20**(8):806-815

[11] Lindgren S, Janzon L. Prevalence of swallowing complaints and clinical findings among 50-79-year-old men and women in an urban population. Dysphagia. 1991;**6**:187-192

[12] Carrión S, Cabré M, Monteis R, Roca M, Palomera E, Serra-Prat M, et al. Oropharyngeal dysphagia is a prevalent risk factor for malnutrition in a cohort of older patients admitted with an acute disease to a general hospital. Clinical Nutrition. 2015;**34**(3):436-442

[13] Penalva-Arigita A, Prats R, Lecha M, Sansano A, Vila L. Prevalence of dysphagia in a regional hospital setting: Acute care hospital and a geriatric sociosanitary care hospital: A cross-sectional study. Clinical Nutrition ESPEN. 2019;**33**:86-90

[14] Melgaard D, Rodrigo-Domingo M, Morch MM. The prevalence of oropharyngeal dysphagia in acute geriatric patients. Geriatrics (Basel). 2018;**3**(2):15

[15] Tian L, Hu Z, Yang L, Xiang Y. The prevalence of dysphagia at risk among older adults in nursing homes:

A meta-analysis. Psychogeriatrics. 2024;**24**(1):127-137

[16] Chen PH, Golub JS, Hapner ER, Johns MM 3rd. Prevalence of perceived dysphagia and quality-of-life impairment in a geriatric population. Dysphagia. 2009;**24**(1):1-6

[17] Wilkinson T, de Picciotto J. Swallowing problems in the normal ageing population. The South African Journal of Communication Disorders. 1999;**46**(1):55-64

[18] Simsek Yurt N, Bocek AE. Dysphagia frequency and associated risk factors in geriatric patients receiving home care. Konuralp Medical Journal. 2023;**15**(2):236-242

[19] Watanabe K, Umegaki H, Huang CH, Arakawa Martins B, Asai A, Kanda S, et al. Association between dysphagia risk and unplanned hospitalization in older patients receiving home medical care. Geriatrics & Gerontology International. 2019;**19**(10):977-981

[20] Koch I, Ferrazzi A, Busatto C, Ventura L, Palmer K, Stritoni P, et al. Cranial nerve examination for neurogenic dysphagia patients. Otolaryngol (Sunnyvale). 2017;7(319):2

[21] Daniels SK, Huckabee M-L, Gozdzikowska K. Dysphagia Following Stroke. San Diego: Plural Publishing, Inc; 2019

[22] Kim SB, Lee SJ, Lee KW, Lee JH, Kim DW. Usefulness of early Videofluoroscopic swallowing study in acute stroke patients with dysphagia. Annals of Rehabilitation Medicine. 2018;**42**(1):42-51

[23] Thiyagalingam S, Kulinski AE, Thorsteinsdottir B, Shindelar KL, Takahashi PY. Dysphagia in older adults. Mayo Clinic Proceedings. 2021;**96**(2):488-497

[24] Dziewas R, Glahn J, Helfer C, Ickenstein G, Keller J, Ledl C, et al. Flexible endoscopic evaluation of swallowing (FEES) for neurogenic dysphagia: Training curriculum of the German Society of Neurology and the German stroke society. BMC Medical Education. 2016;**16**:70

[25] Rogus-Pulia N, Wirth R, Sloane PD. Dysphagia in frail older persons: Making the most of current knowledge. Journal of the American Medical Directors Association. 2018;**19**(9):736-740

[26] Giraldo-Cadavid LF, Leal-Leano LR, Leon-Basantes GA, Bastidas AR, Garcia R, Ovalle S, et al. Accuracy of endoscopic and videofluoroscopic evaluations of swallowing for oropharyngeal dysphagia. Laryngoscope. 2017;**127**(9):2002-2010

[27] Takizawa C, Gemmell E, Kenworthy J, Speyer R. A systematic review of the prevalence of oropharyngeal dysphagia in stroke, Parkinson's disease, Alzheimer's disease, head injury, and pneumonia. Dysphagia. 2016;**31**(3):434-441

[28] Molfenter SM, Lenell C, Lazarus CL. Volumetric changes to the pharynx in healthy aging: Consequence for pharyngeal swallow mechanics and function. Dysphagia. 2019;**34**(1):129-137

[29] Sakai K, Nakayama E, Tohara H, Kodama K, Takehisa T, Takehisa Y, et al. Relationship between tongue strength, lip strength, and nutrition-related sarcopenia in older rehabilitation inpatients: A cross-sectional study. Clinical Interventions in Aging. 2017;**12**:1207-1214

[30] Morita K, Tsuka H, Kato K, Mori T, Nishimura R, Yoshida M, et al. Factors

related to masticatory performance in healthy elderly individuals. Journal of Prosthodontic Research. 2018;**62**(4):432-435

[31] Affoo RH, Foley N, Garrick R, Siqueira WL, Martin RE. Meta-analysis of salivary flow rates in young and older adults. Journal of the American Geriatrics Society. 2015;**63**(10):2142-2151

[32] Espinosa-Val MC, Martin-Martinez A, Graupera M, Arias O, Elvira A, Cabre M, et al. Prevalence, risk factors, and complications of oropharyngeal dysphagia in older patients with dementia. Nutrients. 2020;**12**(3):863

[33] Banda KJ, Chu H, Chen R, Kang XL, Jen HJ, Liu D, et al. Prevalence of oropharyngeal dysphagia and risk of pneumonia, malnutrition, and mortality in adults aged 60 years and older: A meta-analysis. Gerontology. 2022;**68**(8):841-853

[34] Cabre M, Serra-Prat M, Palomera E, Almirall J, Pallares R, Clave P. Prevalence and prognostic implications of dysphagia in elderly patients with pneumonia. Age and Ageing. 2010;**39**(1):39-45

[35] Holland G, Jayasekeran V, Pendleton N, Horan M, Jones M, Hamdy S. Prevalence and symptom profiling of oropharyngeal dysphagia in a community dwelling of an elderly population: A self-reporting questionnaire survey. Diseases of the Esophagus. 2011;**24**(7):476-480

[36] Nagy A, Peladeau-Pigeon M, Valenzano TJ, Namasivayam AM, Steele CM. The effectiveness of the head-turn-plus-chin-down maneuver for eliminating vallecular residue. In: Codas. Brasil: SciELO; 2016

[37] Flynn E, Smith CH, Walsh CD, Walshe M. Modifying the consistency of food and fluids for swallowing difficulties in dementia. Cochrane Database of Systematic Reviews. 2018;**9**(9):CD011077

[38] Wirth R, Dziewas R, Beck AM, Clave P, Hamdy S, Heppner HJ, et al. Oropharyngeal dysphagia in older persons–from pathophysiology to adequate intervention: A review and summary of an international expert meeting. Clinical Interventions in Aging. 2016;**11**:189-208

[39] Manabe T, Teramoto S, Tamiya N, Okochi J, Hizawa N. Risk factors for aspiration pneumonia in older adults. PLoS One. 2015;**10**(10):e0140060

[40] Clark HM, Shelton N. Training effects of the effortful swallow under three exercise conditions. Dysphagia. 2014;**29**(5):553-563

[41] Lazarus C. Mendelson maneuver and masako maneuver. In: Manual of Diagnostic and Therapeutic Techniques for Disorders of Deglutition. Verlag, New York: Springer, Inc; 2012. pp. 269-280

[42] Lazarus C, Logemann JA, Gibbons P. Effects of maneuvers on swallowing function in a dysphagic oral cancer patient. Head & Neck. 1993;**15**(5):419-424

[43] Bath PM, Lee HS, Everton LF. Swallowing therapy for dysphagia in acute and subacute stroke. Cochrane Database of Systematic Reviews. 2018;**10**(10):CD000323

Chapter 5

# Perspective Chapter: Radiology in Swallowing Problems

*Liam D. Hyland*


## Abstract

This chapter focuses on the radiological investigations performed in patients with swallowing problems. It outlines the different imaging modalities used when assessing patients with dysphagia to include ultrasound, computed tomography, magnetic resonance imaging, dynamic studies and X-ray, and highlights some of the key structural pathologies seen on different scans. It explores the different applications, techniques, clinical implications, advantages and limitations of these modalities, whilst considering the fact that that imaging itself comes secondary to the clinical evaluation of patients by means of a thorough history and examination. This chapter not only outlines the benefits of radiology in diagnosing conditions that affect the function of swallowing; it also explains how radiology can provide guidance and work up for surgical procedures and allow monitoring of conditions following surgical procedures to help improve swallowing.


**Keywords:** swallowing, radiology, anatomical, functional, dynamic, resolution, pharyngeal, enhancement, signalling

## 1. Introduction

Radiology is an ever-expanding specialty within ear, nose and throat (ENT) and is a significant cornerstone in the diagnosis and management of swallowing disorders. Its application within ENT not only provides detailed insights into the anatomical and pathological conditions affecting these regions but also helps to facilitating accurate diagnosis and effective treatment planning to patients with dysphagia [1]. Radiology can be used to diagnose structural pathology, stage head and neck tumours, allow follow-up of a particular condition following intervention, and provide guidance for procedures.

There are a variety of imaging modalities used to help in the assessment of swallowing problems; the most frequently used are ultrasound (US), computed tomography (CT), magnetic resonance imaging (MRI), dynamic studies and X-ray [2].

In all clinical cases, it is important to remember that imaging comes secondary to the evaluation of patients by means of a thorough history and examination. Indeed, in the emergency setting, it is imperative that patients are stabilised from a clinical perspective before imaging is considered [3].

This chapter will explore the applications, techniques, clinical implications, advantages and limitations of all of these imaging modalities in the context of swallowing problems.

## 2. Ultrasound (US)

US provides real-time, dynamic imaging of the anatomical structures involved in swallowing. It is a non-invasive, cost-effective imaging modality that is useful for assessing the movement and function of muscles and soft tissues, making it an excellent tool for evaluating swallowing disorders.

Ultrasound uses high-frequency sound waves to create images of the inside of the body. It does this via the use of a small probe that is placed on the surface of the skin after a thin layer of gel is applied. US uses sound waves with frequencies greater than 20 kHz and diagnostic US typically uses frequencies between 2 and 20 MHz.

The probe sends out sound waves which reverberate off of different body tissues and organs, creating echo signals that are detected by the probe and subsequently converted into electrical signals. A computer then turns the electrical signals into a moving image that appears on a screen or monitor.

The image produced is based on the strength of the sound signal and how long it takes to travel through the body. Different types of tissue reflect sound waves differently, which helps the computer determine the shape, structure, and position of organs. Some ultrasounds can also measure the speed and direction of blood flow.

### 2.1 US serves a number of general applications

*Anatomical assessment*: US can visualise the tongue, hyoid bone, suprahyoid and infrahyoid muscles which are all involved in the oral and pharyngeal phases of deglutition.

*Functional evaluation*: Dynamic US can assess the movement of the previously mentioned swallowing-related muscles and structures, in order to identify functional impairments.

*Guided interventions*: US can guide therapeutic interventions, such as the precise injection of botulinum toxin into spastic muscles [4].

### 2.2 US imaging for swallowing disorders involves specific techniques and protocols to optimise the visualisation of relevant structures

*B-mode US*: Provides static images of the anatomical structures involved in swallowing.

*M-mode US*: Captures motion over time, allowing for the assessment of dynamic movements during swallowing.

*Doppler US*: Evaluates blood flow in swallowing-related structures, which can be useful in assessing vascular abnormalities such as carotid artery aneurysms (see **Figure 1**) [5].

*3D US*: Offers three-dimensional visualisation of swallowing structures, providing detailed anatomical information.

*Sonoelastography*: Calculates tissue stiffness, which can help in identifying pathological changes in the muscles involved in swallowing [6].

### 2.3 US has a wide range of specific clinical applications in the evaluation and management of swallowing disorders

*Detection and staging*: US can detect tumours within the head and neck in areas such as pharynx, larynx and salivary glands (see **Figure 2**) as well as the

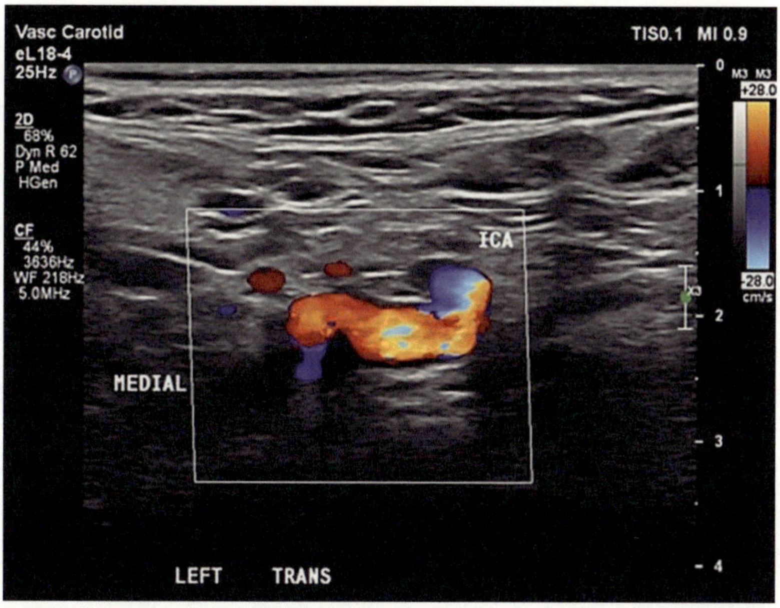


**Figure 1.**
*US Doppler of left internal carotid artery with a saccular aneurysm and partial thrombosis.*

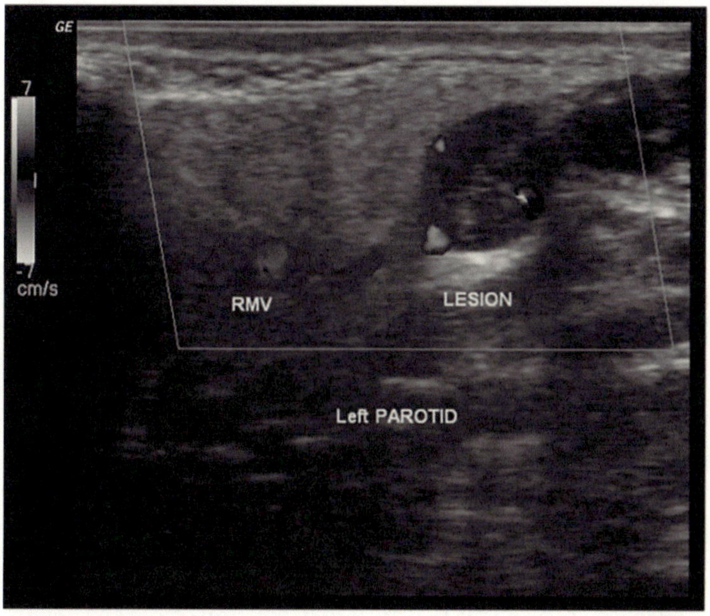


**Figure 2.**
*US of left parotid gland demonstrating a well-defined hypoechoic lesion within the superficial lobe with adjacent retromandibular vein (RMV); this was ultimately confirmed as a Warthin's tumour on FNA and excision biopsy.*

oesophagus; this helps to subsequently assess the impact of these structures on swallowing function from the degree of pressure they may be exerting on surrounding structures (see **Figure 3**) [7].

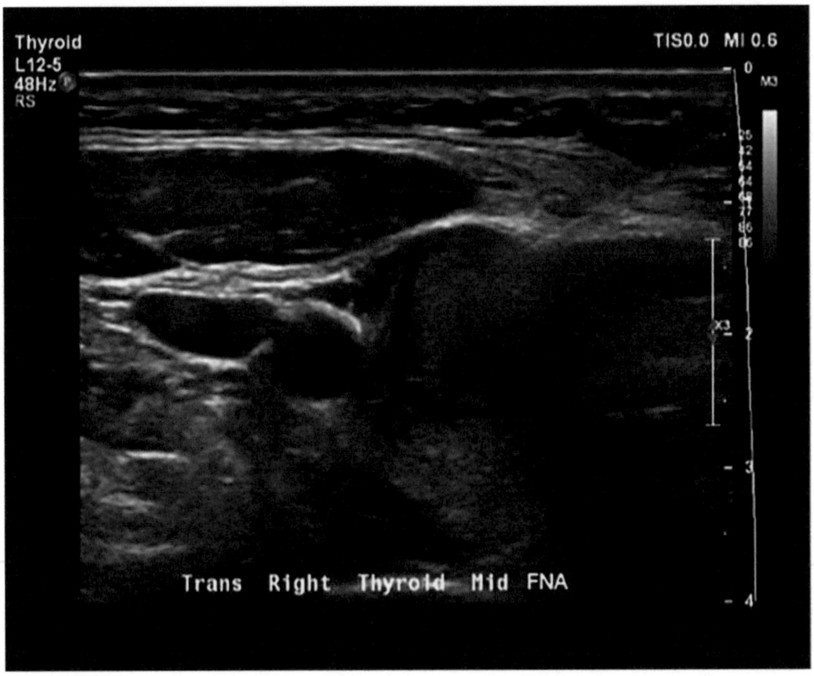


**Figure 3.**
*US of right thyroid isoechoic nodule undergoing FNA with a 25-gauge needle.*

*Guided biopsies*: US can guide fine-needle aspiration biopsies of suspicious lesions, such as those in the thyroid gland (see **Figure 4**), which can ultimately aid in the diagnosis of malignancy and allow planning for operative management [8].

*Abscesses and collections*: US is useful as an initial form of imaging to help ascertain whether fluid is present in a particular space of the head and neck, to suggest presence of an abscess (see **Figure 4**) or collection, which could impact on swallowing.

## 2.4 US has a number of advantages within the clinical setting for patients with dysphagia, however, there are also limitations that should be considered

### 2.4.1 Advantages

*Non-invasive*: US is a non-invasive procedure, making it suitable for repeated use and for patients who may not tolerate procedures that are more invasive e.g. MRI [9].

*No radiation*: Unlike other imaging modalities, US does not involve exposure to ionising radiation, making it comparatively safer for use in certain patient populations such as paediatrics and pregnant patients.

*Real-time imaging*: US provides real-time visualisation of the swallowing process, allowing for dynamic assessment of swallowing mechanics [10].

### 2.4.2 Limitations

*Operator-dependent*: The quality of US imaging is highly dependent on the skill and experience of the operator who manoeuvres the probe and orchestrates the properties of the machine.

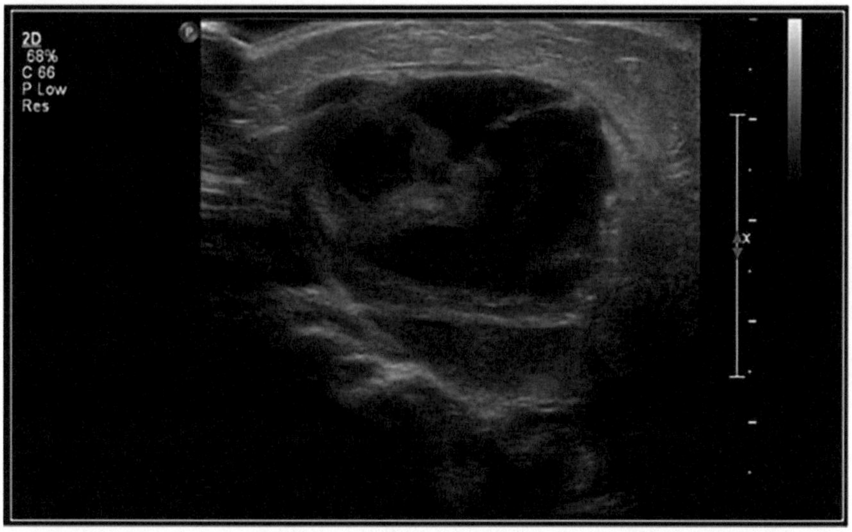


**Figure 4.**
*US of right enlarged neck node with surrounding abscess formation suggested by areas of liquefaction.*

*Limited penetration*: US has limited tissue penetration compared to other imaging modalities when used in patients with a high BMI or those with extensive subcutaneous fat.

*Limited soft tissue contrast*: While US provides good soft tissue contrast, it may not be as detailed as CT or MRI in assessing certain deeper level structures.

### 2.5 Advancements in US technology

*High-frequency US*: This technology allows for higher resolution imaging of superficial structures which can improve diagnostic accuracy.

## 3. Computed tomography (CT)

CT provides detailed cross-sectional imaging that visualises soft tissue and bony anatomy with high resolution, which can help in the detailed assessment of structures involved in swallowing. It is particularly useful for identifying structural abnormalities and guiding further diagnostic and therapeutic interventions.

CT involves an X-ray source that rotates around the body of a patient and emits a fan shaped X-ray beam that is projected through a particular slice of the body to be imaged; the penetrating radiation is captured and measured by a detector on the opposite side of the X-ray source. As the X-ray beam rotates around the patient, multiple snapshot images are obtained which are reconstructed into cross-sectional slices by a computer; the slices are subsequently stacked together in order to create a 3D image.

The unit of measurement for the degree of tissue penetration is the Hounsfield Unit (HU). Water has a HU of 0 which is represented by a particular shade of grey within a pixel in the image generated. Values higher than water are positive e.g. bone and soft tissue. Values lower than water are negative e.g. air and fat.

### 3.1 CT serves a number of general applications

*Anatomical assessment*: CT can help to identify structural abnormalities such as tumours, strictures and diverticula, all of which can cause dysphagia.

*Functional evaluation*: There are advanced CT techniques, including dynamic swallowing CT, that allow for observing the mechanics of swallowing and the identification of functional problems.

*Preoperative planning*: CT provides detailed anatomical head and neck information that is crucial for surgical planning, especially in cases that involve tumours or complex structural abnormalities.

### 3.2 CT imaging for swallowing disorders involves the use of different CT properties to help detect relevant anatomical structures and pathology

*Non-contrast CT*: Useful for initial assessment and for identifying calcifications or foreign bodies. Can be of benefit to those patients in whom contrast media is contraindicated such as in kidney disease, allergy and pregnancy.

*Contrast-enhanced CT*: Enhances the visualisation of soft tissues and vascular structures, aiding in the detection of tumours and inflammatory conditions.

*Dynamic swallowing CT*: This technique involves capturing live images during the act of swallowing itself, providing real-time assessment of the swallowing process and identifying functional impairments [11].

*3D reconstruction*: Advanced software on healthcare systems allows for the creation of three-dimensional reconstructions of CT images, offering detailed anatomy which is essential in surgical planning [12].

### 3.3 CT has a number of clinical applications that help in assessing and treating swallowing disorders

*Detection and staging*: CT is essential for detecting tumours in the head and neck region such as those in the nasopharynx (see **Figure 5**), oral cavity, oropharynx, hypopharynx, larynx (see **Figure 6**) and oesophagus, as well as for staging malignancies by assessing the extent to which the tumour has spread locally and distally [13]. This can be of great benefit to patients in whom MRI is contraindicated.

*Surgical planning*: Detailed anatomical information from a CT helps in planning surgical interventions, ensuring precise removal of tumours while preserving vital structures such as nerves and vessels [14].

*Strictures, diverticula and collections*: CT can identify strictures and diverticula as well as parapharyngeal and retropharyngeal collections (see **Figure 7**) that may cause dysphagia, guiding appropriate therapeutic interventions [15].

### 3.4 CT offers numerous advantages in the evaluation of swallowing disorders; however, it also has certain limitations that need to be considered

#### *3.4.1 Advantages*

*High resolution*: CT provides high-resolution images that offer detailed soft tissue and bony anatomical visualisation.

*Rapid imaging*: CT scans can be performed quickly, making them suitable for use in emergency settings [13].

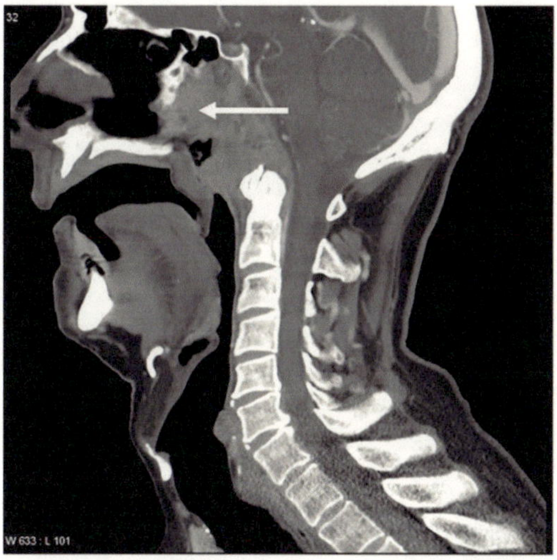


**Figure 5.**
*CT neck with contrast in sagittal view, demonstrating a large heterogeneously enhancing mass of the nasopharynx (arrow) extending into and through the clivus and down to the level of C1.*

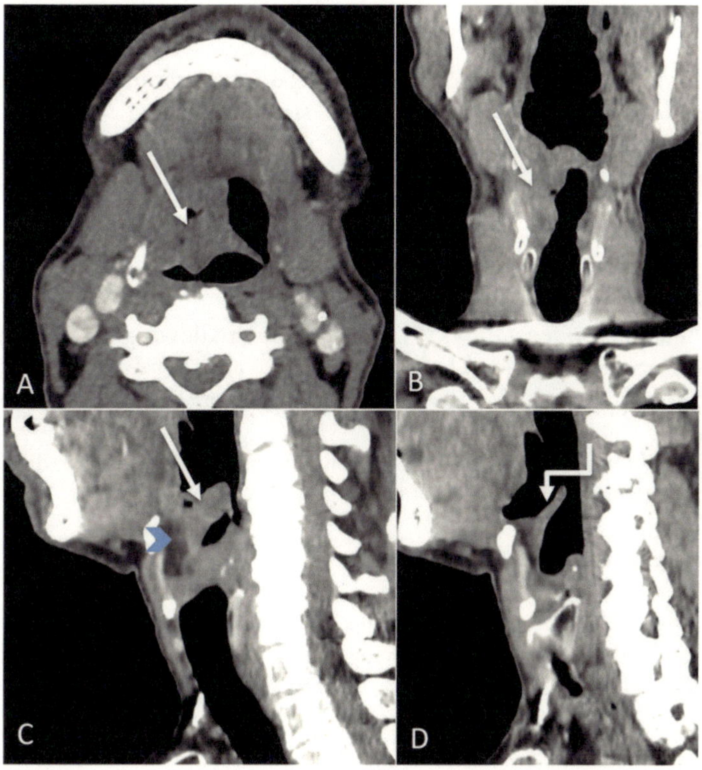


**Figure 6.**
*CT neck with contract in axial, coronal and sagittal views. Shows a proliferative irregular mass (straight arrows) involving the right vallecula and epiglottis with involvement of the median glosso-epiglottic fold. There is also involvement of the pre-epiglottic space also (blue arrowhead) with normal uninvolved epiglottis on the left side (shouldered arrow). This is consistent with a supraglottic laryngeal carcinoma.*

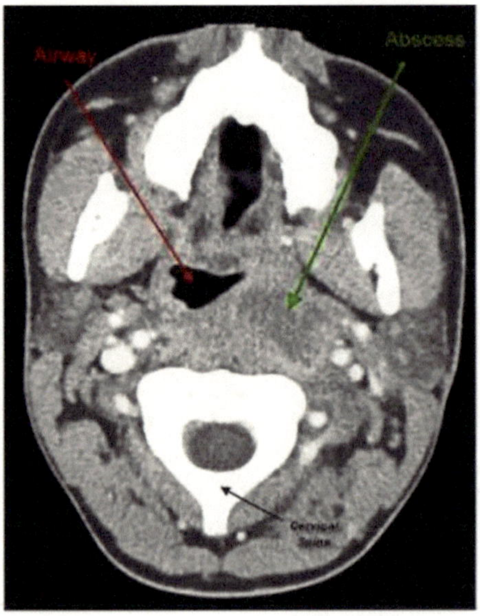


**Figure 7.**
*CT neck with contrast in axial view, outlining a low attenuation fluid collection with peripheral enhancement within the parapharyngeal space representing a deep neck space abscess. Note deviation and compression of the airway.*

*3D visualisation*: Advanced reconstruction modifications and techniques allow for three-dimensional visualisation of anatomical structures.

#### *3.4.2 Limitations*

*Radiation exposure*: CT involves exposure to ionising radiation, which is a significant consideration for patients, especially paediatrics, pregnant patients and those requiring repeat imaging.

*Limited functional information*: While dynamic swallowing CT provides some functional information, it is not as comprehensive as other dynamic studies such as videofluoroscopy [13]. CT is also less effective at soft tissue delineation compared to MRI.

*Cost and availability*: CT scans can be expensive and may not be readily available in all healthcare settings.

### 3.5 Advancements in CT technology

*Area-detector CT*: This technology allows for rapid acquisition of volumetric data, enabling detailed assessment of swallowing mechanics and improving diagnostic accuracy through multi-planar reconstruction of CT images [16].

## 4. Magnetic resonance imaging (MRI)

MRI provides high-resolution images and superior soft tissue contrast compared to other imaging modalities, making it particularly useful for evaluating complex anatomical regions and soft tissue areas involved in the swallowing process. It does not involve exposure to ionising radiation, making it a safer modality for repeated use if necessary.

MRI scans use radio waves and strong magnetic fields to create detailed images of the inside of the body. The MRI machine involves an electric current that passes through sets of coiled wires in order to create powerful magnets. A transmitter and receiver in the machine send and receive radio waves respectively. The magnetic field created by the magnets interacts with hydrogen atoms in the body.

It is the combined interaction between the magnetic field, radio waves and hydrogen atoms that forms cross-sectional slices which are subsequently converted into digital images by a computer.

### 4.1 MRI serves a number of general applications

*Anatomical assessment*: MRI can visualise the muscles, tendons, ligaments, vessels and nerves involved in swallowing which can help to identify abnormalities.

*Functional evaluation*: Advanced MRI techniques, such as real-time MRI, allow for the assessment of swallowing mechanics and see whether there is any functional impairment present [17].

*Preoperative planning*: Just like CT, MRI is crucial for surgical planning as it provides detailed anatomical information which are of a higher degree than CT, due to more optimal soft tissue delineation [18].

### 4.2 There are several MRI weightings and sequences, all of which can be used to tailor swallowing problems to a specific diagnosis

*Diffusion-weighted imaging (DWI)*: This technique uses the diffusion of water molecules to generate contrast. Diffusion-weighted imaging is useful in differentiating tumour recurrence from post-radiation changes. Overall, it helps to evaluate tissue integrity and can help in identifying areas of inflammation or tumour infiltration [19].

*T1-weighted (T1W) imaging*: In these images, the fluid signal in cerebrospinal fluid or orbital fluid appears dark, whereas fat appears bright or white (see **Figure 8**). T1W images are useful for looking at the extent of tumour spread as they tend to grow through and obliterate the fat planes. The loss of the normal fat in the bone marrow of the mandible and in the skull base is particularly useful in staging.

*T2-weighted (T2W) imaging*: In these images, fluid appears to be of high signal and fat is also bright or white (see **Figure 8**). T2W images are useful for looking at high signal fluid necrosis in metastatic lymph nodes from a squamous cell carcinoma and for distinguishing a sinus tumour from surrounding fluid secretions. This type of imaging highlights differences in tissue composition, useful for identifying pathological changes.

*Gadolinium*: This is a paramagnetic contrast agent that is used in MRI. It acts in the same way as iodine-based contrast media used in CT scans. Post-gadolinium fat-saturated T1W images are used to show enhancement (an increase in signal) and are useful for demonstrating necrotic lymph nodes and enhancing tumours. Fat saturated means that the bright fat signal is suppressed or removed from the image, leaving the pathology more visible.

*Short-tau inversion recovery (STIR) sequence*: This is a T2W scan with fat signal suppression. This shows pathology and fluid as white or bright in the image and is therefore more visible than in an ordinary T2W image. It is an imaging technique that is of great value in delineating head and neck cancers.

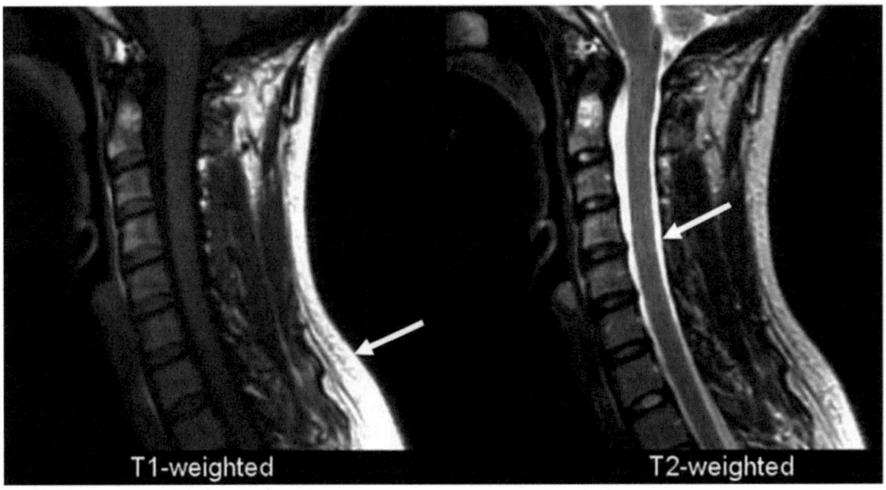


**Figure 8.**
*MRI scans in sagittal views showing contrast differences between T1W and T2W imaging. Note the difference in brightness of the subcutaneous fascia (fat) indicated by the arrow in the T1W image AND the cerebrospinal fluid (water) indicated by the arrow in the T2DW image.*

*Dynamic MRI*: This technique captures images during the act of swallowing, providing real-time assessment of swallowing mechanics [20].

*Functional MRI (fMRI)*: This modality assesses brain activity related to swallowing, helping to identify neurological causes of dysphagia [21].

### 4.3 MRI has a wide range of clinical applications in the assessment and management of patients with dysphagia

*Detection and staging*: MRI is vital for detecting tumours in the head and neck region such as those in the nasopharynx, oral cavity (see **Figure 9**), oropharynx, hypopharynx (see **Figure 10**), larynx and oesophagus can assist in for staging malignancies by assessing the extent of tumour spread [22].

*Surgical planning*: Detailed anatomical information from MRI scans aids in planning surgical interventions, ensuring precise removal of tumours while preserving vital structures [23].

*Strictures, diverticula and cricopharyngeal dysfunction*: MRI can assess for strictures and diverticula whilst dynamic MRI can assess the function of the cricopharyngeal muscle and identify dysfunctions that may cause swallowing difficulties [24, 25].

### 4.4 While MRI offers numerous advantages in the evaluation of swallowing disorders, it also has some limitations that need to be considered

#### *4.4.1 Advantages*

*High resolution*: MRI provides high-resolution images with excellent soft tissue contrast.

*No radiation*: MRI does not involve exposure to ionising radiation, making it comparatively safer for repeated use and for paediatric and pregnant patients.

*Multiplanar imaging*: MRI can capture images in multiple planes, providing comprehensive anatomical information.

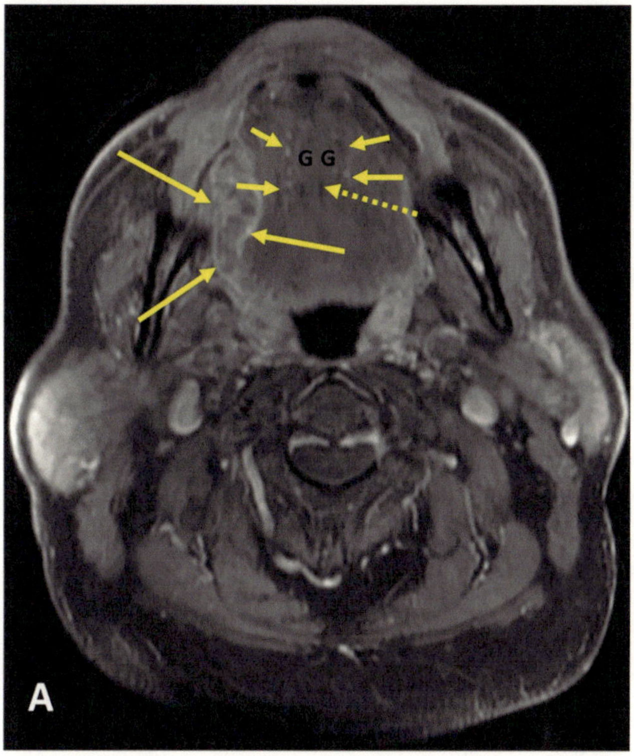


**Figure 9.**
*T1DW fat saturated MRI neck with contrast in axial view, demonstrating a 4.3 cm heterogeneously enhancing mass (solid long arrows) occupying the right lateral edge of the tongue and floor of the mouth. The hypointense fatty lingual septum (dashed arrow), marking the midline floor of the mouth, is intact. Paired genioglossus (G) muscles are situated lateral to the midline septum. The sublingual space containing the neurovascular bundles (solid short arrows) is lateral to the genioglossus muscles. This is consistent with a right tongue squamous cell carcinoma.*

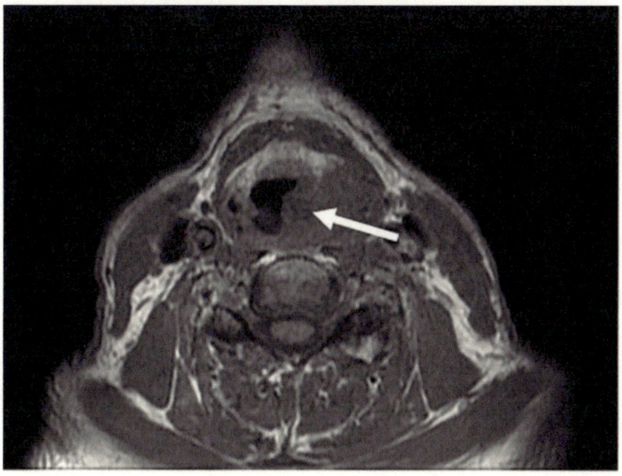

**Figure 10.**
*T2DW MRI neck with contrast in axial view, outlining abnormal enhancing mucosal thickening centred on the left piriform sinus (arrow) extending into the ipsilateral aryepiglottic fold and posterior wall of the hypopharynx. This is consistent with a hypopharyngeal squamous cell carcinoma.*

#### *4.4.2 Limitations*

*Cost and availability*: MRI scans can be expensive and may not be readily available in all healthcare settings.

*Longer acquisition times*: MRI scans take longer to perform compared to other imaging modalities, which can be challenging for some patients.

*Contraindications*: MRI is contraindicated in patients with certain implants or devices (e.g., pacemakers, iron-containing brain clips, cardiac prosthetic valves). Gadolinium should be used cautiously in those patients with known kidney disease. Patients can have anaphylactic reactions to IV gadolinium; however, this is less common than with IV iodinated contrast.

### 4.5 Advancements in MRI technology

*Real-time 3D MRI*: This technology allows for real-time volumetric imaging, providing detailed assessment of swallowing mechanics [26].

## 5. Dynamic studies and X-ray

Dynamic studies provide real-time detailed visualisation of the swallowing process. Alongside use of X-ray for techniques such as fluoroscopy and barium swallow studies, the images produced are invaluable for the assessment of both anatomical structures and functional movements. These help to identify the underlying causes of dysphagia and guide appropriate treatment strategies.

The quality of the images produced by fluoroscopy can be further enhanced by the use of image intensifiers, which amplify X-ray beams whilst keeping the radiation dose as low as possible.

Lateral soft-tissue X-rays of the neck are of limited value in isolation. They may demonstrate opaque foreign bodies; however, many foreign bodies are likely to be non-opaque and therefore, contrast swallows are more accurate in this situation [27].

A contrast swallow is not only indicated in the investigation of dysphagia but also if in cases where symptoms are suggestive of a motility disorder.

### 5.1 Dynamic studies and X-ray imaging serve a number of general applications

*Anatomical assessment*: Dynamic studies can identify structural abnormalities such as tumours, strictures and diverticula that may cause swallowing problems.

*Functional evaluation*: These studies assess the coordination and timing of swallowing-related muscles and structures which are invaluable for outlining functional impairments.

*Preoperative planning*: Dynamic studies provide detailed anatomical and functional information that is crucial for surgical planning, especially in cases involving tumours or complex structural abnormalities [28].

### 5.2 There are a number of different dynamic methods through which the act of swallowing can be visually assessed

*Videofluoroscopic swallow study (VFSS)*: VFSS, also known as a modified barium swallow study, involves the patient swallowing a barium-coated substance while

X-ray images are captured in real-time and in rapid succession, creating a video of the swallowing process. This study provides a dynamic view of the swallowing process, highlighting both anatomical and functional aspects [29]. VFSS is particularly useful for assessing the timing and coordination of the oral and pharyngeal phases of swallowing, identifying issues such as aspiration, penetration, and residue [30].

*Fibreoptic endoscopic evaluation of swallowing (FEES)*: FEES involves the insertion of a flexible endoscope through the nose to visualise the pharynx and larynx during swallowing. This study provides real-time images of the swallowing process without the use of radiation [31]. FEES is useful for assessing the pharyngeal phase of swallowing, identifying structural abnormalities, and evaluating the effectiveness of therapeutic interventions [32].

*Barium swallow*: This involves the patient swallowing a barium solution, which coats the oesophagus and provides clear images on X-ray. It helps in identifying structural abnormalities and assessing the movement of the barium through the oesophagus [33]. Barium swallows are more sensitive in visualising pharyngeal pouches, pharyngeal webs and cricopharyngeal hypertrophy. Image acquisition is preferably at the rate of 2 frames per second during a bolus swallow.

*Double-contrast studies*: These involve the use of both barium and air to provide detailed images of the mucosal surface of the oesophagus, helping to identify subtle abnormalities [34].

*Dynamic swallowing studies*: These studies capture images during the act of swallowing, providing real-time assessment of the mechanics of swallowing and identifying functional impairments [35]. Water soluble contrast swallows use non-ionic relatively inert contrast media to outline structural pathology in swallowing and are preferentially indicated when there is a high risk of aspiration or when perforation of the oesophagus is suspected.

### 5.3 Dynamic studies and X-ray have a wide range of clinical applications in the evaluation and management of swallowing disorders

*Strictures and diverticula*: Dynamic imaging can identify strictures, diverticula (see **Figure 11**) and other structural abnormalities that may cause dysphagia, guiding appropriate therapeutic interventions [36].

*Foreign bodies*: X-ray imaging is effective in locating and assessing the impact of foreign bodies in the aerodigestive tract (see **Figure 12**) [37]. X-ray will help identify the nature and location of the foreign body. Lateral soft tissue X-ray view of the neck is essential in showing whether the foreign body has passed into the oesophagus or through the larynx (see **Figure 13**). In addition to a foreign body shadow, particular signs to look out for on X-ray may include prevertebral widening, loss of cervical lordosis and surgical emphysema.

*Cricopharyngeal dysfunction*: Videofluoroscopy can assess the function of the cricopharyngeal muscle and identify dysfunctions that may cause swallowing difficulties.

*Achalasia*: Dynamic studies can help in assessing overall swallowing function and diagnosing achalasia by visualising the peristaltic waves of the oesophagus with characteristic features on barium swallow being that of a rat‘s tail or bird’s beak appearance (see **Figure 14**).

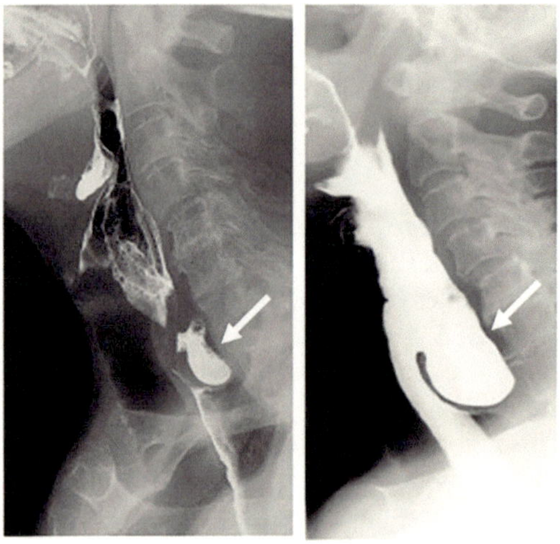

**Figure 11.**
*Barium swallow study demonstrating a smaller diverticulum (left image arrow) and a larger pharyngeal pouch (right image arrow).*

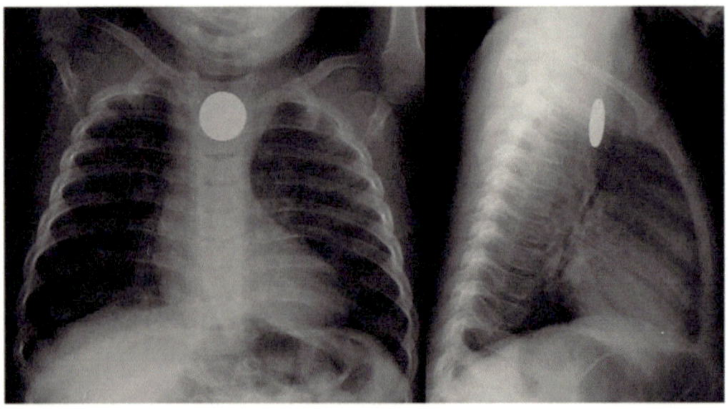

**Figure 12.**
*Plain X-ray radiograph in AP and lateral views showing a coin lodged in the oesophagus at the lower cervical/ upper thoracic level.*

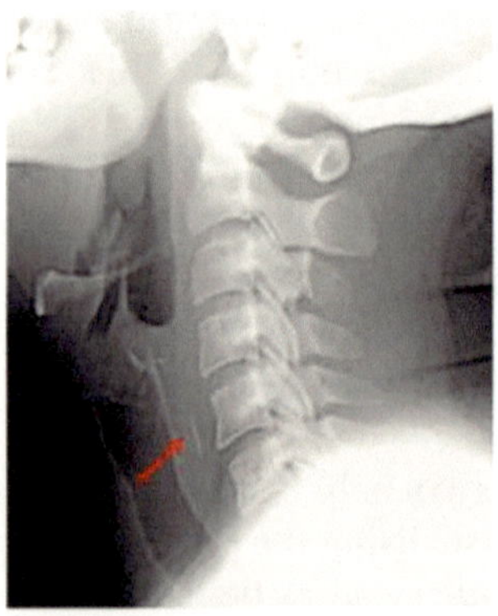

**Figure 13.**
*Plain X-ray radiograph in lateral soft tissue view showing a piece of chicken bone impacted in the oesophagus (red arrow).*

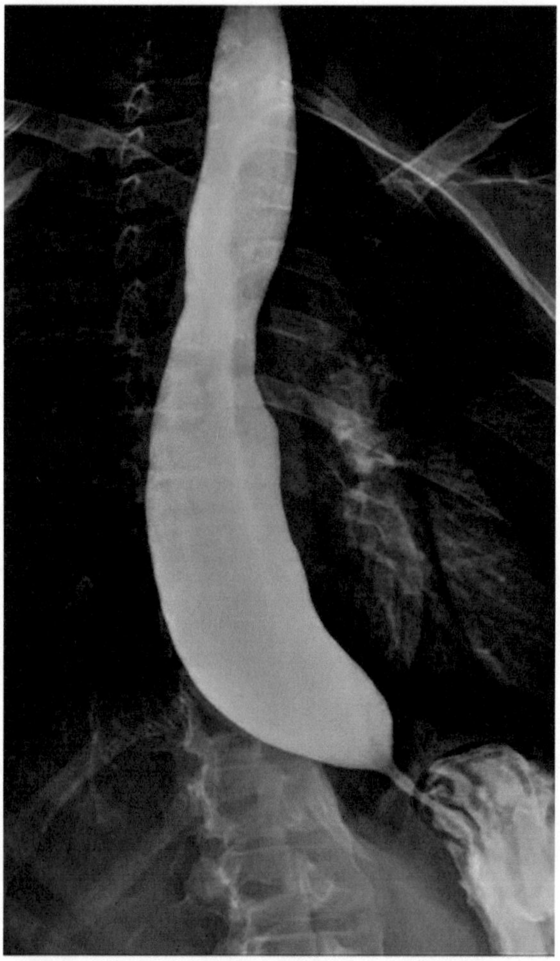

**Figure 14.**
*Barium swallow study outlining dilatation and stasis in the oesophagus with tapering at the lower oesophageal sphincter and narrowing at the gastro-oesophageal junction consistent with bird beak sign or rat-tail sign seen in achalasia.*

## 5.4 While dynamic studies and X-rays offer numerous advantages in the evaluation of swallowing disorders, it also has certain limitations that need to be considered

### *5.4.1 Advantages*

*Dynamic assessment*: Techniques like videofluoroscopy provide real-time visualisation of the swallowing process, allowing for dynamic assessment of swallowing mechanics.

*Detailed visualisation*: X-ray imaging provides detailed images of the oesophagus and surrounding structures, aiding in the identification of structural abnormalities.

*Non-invasive*: X-ray imaging is a non-invasive procedure, making it suitable for repeated use and for patients who may not tolerate more invasive procedures.

### 5.4.2 Limitations

*Radiation exposure*: X-ray imaging involves exposure to ionising radiation, which is a consideration, especially in paediatric and repeated imaging.

*Limited soft tissue contrast*: X-ray imaging provides limited soft tissue contrast compared to other modalities like MRI, which may limit its effectiveness in certain cases.

## 5.5 Advancements in dynamic studies and X-ray technology

*High-resolution manometry*: This technology allows for detailed assessment of oesophageal pressure patterns during swallowing, improving diagnostic accuracy [38].

*Digital radiography*: This technology allows for rapid acquisition of high-resolution images, improving diagnostic accuracy and reducing radiation exposure.

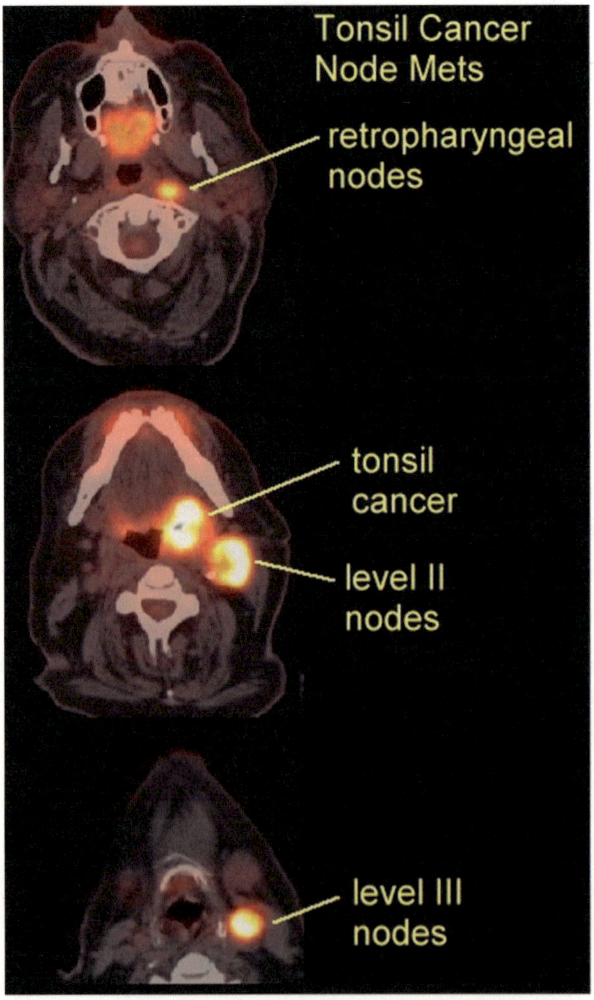


**Figure 15.**
*PET-CT scan in axial view demonstrating asymmetrical contrast medium enhancement of the left tonsil with associated uptake in ipsilateral lymph nodes.*

## 6. Advanced imaging techniques

Advancements in imaging technology have introduced several sophisticated techniques that enhance diagnostic accuracy and therapeutic planning in patients with swallowing problems.

*Positron emission tomography (PET)*: PET provides functional information about metabolic activity which is crucial for imaging of head and neck cancers, aiding in staging of tumours, providing scope for treatment planning and monitoring response to therapy.

PET–CT scan uses radioactive glucose in the form of fluorodeoxyglucose (FDG) as the tracer. The FDG is injected into the patient and accumulates in areas of high metabolic activity (see **Figure 15**). This will include normal structures such as the brain and heart. The tracer is excreted by the kidneys and therefore the urinary tract will also show increased activity. Increased activity is also a feature of tumours, referred to as PET positive lesions. FDG values can be useful in differentiating between inflammation and tumour with inflammation giving values of 2.32 ± 1.00, tumour 1.66 ± 0.34, and inflammation with tumour 0.78 ± 0.05 [39].

PET and CT images are acquired during the scan and fused together by software to allow a map of functional activity onto structural landmarks. In head and neck surgery, the main indications to perform a PET scan are investigating primary cancer of unknown origin and suspected recurrent head and neck cancer. FDG PET-CT is expensive and involves a high radiation dose being administered to the patient; however, the advantage over structural imaging alone outweighs this, particularly in advanced metastatic head and neck malignancies [40].

*3D imaging*: 3D imaging is used in surgical planning and reconstruction, providing detailed anatomical visualisation that aids in precise surgical interventions (see **Figure 16**). Not only does it enhance surgical precision and outcomes, but it also allows for patient education and preoperative planning. 3D imaging requires highly specialised software and operator expertise; it confers a significantly higher cost when compared with other standard imaging modalities [41].

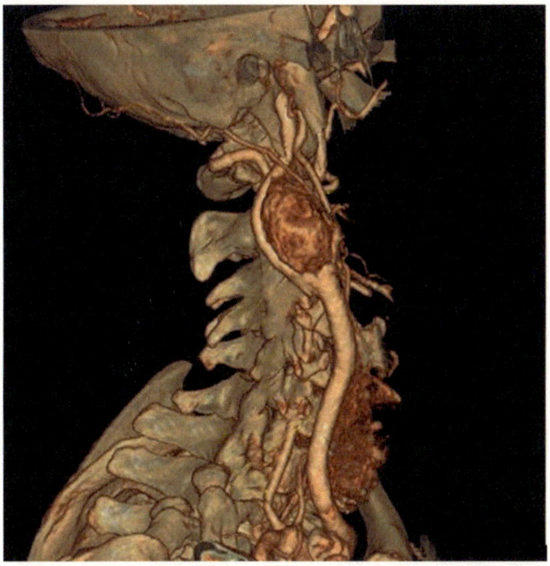

**Figure 16.**
*3D volume rendering of a right carotid body mass with marked enhancement that is splaying the ICA and ECA.*

## 7. Conclusion

Imaging is an integral part of ENT practice which enhances diagnostic accuracy and guides therapeutic decisions in patients with swallowing problems. From plain radiography to advanced techniques like PET and 3D imaging, each modality has its own unique applications and indications. Effective imaging interpretation and clinical correlation requires a collaborative approach between radiologists, ENT surgeons, oncologists and other specialists to ensure comprehensive patient care and optimal outcomes.

Advances in imaging technology continue to improve patient outcomes, making it an exciting and evolving field in the management of swallowing disorders. Currently, AI algorithms are being developed to assist in the interpretation of US, CT and MRI images, which ultimately enhances diagnostic precision and reduces burden on radiologists [42].

## 8. Common clinical presentations: Which investigation to do?

Please see the below **Figure 17** which gives a rough guide as to which investigations to consider or perform for specific presenting complaints and pathologies relating to swallowing problems.

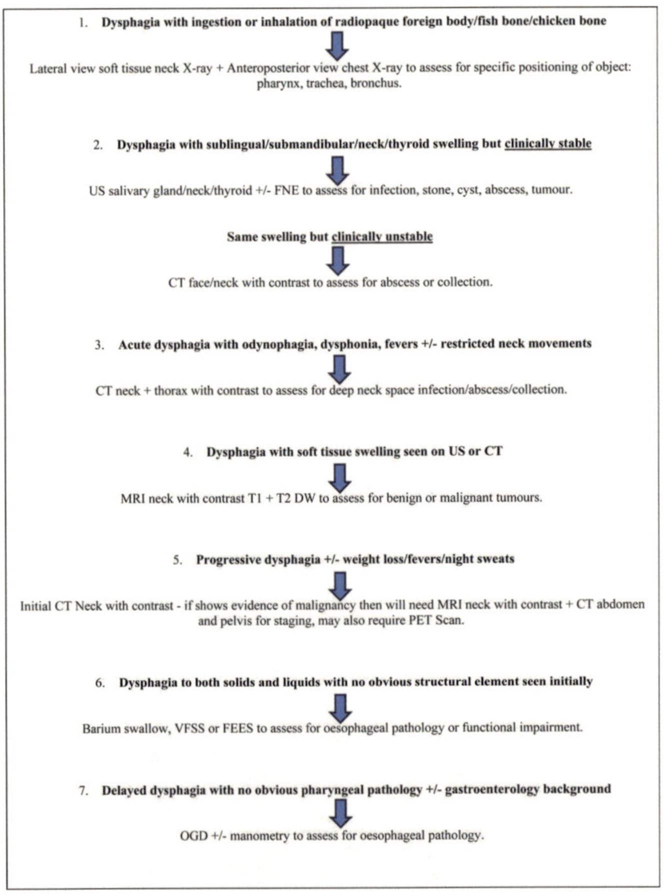


**Figure 17.**
*Guide on which imaging modality is most suitable based upon clinical presentation.*

## Author details

Liam D. Hyland
CT2 ENT, Nottingham University Hospitals NHS Trust, United Kingdom

*Address all correspondence to: liam.hyland@nhs.net

## References

[1] Ear Nose and Throat: The Official Handbook for Medical. Available from: https://www.entuk.org/_userfiles/pages/files/groups/ear_nose_and_throat_the_offici_sfo_uk_compressed.pdf [Accessed: September 16, 2024]

[2] Koch BL, Hamilton BE, Hudgins PA, Ric HH. Diagnostic Imaging: Head and Neck. Elsevier; 2017. 1247 p. DOI: 10.1016/B978-0-323-44301-2.50421-3

[3] Wilson G, Turner H, Dwiddar N, Charlton A, Cole S, Allam A. Basic ENT Skills Training (B.E.S.T.) Course Handbook, Nottingham University Hospitals NHS Trust. 2020

[4] Hsiao M-Y, Wu C-H, Wang T-G. Emerging role of ultrasound in dysphagia assessment and intervention: A narrative review. Frontiers in Rehabilitation Sciences. 2021;**11**:2

[5] Use-of-Ultrasound-for-Swallowing-and-Upper-Airway. Available from: https://www.rcslt.org/wp-content/uploads/2022/05/Use-of-ultrasound-for-swallowing-and-upper-airway-assessment-May-2022.pdf [Accessed: September 16, 2024]

[6] de Andrade RA, de Pernambuco L, de Almeida AN, Mulatinho ME, dos Santos EN, da Silva HJ. Methodological procedures to acquire and analyze ultrasound images of swallowing: A scoping review. Dysphagia. 2024

[7] Potente P, Buoite Stella A, Vidotto M, Passerini M, Furlanis G, Naccarato M, et al. Application of ultrasonography in neurogenic dysphagia: A systematic review. Dysphagia. 2022;**38**(1):65-75

[8] McIvor NP, Freeman JL, Salem S, Elden L, Noyek AM, Bedard YC. Ultrasonography and ultrasound-guided fine-needle aspiration biopsy of head and neck lesions: A surgical perspective [Internet]. The Laryngoscope. 1994. Available from: https://pubmed.ncbi.nlm.nih.gov/8196441/;**104**(6 Pt 1):669-674 [Accessed: September 16, 2024]

[9] Iowa Radiology. MRI vs. Ultrasound: What's the Difference? [Internet]. Iowa Radiology Blog. Iowa Radiology; 2024. Available from: https://info.iowaradiology.com/mri-vs.-ultrasound-whats-the-difference [Accessed: September 16, 2024]

[10] Ota T, Madokoro S, Shimizu K, Yoneda M. Reliability of ultrasound real-time tissue elastography in evaluating swallowing-related muscle elasticity and effects of swallowing exercises. Sonography. 2024

[11] Inamoto Y, Ueha R, Gonzalez-Fernandez M. Emerging dysphagia technologies: Swallowing CT. Current Otorhinolaryngology Reports. 2023;**11**(2):154-160

[12] Inamoto Y, González-Fernández M, Saitoh E. 3D-CT evaluation of swallowing: Metrics of the swallowing response using swallowing CT. Dysphagia. 2021;**37**(2):237-249

[13] Inamoto Y, Ueha R, Gonzalez-Fernandez M. Use of CT for dysphagia evaluation: Advantages and disadvantages in the study of swallowing. Current Physical Medicine and Rehabilitation Reports. 2024;**12**(3):250-255

[14] Swallowing Disorders Update [Internet]. The Radiology Assistant: Swallowing disorders update. Available from: https://radiologyassistant.nl/

head-neck/swallowing/swallowing-disorders-update [Accessed: September 16, 2024]

[15] NHS Choices. NHS. Available from: https://www.nhs.uk/conditions/swallowing-problems-dysphagia/ [Accessed: September 16, 2024]

[16] Kang EJ. Clinical applications of wide-detector CT scanners for cardiothoracic imaging: An update [Internet]. Korean Journal of Radiology. 2019;**20**(12):1583-1596. Available from: https://www.ncbi.nlm.nih.gov/pmc/articles/PMC6923215/ [Accessed: September 16, 2024]

[17] Zu Y, Narayanan SS, Kim Y-C, Nayak K, Bronson-Lowe C, Villegas B, et al. Evaluation of swallow function after tongue cancer treatment using real-time magnetic resonance imaging. JAMA Otolaryngology–Head & Neck Surgery. 2013;**139**(12):1312

[18] Kulinna-Cosentini C, Arnoldner MA, Kristo I, Jomrich G, Schima W, Riegler M, et al. Swallowing MRI for gerd—Diagnosis and treatment monitoring. European Surgery. 2019;**51**(5):231-238

[19] Baliyan V, Das CJ, Sharma R, Gupta AK. Diffusion weighted imaging: Technique and applications [Internet]. World Journal of Radiology. 2016. Available from: https://www.ncbi.nlm.nih.gov/pmc/articles/PMC5039674/

[20] Voskuilen L, Schoormans J, Gurney-Champion OJ, Balm AJ, Strijkers GJ, Smeele LE, et al. Dynamic MRI of swallowing: Real-time volumetric imaging at 12 frames per second at 3 T. Magnetic Resonance Materials in Physics, Biology and Medicine. 2021;**35**(3):411-419

[21] Malandraki GA, Johnson S, Robbins J. Functional MRI of swallowing: From neurophysiology to neuroplasticity [Internet]. Head & Neck. 2011;**33 Suppl 1**: S14-S20. Available from: https://www.ncbi.nlm.nih.gov/pmc/articles/PMC3747973/ [Accessed: September 16, 2024]

[22] Pigorsch SU, May C, Kessel KA, Graf S, Bier H, Nüsslin F, et al. MRI- and CT-determined changes of dysphagia/aspiration-related structures (dars) during and after radiotherapy [Internet]. PLoS One. 2020. Available from: https://www.ncbi.nlm.nih.gov/pmc/articles/PMC7467287/ [Accessed: September 16, 2024]

[23] Jansen JFA, Parra C, Lu Y, Shukla-Dave A. Evaluation of head and neck tumors with functional MR imaging [Internet]. Magnetic Resonance Imaging Clinics of North America. 2016. Available from: https://www.ncbi.nlm.nih.gov/pmc/articles/PMC4663682/ [Accessed: September 16, 2024]

[24] Biggemann L, Uhlig J, Gliem N, Al-Bourini O, Wedi E, Ellenrieder V, et al. Assessment of esophageal motility disorders by real-time MRI. European Journal of Radiology. 2020;**132**:109265

[25] Neil BM, Cricopharyngeal myotomy workup [Internet]. Imaging studies, other tests, histologic findings. Medscape. 2023. Available from: https://emedicine.medscape.com/article/836966-workup [Accessed: September 16, 2024]

[26] Engwall O. From real-time MRI to 3D tongue movements. Interspeech. 2004;**2004**:1109-1112

[27] McCrory D, Smith C, Hampton S. Foiling the barium swallow! BMJ Case Reports. 2019;**12**(1)

[28] Dysphagia [Internet]. Mayo Clinic. Mayo Foundation for Medical Education and Research; 2024. Available from: https://www.mayoclinic.org/

diseases-conditions/dysphagia/diagnosis-treatment/drc-20372033 [Accessed: September 16, 2024]

[29] Vishak MS, Ramasamy K. Swallowing rehabilitation: Tracing the evolution of assessment and intervention approaches for dysphagia over 30 years. Indian Journal of Otolaryngology and Head & Neck Surgery. 2023;**76**(2):2171-2175

[30] Videofluoroscopic Swallowing Study (VFSS). Available from: https://www.asha.org/public/speech/swallowing/videofluoroscopic-swallowing-study/ [Accessed: September 16, 2024]

[31] Fiberoptic Endoscopic Evaluation of Swallowing (fees) - asha. Available from: https://www.asha.org/practice-portal/clinical-topics/adult-dysphagia/fiberoptic-endoscopic-evaluation-of-swallowing/ [Accessed: September 16, 2024]

[32] What is fees?: Fiberoptic Endoscopic Evaluation of Swallowing - Advanced dysphagia [Internet]. Diagnostics. Available from: https://www.dysphagia-diagnostics.com/what-is-fees [Accessed: September 16, 2024]

[33] Barium Swallow and Barium Meal [Internet]. Available from: https://www.spirehealthcare.com/treatments/bowel-treatments/barium-swallow-and-barium-meal/ [Accessed: September 16, 2024]

[34] Double-Contrast Barium Swallow Guide. Available from: https://geiselmed.dartmouth.edu/radiology/wp-content/uploads/sites/47/2019/04/Normal_Barium_Swallow.pdf [Accessed: September 16, 2024]

[35] Carbo AI, Brown M, Nakrour N. Fluoroscopic swallowing examination: Radiologic findings and analysis of their causes and pathophysiologic mechanisms. Radiographics. 2021;**41**(6):1733-1749

[36] Patel R. Assessment of swallowing disorders. In: Swallowing – Physiology, Disorders, Diagnosis and Therapy. Springer; 2015. pp. 49-60

[37] Barbon CE, Warneke CL, Ledger B, Rogus-Pulia N, Cunningham L, Coyle JL, et al. Reliability and confidence of dynamic imaging grade of swallowing toxicity (digest) rating among research and clinical speech pathologists before and after implementation of a training manual: A multi-site study. Dysphagia. 2024

[38] Conklin JL. Evaluation of esophageal motor function with high-resolution manometry. In: Dysphagia Evaluation and Management in Otolaryngology. Elsevier; 2019. pp. 87-98

[39] Yang Z, Zan Y, Zheng X, Hai W, Chen K, Huang Q, et al. Dynamic FDG-PET imaging to differentiate malignancies from inflammation in subcutaneous and in situ mouse model for non-small cell lung carcinoma (NSCLC). PLoS One. 2015;**10**(9)

[40] Ayesa SL, Murphy A. Positron emission tomography: Evolving modalities, radiopharmaceuticals and professional collaboration. Journal of Medical Radiation Sciences. 2022;**69**(4):415-418

[41] Portnoy Y, Koren J, Khoury A, Factor S, Dadia S, Ran Y, et al. Three-dimensional technologies in presurgical planning of bone surgeries: Current evidence and future perspectives. International Journal of Surgery. 2023;**109**(1):3-10

[42] Panayides AS, Amini A, Filipovic ND, Sharma A, Tsaftaris SA, Young A, et al. AI in medical imaging informatics: Current challenges and future directions [Internet]. IEEE Journal of Biomedical and Health Informatics. 2020;**24**:1837-1857. Available from: https://www.ncbi.nlm.nih.gov/pmc/articles/PMC8580417/ [Accessed: September 16, 2024]

Section 2

# Swallowing Disorders

Chapter 6

# Swallowing Disorder in Cleft Lip and Palate: An Otorhinolaryngologist's Perspective

*Hardip Singh Gendeh, Ronik Kothari and Mawaddah Azman*

## Abstract

Swallowing disorders is a spectrum of conditions due to anatomical, physiological and iatrogenic causes. Craniofacial abnormalities contribute to swallowing disorders, respiratory disorders, lack of nutrition, weight loss and failure to thrive. Cleft lip and palate, either unilateral or bilateral, involves the lips and/or palate and is the most common craniofacial disorder and has the potential to cause significant swallowing disorders. The process of swallowing begins with the oral preparatory phase, followed by oral propulsion, pharyngeal and oesophageal phases. The oral preparatory phase involves the three groups of muscles of mastication. The propulsion phase transports food from the oral cavity to the pharynx, while the pharyngeal phase transports food to the oesophagus while protecting the airway. Dysphagia, which defines a swallowing disorder, is the inability or difficulty faced in swallowing. There are many aetiologies of dysphagia, and common otorhinolaryngological causes were discussed. Patients with a cleft lip may have suckling and feeding issues. A cleft palate often results in disruption to the first three phases of swallowing, resulting in nasal regurgitation and predisposing to aspiration. Therefore, the chapter discusses in detail how this swallowing process is dysfunctional or disturbed. In conclusion, a tailored approach by a multidisciplinary team with timely feeding intervention, lip and palate correction, and post-procedural dental and swallowing assessment is essential.

**Keywords:** dysphagia, odynophagia, aspiration, palatoplasty, velopharyngeal insufficiency

## 1. Introduction

> *"A man must not swallow more beliefs than he can digest."*
> *- Havelock Ellis*

Swallowing disorders cover a spectrum of disease including difficulty in swallowing (dysphagia) and painful swallowing (odynophagia). These may be due to anatomical, physiological or iatrogenic aetiology [1].

Patients with swallowing disorders may present to a variety of specialities ranging from the general practitioner, family physician, dentist, otorhinolaryngologist, oral maxillofacial surgeon, gastroenterologist, upper gastrointestinal surgeon or even the neurologist. As the author of the chapter is from an otorhinolaryngologist background, we will dwell on the otorhinolaryngology perspective of dysphagia.

Craniofacial abnormalities, either congenital or acquired may cause swallowing disorders in addition to respiratory, nutritional and weight gain and ultimately thriving failures (**Figure 1**). In more severe cases, one may lose the ability to protect the airway during swallowing. Cleft lip and/or palate is the commonest of craniofacial disorders, with an incidence of up to 1 in 700. It is more common among Caucasians and Asians and less so among Africans [2, 3]. Cleft lip and/or palate can be isolated or in association with a craniofacial abnormality. It can manifest as a unilateral cleft or bilateral cleft, involving just the lips or palate or in combination. The extreme end involves the face and is termed an orofacial cleft, whereby the defect extends into the facial regions of the maxilla and orbit [4].

Holding true to the words of Mr. Ellis, there are many aetiologists of dysphagia. Therefore, this chapter aims to describe the head and neck anatomy and physiology of swallowing, common otorhinolaryngological causes of dysphagia and its management and discuss the role of cleft lip and/or palate in causing swallowing disorders.

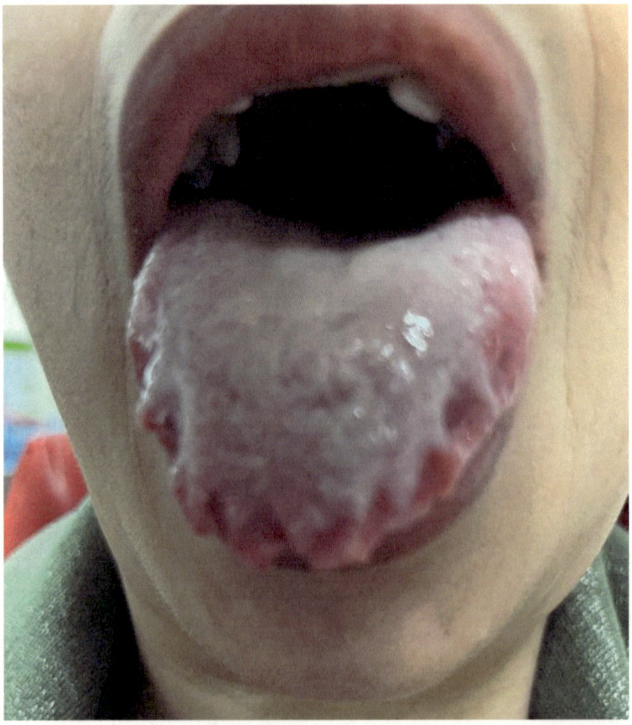

**Figure 1.**
*Cranial abnormalities may cause midface hypoplasia and oropharyngeal crowding which affects swallowing. Note the lingual displacement as evident by scalloping at the edges of the tongue due to dental compression.*

## 2. Anatomy of swallowing

The process of swallowing begins within the realm of otorhinolaryngology. It begins with the oral preparation stage. When food first enters the mouth, it is chewed and prepared for swallowing with the muscles of mastication. This group of muscles includes the temporalis, masseter, medial pterygoid, and lateral pterygoid muscles.

The temporalis arises from the temporal fossa and travels deep to the zygomatic arch to attach to the medial surface of the coronoid process. With innervation by the deep temporal branches of the mandibular nerve, the temporalis allows for elevation and retraction of the mandible. The masseter muscle arises from the maxillary process of the zygomatic bone and attaches to the lateral surface of the angle of the mandible. Through innervation from the masseteric nerve, the masseter functions to elevate the mandible. The medial pterygoid has a deep and superficial head, originating from the medial surface of the lateral pterygoid plate of the sphenoid bone and the maxillary tuberosity, respectively. With innervation from the medial pterygoid branch of the mandibular nerve, the medial pterygoid functions to elevate the mandible and facilitate side-to-side movement. Lastly, the lateral pterygoid has a superior head and inferior head arising from the infratemporal crest of the sphenoid bone and the lateral pterygoid plate of the sphenoid bone, respectively. The lateral pterygoid inserts onto the pterygoid fovea on the neck of the mandible. Through innervation from the lateral pterygoid branch of the mandibular nerve, the muscle is responsible for protrusion and depression of the mandible [5].

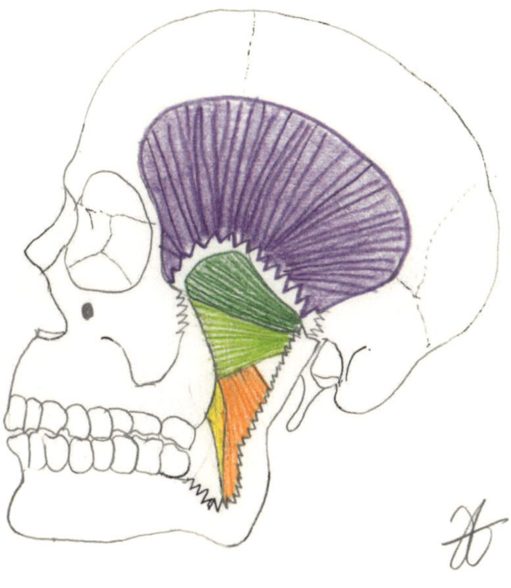

**Figure 2.**
*The three muscles of mastication. The temporalis is a fan-shaped muscle (purple), and its insertion into the medial surface of the coronoid inferiorly is not shown. The superior head (dark green) and inferior head (light green) of the lateral pterygoid insert into the fibrous capsule and articular disc of the temporomandibular joint. The deep head (orange) and superficial head (yellow) of the medial pterygoid insert into the medial surface of the ramus of the mandible. Part of the zygoma and mandibular ramus had been subtracted (saw lines) to better visualise the medial and lateral pterygoids. (Image drawn by author.)*

These are the four main muscles that work together in order to allow for the complex movements involved in grinding of teeth and chewing of food (**Figure 2**). Coordination between other muscles in the oral cavity allows for mastication to occur efficiently. A labial seal is formed after accepting a food bolus, keeping food within the oral cavity. Likewise, coordinated movements of the tongue allow food boluses to be placed in line with dentition for mastication. In addition to the mechanical digestion that occurs in the mouth, there is a small degree of chemical digestion that begins with salivary amylase. The bulk of this enzyme is produced in the pancreas; however, the salivary glands begin the digestion of carbohydrates with the release of ptyalin, or salivary amylase. The saliva in the oral cavity also helps to soften the food and prepare for the next steps of swallowing [6].

Just prior to the next stage in swallowing, the food bolus that has been prepared through mechanical and chemical digestion in the oral cavity is sealed posteriorly by the soft palate and tongue. This seal, formed with coordinated contractions of the tongue and soft palate, prevents leakage of the bolus into the oropharynx. When a bolus is ready, the food is propelled through the fauces of the oropharynx in the oral propulsive stage. The area of tongue-palate contact gradually expands backward, squeezing the food along towards the oropharynx [7].

This propulsion brings the next stage, known as the pharyngeal stage. The pharynx is a tubular structure, and its anatomy is described in **Figure 3**. There are two essential components to this stage. The first, of course, involves the swallowing and passage of food through the pharynx. The second involves protection of the larynx and trachea of the airway. Through elevation of the soft palate, the nasopharynx is

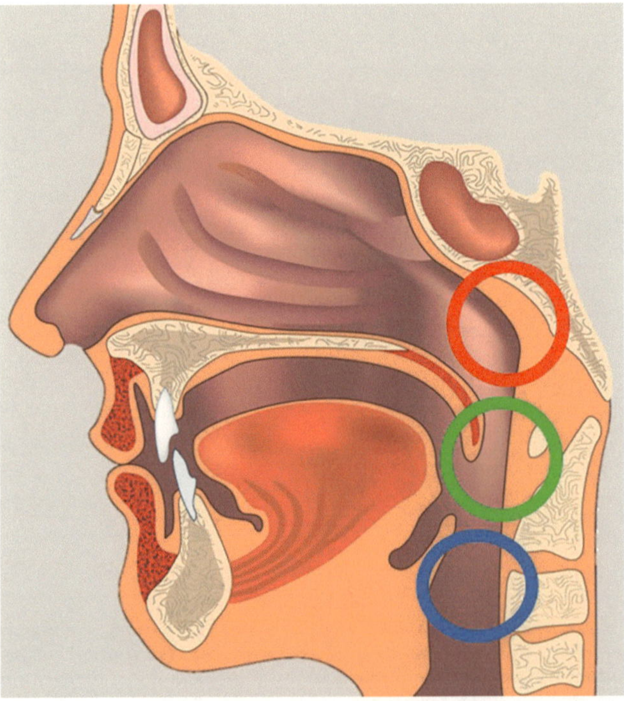

**Figure 3.**
*The pharynx can be classified into the nasopharynx (red circle), oropharynx (green circle) and laryngopharynx (blue circle). The nasopharynx is separated from the oropharynx below by the soft palate, while the oropharynx is separated from the laryngopharynx by the lower border of the epiglottis (laryngeal attachment).*

closed, preventing aspiration of solids, liquids, or saliva. As the larynx is displaced upward and forward, the epiglottis tilts backward, leaving only one direction for a bolus to move while providing airway protection [8, 9].

The pharyngeal stage specifically presents problems for individuals with loss of control of these muscles. When the larynx cannot be adequately closed, there is a high level of risk for aspiration. Dysphagia at this stage is one of the common causes of aspiration pneumonia. A few other presentations of aspiration pneumonia are in older patients undergoing anaesthesia or with a history of Parkinsonian disease or alcohol use disorder [9, 10]. There are a number of different aetiologies for the dysphagia that occurs at this stage. Up to 70% of head and neck cancer patients, 50% of stroke patients, and 11% of Parkinson's patients develop aspiration pneumonia [11].

The propulsion of food from the pharynx to the oesophagus leads to the final stage of swallowing, the oesophageal stage. The details of this process will be covered in the gastroenterology chapter.

Deficiencies at any stage of the swallowing process can lead to dysphagia, or difficulty with swallowing. Dysphagia is most apparent with an inability to swallow or extensive time required to swallow. It may also be present with frequent choking or hesitancy with swallowing food. Coughing while eating may be confused with symptoms of GERD, but when it occurs during or immediately after eating or drinking, it is more likely to be dysphagia. Drooling and inability to manage secretions is a serious sign that can lead to more problems as well. Other non-specific signs include recurrent pneumonia, unexplained weight loss, regurgitation, or heartburn. Dysphagia is a serious condition that can cause a number of uncomfortable symptoms [12].

## 3. Otorhinolaryngology aetiologies of dysphagia

Dysphagia can result from a number of otorhinolaryngology issues (**Table 1**). Age-related weakness of the muscles of mastication is the most benign of these conditions.

| Cause | Dysphagia symptoms | Diagnostics |
|---|---|---|
| CNS disorders | • Dysphagia with liquids<br>• Acute onset in stroke<br>• Insidious onset in neurodegenerative disorders | • Barium swallow showing difficulty in initial swallowing phases<br>• Neuroimaging showing stroke or neurodegeneration |
| Muscular disorders | • Dysphagia with liquids<br>• Associated with progressive weakness<br>• Subacute onset | • Flexible Endoscopic Evaluation of Swallowing (FEES) showing weak pharyngeal contraction<br>• Manometry showing ineffective swallow |
| Head and neck malignancies | • Chronic dysphagia with odynophagia and hoarseness<br>• Insidious onset | • Endoscopy showing tumour<br>• Radioimaging for localising tumour and extension |
| Iatrogenic | • Prior surgery or radiotherapy for head and neck malignancy | • Clinical diagnosis |
| Zenker diverticulum | • Regurgitation<br>• Halitosis | • Barium swallow showing contrast filled pouch |

**Table 1.**
*ENT related aetiology for dysphagia with common clinical associations and initial diagnostics.*

As with any other muscle, with advanced age, an individual's temporalis, masseter and pterygoids lose their strength. Individuals may have difficulty with chewing and preparing a food bolus for swallowing. When all other conditions have been ruled out, these muscles can be rehabilitated through regular exercise and physical and occupational therapy [13].

Pathologic processes such as throat infection are common in all age groups. Tonsillitis and spreading infection in the area can lead to inflammation and irritation of the soft palate and other muscles in the oral cavity. These are typically acute conditions that resolve quickly with symptomatic treatment of viral in aetiology or a short course of antibiotics of bacterial in aetiology. Through treatment of underlying infection, dysphagia should also be resolved [14].

Throat, lung and oesophageal cancer can cause dysphagia at every point of presentation and treatment. To begin, there can be mass effect and extraluminal compression. Oesophagal tumours may be intraluminal and result in a mechanical obstruction, presenting with dysphagia. However, initial stages of oesophageal tumours may be small, presenting only a globus sensation or foreign body sensation within the throat. This is a non-specific presentation, as globus may also occur in a myriad of laryngeal pathologies such as GERD or laryngo-pharyngeal reflux, as stated in the section mentioned before [15]. Depending on tumour grading and staging, various treatment protocols will be implemented. Surgery may initially lead to improvement of mass effect from tumour. However, the resulting scar may also cause mass effect or weakness of muscle strength or movement. A second surgery may be warranted in cases of severe dysphagia due to hypertrophic scarring. Chemotherapy and radiation are often used neoadjuvantly with surgery. Depending on radiation dosing and location, the muscles and processes involved in swallowing may also be affected. These deficiencies are usually temporary and typically resolve within weeks or months of completing radiotherapy treatment [16, 17].

Nerve disease may also be responsible for dysphagia. This can be paraneoplastic syndromes, such as Lambert-Eaton myasthenic syndrome, or primary causes. Primary causes of nerve dysfunction include Parkinsonian diseases, multiple sclerosis, amyotrophic lateral sclerosis, myasthenia gravis, or stroke. These all have their own respective treatments, which may or may not resolve dysphagia symptoms [18].

In some cases, iatrogenic injury in otorhinolaryngology cases may also lead to dysphagia. This is possible during thyroid and parathyroid surgeries due to the anatomic proximity of the various branches of the laryngeal nerve. Trauma to the recurrent laryngeal nerve results in ipsilateral vocal cord immobility, predisposing to aspiration. The external branch of the superior laryngeal nerve runs in proximity to the superior thyroid artery; injury to it results in loss of supraglottic sensation. Measures during operation, such as continuous nerve stimulation and avoidance of the nerve, are taken to prevent complications from necessary surgery.

Vocal cord paralysis can result from this iatrogenic injury or idiopathically. Surgery with vocal fold medialisation is an option to correct this paralysis. During this procedure, the paralysed vocal cord is pushed to the middle so the contralateral functioning vocal fold can close properly. The medialisation is achieved through injection laryngoplasty, medialisation laryngoplasty, or arytenoid adduction.

## 4. Bedside investigations of swallowing disorders

There are a number of diagnostic procedures to identify the presence of dysphagia. A flexible naso-pharyngo-laryngo-scopy (FNPLS) with a distal tip videography allows the visualisation of the nasal pathways up to the level of the vocal cords. An angled rod scope can do the job just well but requires adequate anaesthesia to the oropharynx to prevent gagging (**Figure 4**). These have replaced the traditional indirect laryngoscopy utilising a dental mirror to visualise the laryngopharynx (if the mirror is faced inferiorly, **Figure 5**) or nasopharyngeal structures (if the mirror is faced upwards). A good view of the oral cavity and oropharynx using a headlight and tongue depressor is essential. Fiberoptic endoscopic evaluation of swallowing (FEES) is another option in which a flexible endoscope is inserted through the nose while various liquids and solids are swallowed. With distal chip endoscopy, detailed images are taken of the swallowing process through endoscopic photography. Other options for imaging include swallowing fluoroscopy and

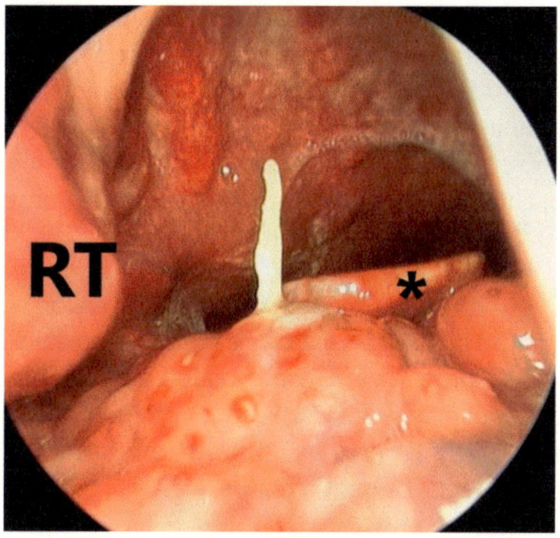


**Figure 4.**
*A 70-degree rod Hopkins scope (indirect laryngoscopy) used to investigate a patient presenting with odynophagia and dysphagia. The culprit was a fishbone (white) at the lingual tonsils. Appreciate the right tonsils (RT) and tip of the epiglottis (*).*

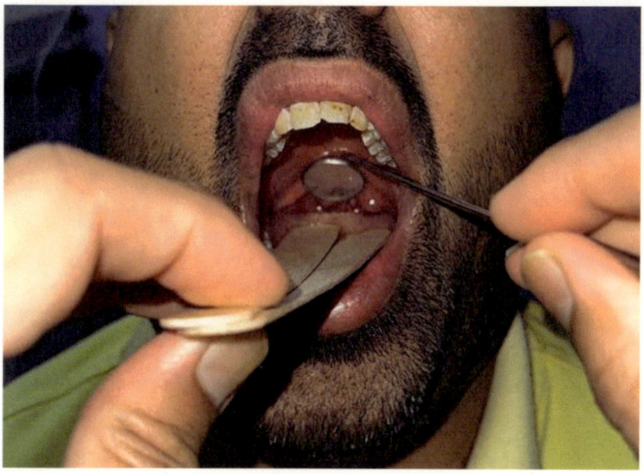

**Figure 5.**
*Indirect laryngoscopy to visualise the laryngopharynx and the larynx in the absence of a scope. Note the mirror is tilted downwards.*

oesophageal manometry. While some of these procedures have possible complications, they are the best form of evaluation for swallowing disorders. Some otorhinolaryngologists have progressed into performing a transnasal esophagoscopy (TNE) under local anaesthesia, which often comes with insufflation required for better visualisation of the oesophageal mucosa.

## 5. Cleft disorders

Cleft disorders are discontinuities of the lips, hard palate, soft palate and alveolar bones, respectively, or in combination. This often occurs during the first trimester of life, between the 4th and 9th weeks of gestation [19]. At times the surface mucosa is well formed while the underlying muscles fail to fuse, resulting in a submucosal cleft [20]. A submucosal cleft has triad characteristics: notching of the posterior bony palate at midline, failure of fusion of soft palate muscle at midline (a palpable defect) and a bifid uvula (visualised defect, **Figure 6**) [10].

There is a stark difference between the anatomy and physiology of a newborn and an adult. In newborns, the oropharyngeal space is yet to be voluntary and remains involuntary [21].

- The larynx and hyoid bone sit at a more superior position compared to an adult. As a result, the epiglottis too sits in a more superior position, almost being in contact with the soft palate. This forms a sealed cuff of soft tissue at the oropharynx, closing the airway from the oral cavity during breathing. Therefore, the laryngopharynx is almost non-existent in an infant, with the larynx being in direct connection to the nasopharynx superiorly.

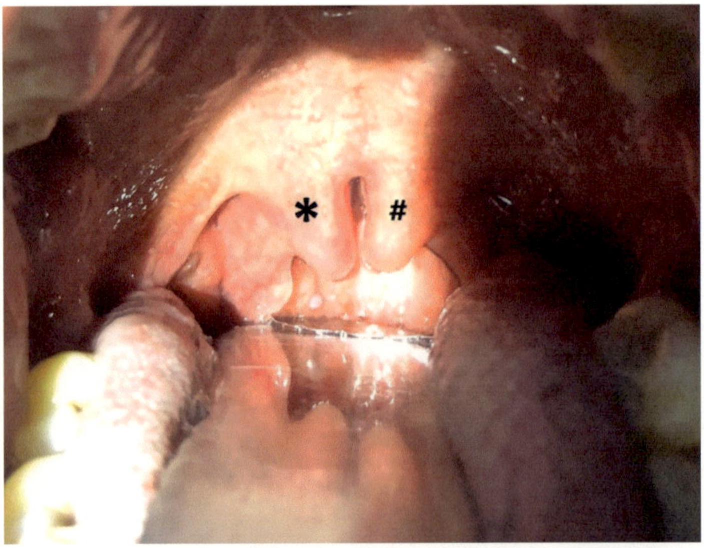


**Figure 6.**
*A patient with a bifid uvula. Note there is a right limb (*) and left limb (#) of the uvula separated at the midline. In the presence of a bifid uvula with a normal appearance of the palate, a submucosal cleft should be suspected and examined for.*

- Not forgetting, newborns lack dentition to help chew and prepare the food bolus for the pharyngeal or oropharyngeal phase of swallowing.
- The hard palate is often flatter, further reducing space within the oral cavity.

In infants, a fine mechanism of control between swallowing and respiration is involuntarily controlled, with precise coordination preventing choking and hypoxia during feeding. In the presence of a cleft palate, fluids and food are diverted into the nasal cavity. When the child inhales, these substances may be directed into the laryngopharynx via abducted vocal cords into the trachea, resulting in penetration and aspiration.

In cleft lip and palate disorders, several of the following mechanisms are impaired.

### 5.1 Suckling

The primitive suckling reflex occurs in children when there is stimulation at the tongue tip or palate, facilitating anterior and posterior movements of the tongue in a horizontal plane. This suckling reflex is true for both liquids and solids and will be replaced by a voluntary suckling after 3–6 months [22].

The presence of a cleft lip and/or palate results in insufficient negative and positive pressure for effective breastfeeding postpartum, required for suckling and nipple compression, respectively [23]. They fail to obtain a good seal with the nipple. Up to 50% of mothers with infants with a cleft lip and/or palate struggle with breastfeeding, and 45% continue with it [24]. Besides, drooling may occur as fluids may easily escape the oral cavity.

### 5.2 Oral preparatory

This phase begins when liquid or solids are being accepted into the oral cavity and consists of mastication, salivation and bolus formation.

Infants with a unilateral or bilateral cleft of the lip may struggle with forming an adequate seal, resulting in not being able to retain food and overflow of oral contents. This may occur when there is an increase in intraoral pressure during chewing. Haque and Alam [25] demonstrated that the most common dental abnormalities were missing teeth, especially of the lateral incisors and the presence of ectopic or supernumerary teeth [26].

Mastication itself is affected by tongue movements, occlusion force, occlusion contact and mandibular movements. Cleft patients may have insufficiency with at least three or four of these factors. In patients with abnormal dentition, the tongue position may be affected during mastication, resulting in lateral overspill of food from the tongue. Thus, this may contribute to premature progression to the oral propulsive phase without adequate chewing to form smaller boluses [25]. Furthermore, larger boluses may delay the oral preparatory phase, requiring more energy for chewing. Absence of detention may also reduce oral proprioception, making it difficult to 'feel' or estimate bolus sizes. Moreover, a palatal defect may reduce the crushing ability of the tongue for solids. The presence of a cleft reduces the tongue's efficiency to push boluses laterally for chewing. Therefore, this affects mastication, or chewing, required for bolus formation. This phase prepares the food to be complete for the pharyngeal phase.

Then, the tongue shall retrieve the chewed food to complete the oral preparatory phase. The tongue tip and its anterior are elevated to be in contact with the alveolar ridge, further depressing the tongue base and allowing contents to slide posteriorly. The elevation of the tongue presses the contents towards the hard palate, forming a glossopalatal sphincter [7]. The connection between the oral cavity and nasal cavity results in nasal regurgitation, thus reducing the volume available for the oral propulsive phase. Insufficient or absent contact between the tongue and hard palate reduces the efficacy of bolus mixing with saliva required for digestion and propulsion [27]. More energy will be required by the child to suckle and feed, resulting in use of accessory respiratory muscles and eventually failure to thrive in severe cases.

### 5.3 Oral propulsive

The propulsive phase pushes the already formed bolus from the oral cavity into the pharyngeal cavity. As in the oral preparatory phase, more of the anterior tongue comes into contact with the hard palate (up to two thirds), therefore pushing the bolus posteriorly. It ends with the jaw being in the inferior position, with its phase ending by retracting the tongue inferiorly and away from the palate [8, 9].

Cleft palate leads to an inadequate volume of bolus for propulsion posteriorly as some would have been lost via nasal regurgitation, an increase in swallowing time affecting the coordination of voluntary and involuntary processes of swallowing and premature propulsion as some content, especially liquid, may disperse faster posteriorly into the pharynx, increasing the risk of aspiration [9, 26].

### 5.4 Pharyngeal

In the pharyngeal phase, a succession of events takes place. Firstly, the tongue moves posteriorly into the pharynx, and the soft palate elevates to propel food posteriorly. The hyoid bone and the larynx elevate with the epiglottis closure and adduction of the vocal cords. Finally, relaxation of the cricopharyngeus, or the upper oesophageal sphincter, allows food to enter the oesophagus [9]. The cricopharyngeus, a circular muscle, when contracts forms the upper oesophageal sphincter.

The soft palate (velum) and its surrounding muscles form the velopharyngeal sphincter. Inadequate closure of the sphincter is termed velopharyngeal insufficiency (VPI) [10]. Ishikki and Beur have discovered that the lateral pharyngeal wall closure plays a significant role in VPI during swallowing [10, 28]. Therefore, in VPI, inadequate closure of the velum and the pharyngeal muscles will fail to isolate the nasopharynx from the oropharynx in activities of swallowing, speech, blowing and breathing [28]. In patients with cleft palate (more so if there is a soft palate cleft), a VPI is bound to occur, resulting in significant nasal regurgitation. Given that the opening of the Eustachian tubes lies at the anterior border of the nasopharynx, there may also be failure of closure of the cartilaginous Eustachian tube during swallowing, resulting in regurgitation of fluids superior laterally into the middle ear via the Eustachian tubes. This renders the Eustachian tubes dysfunctional, predisposing to middle ear effusions and otitis media with effusions [29].

### 5.5 Oesophageal

The oesophageal phase of swallowing is not affected in a cleft lip and/or plate disorder, as it is an involuntary process dependent on the peristaltic mechanisms of the oesophagus.

### 5.6 Complications

The above alterations to swallowing cause a shortened oropharyngeal phase with an increased pharyngeal phase. Therefore, there may be a delayed stimulation of involuntary pharyngeal reflex resulting in residual build-up within the laryngopharynx. In infants, a disruption in the coordination of the suckling, swallowing and breathing cycle increases the risk of penetration and aspiration into the trachea. Vomiting and regurgitation occur independently or in the same instance.

Swallowing disorders do not only consist of issues pertaining to the stages of swallowing but also include aversion to food. Cleft palate and/or lip patients may develop swallowing aversion due to regurgitation from the nose. This may also occur after corrective surgery that may develop into slow eating later in childhood. Parental anxiety occurs early due to poor latching, resulting in unhelpful and negative interactions during mealtime that may manifest as behavioural issues in older ages [30]. Up to 86% of mothers did not attempt breastfeeding in children with cleft lip and/or palate [31].

There are many other sequels of a cleft lip and palate, such as speaking disorders and smell disorders, that will not be discussed within this book.

## 6. Oral cleft swallowing management

The management of a swallowing disorder in a cleft patient is not a one-man show but requires a multidisciplinary team. Identifying and diagnosing an oral cleft during an infant check just after postpartum is crucial. If delivery occurs at home, the infant check should be done by the midwife or community nurse. Different nations have different protocols pertaining to newborn assessments.

### 6.1 Feeding

Early assessment of feeding is required, preferably by the speech and swallowing therapist. In cases of an isolated cleft lip, quite often suckling is not affected, as the infant shall still be able to form a good seal around the nipple and breast with adequate compression. This may also hold true for unilateral lip clefts extending posteriorly to the maxillary alveolar. In cases of palatal clefts in isolation or in combination with the lip, feeding aids will be required.

A feeding bottle with an orthodontic teat is preferred. One with an opening at the bottom of the teat instead of the end is preferred, allowing milk to flow onto the tongue instead of the palatal surface. The bottle teat should be made of a soft material (often silicon), allowing some moulding and avoiding trauma to the palatal perforation and negative pressure during suckling. There are various products with a plethora of teat material, shape and sizes available.

Positioning during feeds is valuable supplementary assistance. Positioning the infant upright (at least 60 degrees) helps with milk flow from gravity and reduces nasal and Eustachian tube regurgitation. Advocates of a chin stabiliser recommend placing the forefinger in the midline of the chin between the lips and lower mandible and the middle finger beneath the chin for jaw control and better swallowing [31].

Pacing of feeds with pauses helps in allowing the return of normal respiratory rhythm and preventing aspiration [31].

Having a more viscous feed has been shown to increase pharyngeal time, allowing more time for airway protection to occur. Besides, the authors are of the opinion that a more viscous feed should reduce nasal regurgitation. However, this still remains anecdotal in value [31].

## 7. Surgery to the lip and palate

Raghavan et al. [32] described three essential procedures for an average cleft lip and palate repair: lip repair (cheiloplasty), palatoplasty and alveolar bone grafting. Other procedures may ensue depending on complexity and outcomes. They are rhinoplasty, maxillary expansion surgery, revision of lip repair, revision palatoplasty and VPI corrections.

Wilhelmsen et al. in 1966 introduced the "rule of tens", which was taken as a staple practice globally. A lip repair can be done at 10 weeks of life with haemoglobin levels of 10 gm% or more, weighing 10 pounds (4.5 kg), and a total leucocyte count of 10,000 cells/cc [33, 34]. With the advancement of medical care and technology, many have done away with the rule of tens with the exception of body weight [33, 34]. In Malaysia, lip repair is often performed between 3 and 6 months and palate repair between 9 and 18 months [35]. However, many have advocated an early lip repair (as early as the first week of life) and palate repair with good outcomes. Palatoplasty in itself may cause intermittent swallowing disturbance post-procedure due to pain. Enhanced Recovery After Surgery (ERAS) protocol for better optimisation of pain control reduces morphine prescription with reduced hospital revisits for pain management [36].

A study performed at a tertiary hospital in Malaysia revealed that conductive hearing loss improved among cleft lip and palate patients if corrective surgery was performed before the age of one. Twenty-five percent (37 of 148 ears) had mild conductive hearing loss post cleft correction [29].

Long-term follow-up of post-procedure is recommended for continuity of care and to intervene when outcomes deviate away from intended results [32].

### 7.1 Prosthesis

Obturators are measured to make devices (often from acrylic raisins) that are placed in the hard palate to create a separation between the nasal and oral cavity [31]. They often help with preventing regurgitation of oral foods (**Figure 7**). However, its use in infants is scarce, as it requires re-adjustments and re-making in accordance with growth, which may be an expensive ordeal. Most infants would have had a lip and/or palatal repair by then. However, it is popular among adults with a persistent palatal defect either from a failed surgery, incomplete surgical correction, or did not seek/refuse surgical correction. Some complain of small amounts of fluid regurgitation into the nasal cavity despite using obturators. In adults or older children, the obturator can be attached to the available dentition for better support. The authors prefer obturators in palatal defects post surgery for tumour clearance if a reconstruction with a flap is not possible or viable.

### 7.2 Others

Orthodontic treatment is essential to ensure proper alignment of dentition. A paediatric dentist or maxillofacial surgeon performs maxillary or mandibular correction surgery if needed. Speech and swallowing therapy is advocated even after corrective surgery.

A multidisciplinary team delivery of healthcare is ideally performed within a single centre. **Table 2** summarises the role of various disciplines within the care

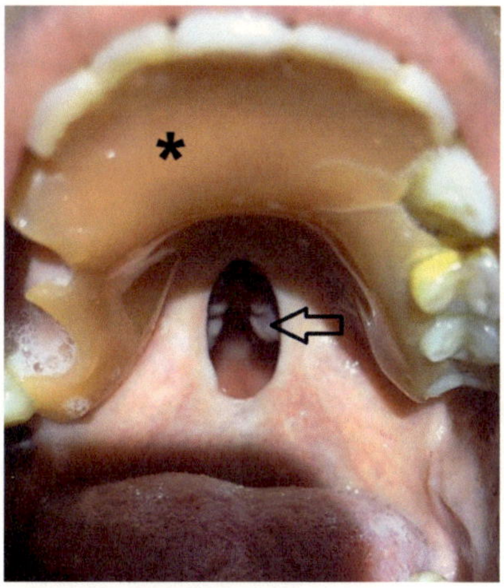

**Figure 7.**
*An intraoral image of an adult patient with a cleft lip and palate. Lip repair was successful, but the patient refused palatal cleft repair. The posterior nasal cavity can be appreciated. The posterior segment of the inferior turbinates (arrow) is seen with a void of a nasal septum. The patient is wearing a denture (*) to compensate for her missing incisors in the upper jaw. She was not able to tolerate a palatal obturator.*

| Discipline | Role | Intervention |
|---|---|---|
| Otorhinolaryngologist | Assess severity of cleft lip and/or palate<br>otology assessment<br>rhinology assessment<br>OSA assessment | Early (neonate)<br>Follow-up |
| Neonatologist/paediatrician | Assess severity of cleft lip and/or palate<br>assess for the presence of any syndrome<br>assess for other developmental disorders | Early (neonate)<br>Early (neonate)<br>1 year onwards |
| Speech & language therapist | Assess feeding and swallowing<br>assess and stimulate speech | Early (neonate)<br>1 year and after |
| Paediatric nurses/community nurses/ occupational therapists | Identification of clefts within the community<br>assess feeding<br>counselling regarding feeding techniques<br>counselling on feeding aids<br>coordinates appointments<br>counselling parents to manage anxiety/uncertainties | Early (neonate) |
| Paediatric dental specialist | General health of teeth<br>palatal extensions for early malocclusions | After 6 months |
| Oral maxillofacial surgeons | Lip and palate repair<br>orthognathic corrective surgery | 1 month onwards |
| Plastic surgeon | Repair of lip<br>repair of nasal aesthetics (rhinoplasty) | 1 month onwards<br>teenagehood |
| Parents | Promote feeding<br>stimulate speech (including articulation) | Early (neonate) |
| Audiologist | Perform early hearing assessment in the form of brainstem evoked response to determine type and severity of hearing loss | Early (neonate)<br>follow-up |
| Orthodontists | Correction of malalignment and dental prosthetics | 6 years onwards |

**Table 2.**
*The various disciplines involved in a cleft patient and their respective roles with intervention within the cleft care pathway.*

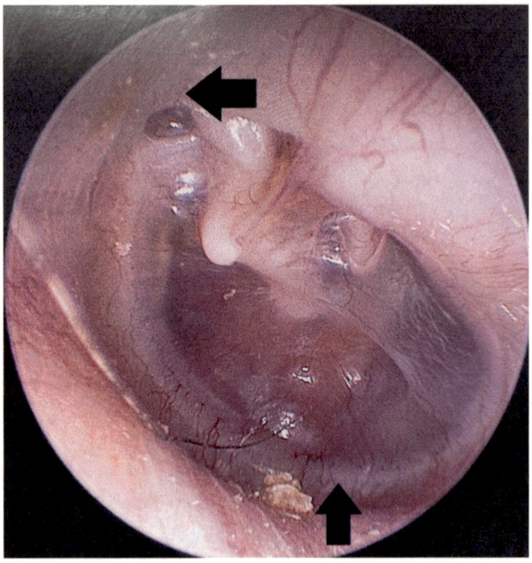

**Figure 8.**
*An adult cleft patient with a retracted tympanic membrane. Although there has not been any fluid behind the tympanic membrane post correction of lip and palate, the patient still suffers from Eustachian tube dysfunction. This is evident by the prominent annulus (lower arrow) and the retracted attic (top arrow). The lateral process of the malleus is prominent too; appreciate the tympanic membrane almost being plastered to the promontory posterior to it.*

team for cleft patients. However, it is not exhaustive, and many roles can be played by other specialities; not all healthcare institutions will have the availability of all disciplines. At the author's centre, a cleft clinic allows for all, if not most, disciplines to meet together and discuss potential issues related to the cleft patient; have a shared goal and expectations via a treatment plan; and reduce the complexity of multiple appointments with different disciplines.

In a patient with a palatal cleft, the tensor veli palatini does not attach to the posterior segment of the hard palate [37]. Instead, it is attached to the free border of the cleft, resulting in significant pneumatic consequences to the Eustachian tube. Often, there is poor control of Eustachian tube dilation during swallowing and yawning. As a result, the cartilaginous part of the Eustachian tube fails to open, preventing secretions from the respiratory epithelium within the middle ear from draining. A middle ear effusion of glue ear develops, contributing to hearing loss (**Figure 8**). Palatal repair may not improve Eustachian tube opening; hence, a follow-up with the ENT or audiologist is pertinent to detect a middle ear effusion, conductive hearing loss and plan for an appropriate intervention. A myringotomy and grommet can be performed for middle ear ventilation. Furthermore, constant reflux of food may cause chronic irritation to the Eustachian tube opening, resulting in hypertrophy of its orifice and obstruction. Gases can be absorbed by the middle ear mucosa, resulting in a negative pressure, further retracting the tympanic membrane more medially [37]. This is known as a retracted tympanic membrane.

## 8. Conclusion

A cleft lip and palate is a common craniofacial abnormality that disrupts three out of the four swallowing mechanisms (oral preparatory, oral propulsion and pharyngeal phase), resulting in nasal regurgitation and an altered suck-swallow-breathe mechanism, which may result in aspiration and failure to thrive. A tailored approach by a multidisciplinary team with timely feeding intervention, lip and palate correction and post-procedural dental and swallowing assessment is required to optimise swallowing and reduce its associated dysfunctions.

## Author details

Hardip Singh Gendeh[1,2*], Ronik Kothari[1,3] and Mawaddah Azman[1]

1 Department of Otorhinolaryngology, Head and Neck Surgery, Faculty of Medicine, Universiti Kebangsaan Malaysia, Kuala Lumpur, Malaysia

2 Allergy Unit, Otorhinolaryngology Clinic, Hospital Canselor Tuanku Muhriz, Kuala Lumpur, Malaysia

3 California University of Science and Medicine, Colton, California, United States

*Address all correspondence to: hardip88@gmail.com

## References

[1] Cook IJ. Oropharyngeal dysphagia. Gastroenterology Clinics of North America. 2009;**38**(3):411-431

[2] Vanderas AP. Incidence of cleft lip, cleft palate, and cleft lip and palate among races: A review. PubMed. 1987;**24**(3):216-225

[3] Murray J. Gene/environment causes of cleft lip and/or palate. Clinical Genetics. 2002;**61**(4):248-256

[4] Gendeh HS. A rare oro-maxillo-ocular facial cleft. Journal of Surgical Academia. 2016;**6**(2):55-55

[5] Basit H, Eovaldi BJ, Siccardi MA. Anatomy, Head and Neck, Mastication Muscles [Internet]. PubMed. Treasure Island (FL): StatPearls Publishing; 2020. Available from: https://www.ncbi.nlm.nih.gov/books/NBK541027/

[6] Breslin PAS, Peyrot des Gachons C. Salivary amylase: Digestion and metabolic syndrome. Current Diabetes Reports. 2016;**16**(10):102

[7] Shaw SM, Martino R. The normal swallow: Muscular and neurophysiological control. Otolaryngologic Clinics of North America [Internet]. 2013;**46**(6):937-956. Available from: https://pubmed.ncbi.nlm.nih.gov/24262952/

[8] Dodds WJ, Stewart ET, Logemann JA. Physiology and radiology of the normal oral and pharyngeal phases of swallowing. American Journal of Roentgenology. 1990;**154**(5):953-963

[9] Palmer JB, Drennan JC, Baba M. Evaluation and treatment of swallowing impairments. American Family Physician [Internet]. 2000;**61**(8):2453-2462. Available from: https://pubmed.ncbi.nlm.nih.gov/10794585/

[10] Hirschberg J. Velopharyngeal insufficiency. Folia Phoniatrica et Logopaedica. 1986;**38**(2-4):221-276

[11] Sanivarapu RR, Gibson J, Vaqar S. Aspiration Pneumonia [Internet]. National Library of Medicine. StatPearls Publishing; 2023. Available from: https://www.ncbi.nlm.nih.gov/books/NBK470459/

[12] Wilkinson JM, Codipilly DC, Wilfahrt RP. Dysphagia: Evaluation and collaborative management. American Family Physician [Internet]. 2021;**103**(2):97-106. Available from: https://pubmed.ncbi.nlm.nih.gov/33448766/

[13] Crary M, Sura L, Madhavan A, Carnaby-Mann G. Dysphagia in the elderly: Management and nutritional considerations. Clinical Interventions in Aging [Internet]. 2012;**7**(1):287. Available from: https://www.ncbi.nlm.nih.gov/pmc/articles/PMC3426263/

[14] Zautner AE. Adenotonsillar disease. Recent Patents on Inflammation & Allergy Drug Discovery [Internet]. 2012;**6**(2):121-129. Available from: https://pubmed.ncbi.nlm.nih.gov/22452646/ [Accessed: 3 January 2022]

[15] Watted A, Watted N, Abu-Hussein M, Muhamad AH. Multidisciplinary treatment in cleft lip and palate patients. International Journal of Dental Research and Oral Health [Internet]. 2020. Available from: https://unisciencepub.com/wp-content/uploads/2020/07/Multidisciplinary-Treatment-in-Cleft-Lip-and-Palate-Patients.pdf

[16] Lakshmipathy D, Allibone M, Rajasekaran K. Dysphagia in head and neck cancer. Otolaryngologic Clinics of North America. 2024;**57**(4):635-647

[17] Strojan P, Hutcheson KA, Eisbruch A, Beitler JJ, Langendijk JA, Lee AWM, et al. Treatment of late sequelae after radiotherapy for head and neck cancer. Cancer Treatment Reviews. 2017;**59**(4):79-92

[18] El Halabi M, Arwani R, Parkman HP. Dysphagia in neurological disorders. Seminars in Neurology. 2023;**43**(04):530-539

[19] Mitic V, Jonovic M, Mitic N, Mitic A, Mitic D, Stojanovic M, et al. Incidence of lip and palate clefts in children in Niš from 1990 to 2007. Srpski Arhiv za Celokupno Lekarstvo. 2011;**139**(5-6):298-303

[20] McMurray JS, Hoffman MR, Braden MN, editors. Multidisciplinary Management of Pediatric Voice and Swallowing Disorders. Cham: Springer International Publishing; 2020

[21] Matsuo K, Palmer JB. Anatomy and physiology of feeding and swallowing: Normal and abnormal. Physical Medicine and Rehabilitation Clinics of North America [Internet]. 2008;**19**(4):691-707. Available from: https://www.ncbi.nlm.nih.gov/pmc/articles/PMC2597750/

[22] Dodrill P. Feeding problems and oropharyngeal dysphagia in children. Journal of Gastroenterology and Hepatology Research [Internet]. 2014. Available from: https://www.semanticscholar.org/paper/Feeding-Problems-and-Oropharyngeal-Dysphagia-in-Dodrill/626bb4b1dc41ce735b0535ab509946405a6df2c7

[23] Masarei AG, Sell D, Habel A, Mars M, Sommerlad BC, Wade A. The nature of feeding in infants with unrepaired cleft lip and/or palate compared with healthy noncleft infants. The Cleft Palate-Craniofacial Journal. 2007;**44**(3):321-328

[24] Eltayeb A, Satti A, Elhadi BH. Mothers' struggle and knowledge towards feeding a child with a cleft lip and palate. Acta Scientific Dental Scienecs. 2022;**6**(1):61-67

[25] Haque S, Alam MK. Common dental anomalies in cleft lip and palate patients. The Malaysian Journal of Medical Sciences: MJMS [Internet]. 2015;**22**(2):55. Available from: https://pmc.ncbi.nlm.nih.gov/articles/PMC4438093/

[26] Todorović J, Zelić M, Jerkić L. Eating and swallowing disorders in children with cleft lip and/or palate. Acta Facultatis Medicae Naissensis [Internet]. 2022;**39**(1):5-13. Available from: https://publisher.medfak.ni.ac.rs/AFMN_1/2022/1-2022/full%20text/1Eating%20and%20Swallowing%20J.Todorovic.pdf

[27] Matsuo K, Palmer JB. Oral phase preparation and propulsion: Anatomy, physiology, rheology, mastication, and transport. Principles of Deglutition [Internet]. 2012:117-131. Available from: https://link.springer.com/chapter/10.1007%2F978-1-4614-3794-9_8

[28] Isshiki N, Honjow I, Morimoto M. Cineradiographic analysis of movement of the lateral pharyngeal wall. Plastic and Reconstructive Surgery [Internet]. 1969;**44**(4):357-363. Available from: https://pubmed.ncbi.nlm.nih.gov/5809005/

[29] Goh BS, Tang CL, Hashim ND, Annamalay T, Abd Rahman FN. Hearing status and behavioural patterns among school aged children with cleft lip and/or

palate. International Journal of Pediatric Otorhinolaryngology. 2019;**118**:1-5

[30] Hasanpour M, Ghazavi Z, Keshavarz S. Feeding behavioral assessment in children with cleft lip and/or palate and parental responses to behavior problems. Iranian Journal of Nursing and Midwifery Research [Internet]. 2017;**22**(2):135-139. Available from: https://www.ncbi.nlm.nih.gov/pmc/articles/PMC5442995/

[31] Miller C. Feeding issues and interventions in infants and children with clefts and craniofacial syndromes. Seminars in Speech and Language. 2011;**32**(02):115-126

[32] Raghavan U, Rao D, Ullas G, Vijayadev V. Postoperative management of cleft lip and palate surgery. Facial Plastic Surgery. 2018;**34**(06):605-611

[33] Wilhelmsen HR, Musgrave RH. Complications of cleft lip surgery. The Cleft Palate Journal [Internet]. 1966;**3**:223-231. Available from: https://pubmed.ncbi.nlm.nih.gov/5220833/

[34] Pendem S, Chandra RB, Selvarasu K, Krishnan M, Muthusekhar MR, Preethi J. Analysis of different facets of the rule of 10 for cleft lip repair for their application in the current era. Curēus [Internet]. 2024. Available from: https://www.ncbi.nlm.nih.gov/pmc/articles/PMC10924625/ [Accessed: 13 April 2024]

[35] CLAPAM. Cleft Management Protocol|Cleft Lip & Palate Association Malaysia [Internet]. Available from: https://clapam.org.my/; https://clapam.org.my/cleft-management-protocol/

[36] Moffitt JK, Cepeda A, Ekeoduru RA, Teichgraeber JF, Nguyen PD, Greives MR. Enhanced recovery after surgery protocol for primary cleft palate repair: Improving transition of care. Journal of Craniofacial Surgery. 2020;**32**(1):e72-e76

[37] Sharma RK, Nanda V. Problems of middle ear and hearing in cleft children. Indian Journal of Plastic Surgery: Official Publication of the Association of Plastic Surgeons of India [Internet]. 2009;**42**(Suppl):S144-S148. Available from: https://www.ncbi.nlm.nih.gov/pmc/articles/PMC2825075/

Chapter 7

# Swallowing Disorders and Eustachian Tube Dysfunction: A Multidisciplinary Perspective

*Hee-Young Kim*


## Abstract

This chapter examines the complex link between swallowing disorders and Eustachian tube dysfunction, highlighting their impact on health and quality of life. It explores the connections between swallowing disorders, Eustachian tube dysfunction, and gastrointestinal disorders such as gastroesophageal reflux disease, laryngopharyngeal reflux disease, and nasopharyngeal reflux. Evidence from both past and present studies suggests that gastrointestinal disorders and Eustachian tube dysfunction affect each other bidirectionally. The chapter emphasizes the role of modern diagnostic tools in improving patient monitoring and demonstrates how a multidisciplinary approach encompassing various medical fields enhances patient outcomes.


**Keywords:** swallowing disorders (SD), Eustachian tube dysfunction (ETD), gastroesophageal reflux disease (GERD), laryngopharyngeal reflux disease (LPRD), nasopharyngeal reflux (NPR)

## 1. Introduction

The objectives of this chapter are to provide comprehensive assessments and integrated treatment options for patients with swallowing disorders (SD) and Eustachian tube dysfunction (ETD). Achieving these objectives requires collaboration among a diverse team of specialists, including otolaryngologists, gastroenterologists, neurologists, speech-language pathologists, audiologists, neuro-vestibular specialists, pulmonologists, cardiologists, ophthalmologists, dietitians/nutritionists, physical therapists, occupational therapists, and psychologists. By working together, these professionals can ensure a holistic and multidisciplinary approach (MDA), ultimately improving patient outcomes and quality of life. This MDA addresses all aspects of ETD and SD, resulting in improved patient outcomes and quality of life [1, 2].

The association between ETD and SD has significant impacts on health and quality of life. This chapter is about how they affect each other, the importance of an MDA, and how diagnostic and therapeutic methods have improved. It also discusses over the anatomy, physiology, and various diagnosis and treatment options for SD and ETD [1–6].

The Eustachian tube (ET) links the middle ear (ME) to the nasopharynx and controls middle ear pressure (MEP) and drainage. SD or dysphagia can make it hard for auditory function. Proper ET function is essential for ear health and hearing, and normal MEP is 0 daPa in both ears [3, 7]. Swallowing activates the throat and soft palate muscles, which influences ET opening and closure. SD can affect MEP, resulting in problems such as barotrauma, otitis media (OM), and chronic ETD. ETD can worsen gastrointestinal (GI) disorders like gastroesophageal reflux disease (GERD), laryngopharyngeal reflux disease (LPRD), and nasopharyngeal reflux (NPR) by disrupting pressure equilibrium, inducing inflammation in the tissues surrounding the ET, and weakening swallowing muscles. Understanding these relationships is crucial for making appropriate diagnosis and treatment [1, 7–10].

## 2. Overview of swallowing disorders (SD)

### 2.1 Anatomy and physiology of swallowing

Swallowing, or deglutition, has two stages: oropharyngeal and esophageal, with muscles regulating ET function [1]. Problems in these stages can affect ET function, leading to ear problems. The Tensor Veli Palatini muscle (mTVP) and Levator Veli Palatini muscle (mLVP) are essential for the key roles in ET function by opening the ET during swallowing, yawning, sneezing, and chewing (**Figure 1**) [11]. This balance is crucial for MEP balance and proper drainage [1–6]. Swallowing involves both voluntary and involuntary brain activities. The cerebral cortex initiates voluntary actions, while the brainstem's swallowing center coordinates involuntary actions. The cranial nerves, specifically the trigeminal (V), facial (VII), glossopharyngeal (IX),

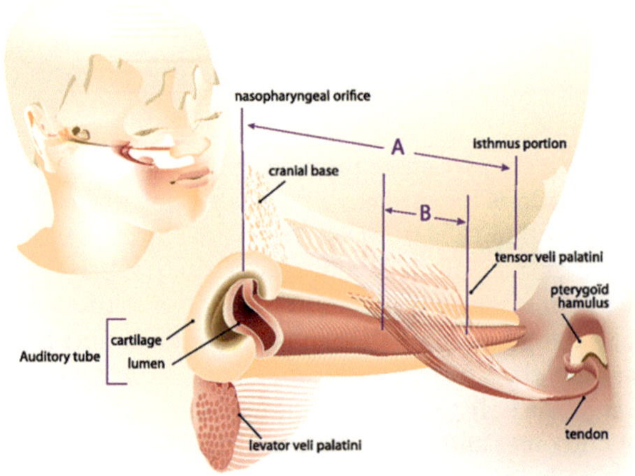


**Figure 1.**
*The tensor veli palatini muscle begins at the cranial base and the lateral side of the auditory tube (Eustachian tube). This figure illustrates the origin of the tensor veli palatini muscle at the cartilaginous and membranous sections of the lateral auditory tube. Before it enters the soft palate, the muscle's tendon wraps around the pterygoid hamulus. Insertion ratio: The insertion ratio is determined by dividing the length of the Eustachian tube cartilage engaged by the tensor veli palatini muscle at the auditory tube (line B) by the total length of the Eustachian tube (line A); this measurement spans from the nasopharyngeal end to the isthmus portion [11] (Figure adapted from the cited study).*

vagus (X), and hypoglossal (XII), play a vital role in delivering signals that regulate the muscles responsible for swallowing [1–5].

### 2.2 Classification of swallowing disorders (SD)

Dysphagia or SD can occur in the oropharyngeal or esophageal stages, or both, because of various factors impacting ear, nose, and throat functions [1]:

#### *2.2.1 Oropharyngeal dysphagia*

Characterized by difficulty initiating swallowing, which can often be triggered by neurological problems (such as stroke or Parkinson's disease), muscular abnormalities, structural concerns, or head and neck tumors. Symptoms include coughing, choking, regurgitation, and the sensation of food stuck in the throat [1].

#### *2.2.2 Esophageal dysphagia*

Defined by the sensation of food sticking in the chest or throat during swallowing. It can be caused by structural anomalies, muscle dysfunction, or disorders such as GERD, LPRD, NPR, and esophageal cancer. Symptoms include regurgitation, chest pain, and difficulty swallowing [1].

### 2.3 Pathophysiological mechanisms: reciprocal relationship

#### *2.3.1 Impact of SD on ET function*

SD can have a considerable impact on ET function due to anatomical and physiological connections to the ME. Impaired swallowing mechanics can produce active muscular ETD (ETD-M), in which the mTVP and mLVP do not operate efficiently, altering nasopharyngeal pressure dynamics and leading to ETD and negative MEP. This negative MEP draws pathogens into the ET and ME, causing inflammatory ETD (ETD-I) and diseases such as OM which may include persistent tympanic membrane (TM) retraction and conductive hearing loss. Proper MEP maintenance is required to avoid ETD-I and OM [6].

#### *2.3.2 Impact of ETD on swallowing function*

The mechanism for SD due to ETD can occur through two pathways:

*Indirect pathway*. ETD can lead to GI disorders [7–10]. GERD, LPRD, and NPR can result in upper esophageal sphincter, laryngeal spasm, and inflammation as well as ETD-I, indirectly causing and exacerbating SD [1].

*Direct pathway*. ETD-M involves muscle disorders around the ET that directly affect swallowing mechanics. Dysfunctional muscles that control the ET, such as the mTVP and mLVP, can disrupt the normal coordination required for swallowing, leading directly to SD [6].

### 2.4 Clinical identification and individual variability

Patients with SD often experience dysphagia or difficulty swallowing, odynophagia or painful swallowing, throat discomfort, sore throat, and a globus sensation or a subjective sensation of a lump or having something stuck in the throat. The variability in symptom perception and expression complicates diagnosis and understanding. Individual differences, linguistic backgrounds, and physical sensations during swallowing necessitate a comprehensive evaluation for accurate diagnosis and treatment [1, 7].

## 3. Overview of Eustachian tube dysfunction (ETD)

### 3.1 ETD: causes, symptoms, and hearing impact

ETD, which can be caused by allergies, colds, sinus infections, anatomical abnormalities, and reflux disorders such as GERD, LPRD, and NPR, has an impact on the ET's ability to balance MEP and discharge ME secretions [2–6]. Symptoms include ear fullness, muffled hearing, popping sounds, itching, discomfort, pain, vertigo, and tinnitus among others. Persistent ETD can cause negative MEP, fluid buildup, and hearing loss, affecting daily activities and quality of life. Uneven MEP causes vertigo and damages the vestibular system [2–10, 12–15]. According to preliminary findings, ETD is a spectrum of disorders with unique pathophysiology [12]. Dr. Hee-Young Kim created novel Patient-Reported Outcome Measures (PROMs) for ETD and proposed using MEP as a surrogate biomarker to increase diagnostic accuracy [7, 13].

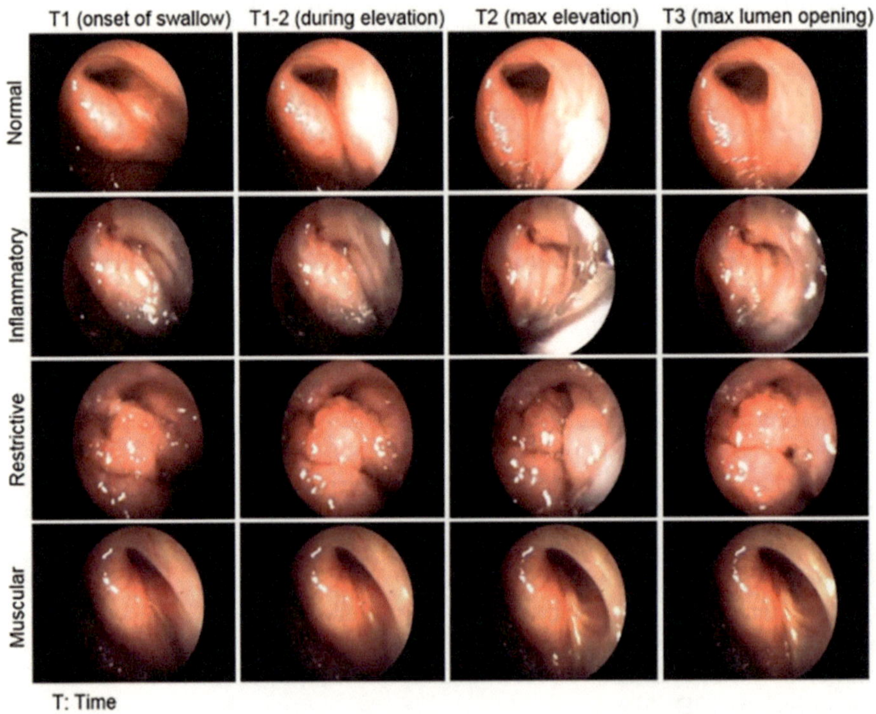


**Figure 2.**
*The appearance of the left Eustachian tube (ET) nasopharyngeal orifice in four different patients, each representing a different endotype: normal ET function, inflammatory ET dysfunction (ETD-I), restrictive ETD (ETD-R), and muscular ETD (ETD-M). These endotypes are shown at various stages of swallowing: soft palate position at rest or onset of swallowing (T1), during the elevation of the soft palate (T1-2), at the peak of elevation (T2), and at the point of maximum lumen ET opening (T3) [6] (Figure adapted from the cited study).*

### 3.2 Endotypes of Eustachian tube dysfunction (ETD)

Understanding the various endotypes of ETD is crucial for accurate diagnosis and treatment (**Figure 2**) [6]:

*Normal Eustachian tube function (ETF-N).* Healthy ME, no significant OM history, clear ME, a neutral TM, and a Type A tympanogram [6]. A tympanogram detects changes in TM movement in response to air pressure. A Type A tympanogram, with a sharp peak within normal limits (WNL) around 0 daPa, indicates normal MEP and TM mobility. Other types include Type Ad (high TM compliance), Type As (reduced TM compliance), and Type C (negative MEP), aiding in diagnosing various ME conditions and ETD [3].

*Patulous ETD (ETD-P):* Constantly open ET, leading to autophony (hearing one's own voice and breathing loudly), low or near-zero opening pressure, steady resistance [6].

*Semi-Patulous ETD (ETD-SP).* Intermittent ET patency, symptoms like ETD-P, occurring occasionally [6].

*Stricture ETD (ETD-S).* Structural abnormalities causing difficulty opening ET, leading to chronic/recurrent OM, high opening pressure, and low pressure equilibration [6].

*Active muscular ETD (ETD-M).* Poor muscle function to open ET, normal passive properties but poor pressure equilibration [6].

*Restrictive ETD (ETD-R).* Lymphoid/adenoid tissue impingement on ET orifice, restricting function [6].

*Inflammatory ETD (ETD-I).* Chronic inflammation from nasal allergies, chronic rhinosinusitis, or GERD, like ETD-S, identified by endoscopic inflammation evidence [6].

*Adhesive ETD (ETD-A).* Difficulty separating ET lumen surfaces due to lack of surfactants/molecular bonds between mucous layers, high opening pressure, and low steady resistance [6].

SD are linked to various ETD endotypes, affecting ET function and patency through muscular and structural impediments. SD often link to ETD endotypes involving muscular function and structural impediment [6].

### 3.3 Diagnostic and therapeutic techniques

A Type A tympanogram typically indicates normal MEP and ET function, but may not necessarily rule out ETD, especially in patients experiencing vertigo [7, 15, 16]. Normal MEP is defined as 0 daPa in both ears [3, 7, 13, 16]. Comprehensive assessment, including Patient-Reported Outcome Measures and additional diagnostic testing, is crucial. Otolaryngologists may miss diagnoses like alternobaric vertigo (AV) and ground-level alternobaric vertigo (GLAV) [6], if relying solely on the term WNL as normal tympanometry readings can still present symptoms, indicating that WNL is not always sufficient [16].

Furthermore, understanding the impact of factors like asymmetric MEP at the same altitude can be critical in diagnosing conditions such as AV and GLAV. In AV, on ascent or descent, the normal tube will not spontaneously, passively open—without the need to swallow and actively dilate the tube—to equalize the relative positive or negative pressure that develops in the ME as the ambient pressure becomes negative or positive. In GLAV, the patients cannot equalize the MEP, even if they attempt to swallow and actively dilate the tube at ground level. Diagnosing such disorders requires careful patient history, symptom correlation, and potentially extra testing beyond standard tympanometry [3, 7–10, 12–15].

The Toynbee phenomenon, reported by Charles Bluestone, describes how nasal or postnasal obstruction impacts the ET during swallowing, exacerbating ETD symptoms such as vertigo. "Sniffing" can increase ETD symptoms by causing negative nasopharyngeal pressure, which impairs ET function [3, 13, 14]. The Toynbee Maneuver involves swallowing while holding both nostrils closed to open the ET and equalize MEP, while the Toynbee Test analyzes MEP changes and assesses ET function [3]. Toynbee maneuvers and tests provide critical information, but they should be performed cautiously, as incorrect performance might exacerbate symptoms no less than the Valsalva maneuver, particularly in severe ETD cases [10]. Individual responses can vary, reflecting the intricacies of ETD and related conditions such as GERD, LPRD, and NPR [17–20].

In addition to non-invasive procedures such as the Toynbee Test, ETC is often employed for both diagnostic and therapeutic techniques [3, 7, 9, 10, 15, 21].

### 3.4 Eustachian tube catheterization (ETC) and traditional treatment

ETC is a traditional treatment involving the insertion of a catheter into the ET to diagnose and treat obstructions or dysfunctions [12]. ETC measures ET patency and functionality, which is critical for recognizing and managing ETD. It aids in the diagnosis of mechanical obstructions and provides therapeutic benefits such as regulating MEP, restoring ambient MEP, reducing ME inflammation, cleaning effusions, and enhancing hearing. Proper ETC technique is essential for accurate diagnosis, effective treatment, and avoiding complications [3, 7–10, 12, 13, 15, 21–24].

Research on ET function in individuals with ventilation tubes shows mixed results. These therapies can have an impact on ET mechanics and SD, enabling for more accurate diagnosis and treatment planning with improved diagnostic methods such as videoendoscopy and sonotubometry [6]. While some research indicates possible benefits, others contend that ventilation tubes may not significantly improve ET function [14]. In my experience, I concur with the viewpoint of the limited effectiveness of ventilation tubes; the benefits of ventilation tubes may be short-lived as they often self-dislodge after several months.

## 4. Reflux-related conditions

### 4.1 Definitions and symptoms of GERD, LPRD, and NPR

GERD, LPRD, and NPR involve reflux affecting the esophagus, hypopharynx, and nasopharynx, respectively:

*Gastroesophageal reflux disease (GERD).* A digestive disorder in which stomach contents often backflow into the esophagus, resulting in heartburn, regurgitation, and esophageal irritation, usually linked with lower esophageal sphincter dysfunction [17, 18].

*Laryngopharyngeal reflux disease (LPRD).* Gastric contents backflow into the hypopharynx and larynx; unlike GERD, it often lacks classic heartburn and is characterized by throat and voice symptoms such as chronic cough, hoarseness, and throat clearing, indicating upper esophageal sphincter [17, 19].

*NPR (nasopharyngeal reflux).* Involves the retrograde flow of gastric contents into the nasopharynx, affecting the upper airway and leading to various upper respiratory and otolaryngologic symptoms [20].

### 4.2 Mechanisms by which GERD and LPRD influence ET function

Reflux can irritate and inflame the ET, disrupting its function and leading to conditions like reflux otitis media (ROM). The mechanisms include:

*Acidic irritation.* Acid reflux into the nasopharynx can inflame tissues around the ET, causing swelling and dysfunction [17–20].

*Neural reflexes.* GERD and LPRD can induce reflexive throat clearing and coughing, disrupting normal ET function [17–20].

*Inflammatory response.* Gastric contents in the upper aerodigestive tract increase inflammatory mediators, exacerbating ET inflammation and resulting in dysfunctions such as barotrauma or otitis media with effusion [17–20].

### 4.3 Reflux otitis media (ROM)

ROM is a ME disease in which nasopharyngeal secretions, including nasal mucoid, refluxed gastric contents, environmental allergens, respiratory pathogens, and other irritants, flow backward into the ME through the ET. Forceful nasal douching may contribute to ROM as well. This leads to inflammation, effusion, and infection in the ME, impairing its function. The ET typically balances air pressure across the eardrum and drains ME secretions, but in ROM, it allows reverse flow, introducing acidic gastric contents and causing irritation [3]. Additionally, the presence of these various secretions and irritants further exacerbates the inflammatory response and effusion within the ME.

Symptoms of ROM include ear pain, pressure, hearing loss, throat discomfort, or a feeling of fullness in the ear, especially after lying down following eating. Treatment involves addressing the underlying reflux with proton pump inhibitors or antacids, improving ET function, and reducing ME inflammation with ETC, steroids, or myringotomy with tympanostomy tubes in severe cases. Understanding NPR and its impact on ROM enables tailored diagnosis and treatment, leading to better patient outcomes [7].

## 5. Historical perspectives: James Yearsley and Peter Allen

### 5.1 Historical perspectives and James Yearsley

James Yearsley (1805–1869) was a pioneering British otolaryngologist and a significant figure in nineteenth-century medicine. He is renowned for his extensive research on the correlation between the condition of the throat and ears. His contributions established the fundamental basis for the contemporary comprehension and treatment of otological disorders. In 1847, Yearsley authored a book titled "Deafness Practically Illustrated," which thoroughly explores the symptoms, origins, and treatments of ear disorders. His insights into the interconnectedness of ENT functions are integral to contemporary MDA in diagnosis and treatment for ENT conditions [22].

#### *5.1.1 Contributions for SD*

Yearsley was also a pioneer in identifying the crucial role that swallowing mechanics play in ear, nose, and throat health. He observed the point, "In those cases where the enlarged glands have an extended base reaching from the vicinity of the

Eustachian tubes to the bottom of the pharynx, and such cases I have frequently seen, we may look for defective speech, hearing, swallowing, and breathing altogether associated, more particularly if the uvula enters into the diseased condition of the parts." This discovery highlighted the multifunctional importance of pharyngeal health, showing how oversized adenoids can simultaneously impact speech, hearing, swallowing, and breathing [22]. Recent studies demonstrated that adenoid tissue could obstruct the ET orifice, both statically and dynamically, impairing its function. This obstruction can lead to restrictive ETD (ETD-R) and active muscular ETD (ETD-M), emphasizing the need to evaluate peri-tubal tissues at rest and during swallowing. Comprehensive care often requires collaboration among otolaryngologists, speech therapists, and gastroenterologists to effectively treat disorders like SD [6].

### *5.1.2 Modern interpretation of "stomach deafness"*

The historical concept of "stomach deafness," originally assumed to describe auditory symptoms caused by GI abnormalities, can now be understood through the lens of modern medicine as a type of ETD connected with NPR. In this disorder, gastric contents reflux into the nasopharynx impairing the ET. This condition resembles what was formerly known as "stomach deafness." This reflux can cause inflammation and dysfunction of the ET, affecting hearing by disrupting pressure regulation and fluid drainage in the ME. Although the term "stomach deafness" is not used in modern terminology, his observations on the impact of throat and nasopharyngeal disorders on ear health set the groundwork for contemporary interpretations of ETD. Yearsley noted as follows: "DEAFNESS FROM of DERANGEMENT of THE STOMACH, (STOMACH DEAFNESS,) must plead guilty to the charge of having had their attention so concentrated on the ear alone in the study of its diseases, as to have left out of view the important relations these bear to the whole system, and the benefit derivable from a treatment embracing all the vital functions, which are so intimately blended and dependent, that none can afford to be put out of consideration even in the management of the most strictly local disease. Even in the writings of and Kramer, the best writers on the subject, not a page is devoted to the intimate connexion existing between the stomach and the ear." This early concept foreshadowed a modern understanding of how systemic disorders can have far-reaching consequences on several body systems, including auditory circuits [21].

### *5.1.3 Low-frequency hearing loss in ETD in Yearsley's observations*

Yearsley observed that patients with ETD could maintain conversations in high tones better than in low tones: "It will be found, that while deafness from tension of the membrane tympani continues, a conversation in a sharp tone is much more audible, than when the sounds are of a graver character. Hence it arises, that in real deafness of this kind, the patient can maintain a conversation with those who talk in a high, better than with others who speak in a low tone of voice." This observation demonstrated the effect of ETD on hearing, as tension on the TM affected low-frequency sounds [22]. Modern research confirms that ETD can result in low-frequency hearing loss due to fluid buildup and MEP changes. Studies using cadaveric human samples showed that hypercontraction of *the* tensor tympani muscle should cause low-frequency hearing loss and a decrease in ME compliance. A proposal suggested that the distorted shape of the TM and ossicular chain impacts the effect of MEP on sound transmission for low frequencies [5].

#### *5.1.4 On the interconnection of body systems*

Yearsley's observations were essential in identifying the multiple links within the human body, particularly between the GI system and auditory function. He noted, "It is surprising how large a proportion of the deaf refer to the stomach as the source of the aural malady; but, on a close examination of the early symptoms, they almost invariably remember a troublesome condition of the throat as constituting an intermediate train of symptoms between the stomach and aural disorders." This statement emphasizes Yearsley's recognition of the intricate connections between unrelated symptoms and systems are intricately linked, emphasizing the importance of a holistic approach to diagnosis and treatment [22].

#### *5.1.5 Focus of medical attention*

"Many writers on the Practice of Medicine have pointed out the stomach as the source of deafness, but none of them ever suspected the frequency of its occurrence. Unfortunately, [medical practitioners] has directed their attention too exclusively to the ear itself, to trace accurately the chain of causation by which the disease approaches the organ of their circumscribed studies." This quote effectively conveys the difficulties and limitations of early medical efforts in diagnosis and treatment for auditory disorders. It criticizes the restricted focus on the ear and advocates for a more holistic understanding of how other body systems, particularly the GI system, might affect auditory function. This viewpoint is consistent with modern approaches to medicine, which emphasizes a more systemic and interdisciplinary technique [22].

#### *5.1.6 Emphasis on symptom complexity*

"In the congested state of the mucous membrane of the throat, Eustachian tube, and ear, there is itching and sometimes pain in the meatus, and the secretion of cerement is either diminished or depraved." James Yearsley's statement emphasizes the complex symptoms of ETD, demonstrating how congestion and inflammation can cause a variety of ear and throat manifestations, including itching [22].

#### *5.1.7 On systemic treatment*

"While I would not for a moment unjustly depreciate the advantage and efficacy of local investigation and treatment, I maintain that some of the most obstinate cases of deafness yield to the continued application of judicious remedies to renovate the stomach and digestive organs; and this I have seen to happen, after having defied the whole range of local treatment in the most skillful hands." This statement supports the concept of systemic treatment, which involves addressing broader health issues to resolve disorders that local treatment alone may not alleviate [22].

#### *5.1.8 Efficiency of ETC*

This elegant line, written by James Yearsley, "It is in this stage of the disorder that catheterism is of the greatest service; the introduction of air breaking down the thick secretion, and occasioning its discharge from the Eustachian tubes, which, by admitting air freely into the tympanum, restores the hearing." wonderfully illustrates the transformative effect of ETC—a treatment that dramatically improves patient outcomes by restoring hearing through rigorous medical intervention [22]. Those with substantial expertise with ETC appreciate the clarity and elegance of this statement. They recognize the significant relief and recovery it provides for patients, and consequently value the depth of ability and understanding required to accomplish such exceptional results. However, those unfamiliar with treating ETD using ETC, on the other hand, should approach this sentence with caution due to the technical and clinical complexities involved. To acknowledge the specialized nature of this medical process, it is advised to refrain from excessive criticism or praise without a thorough clinical experience and understanding.

#### *5.1.9 The role of ETC*

James Yearsley also advocated for the use of ETC to manage AF. He asserted, "Catheterism of the Eustachian passages is safe, painless, and efficient; and it is fortunate that it has such recommendations, inasmuch as, already said, it frequently cannot be dispensed with in the diagnosis and treatment of deafness." Yearsley's recommendation underscores the importance he placed on this method due to its safety, absence of discomfort, and success. He considered it as an essential tool in the otologist's toolbox, particularly when other diagnosis and treatment techniques proved ineffective [22].

#### *5.1.10 Legacy and modern relevance*

Yearsley made substantial contributions to otolaryngology with his early insights into the multisystemic implications of pharyngeal diseases. His research created the groundwork for understanding the interactions between speech, hearing, swallowing, and breathing. Today, his findings continue to inspire an MDA for complicated ENT problems, highlighting the value of holistic medical care [22].

### 5.2 Historical perspectives and Peter Allen

Peter Allen (1826–1874) made notable progress in the field of otolaryngology, particularly in comprehending and managing disorders associated with ET and ME. Allen expanded upon James Yearsley's initial research as his assistant, highlighting the significance of thorough care and providing novel therapeutic methods. His efforts were crucial in promoting the field and establishing an integrated approach to treating otological disorders [23].

#### *5.2.1 Allen's perspective on intralabyrinthine pressure and vestibular symptoms*

Peter Allen suggested that vertigo, common in ETD, could be caused by increased pressure within the inner ear structures, also known as intralabyrinthine pressure. He proposed that increased pressure on the labyrinth fluid or the auditory nerve itself could cause severe vestibular symptoms such as vertigo and vomiting. Allen's perspective was ahead of its time, introducing the idea that mechanical changes in the ME might cause severe disruptions in the delicate balance of the inner ear, affecting both hearing and equilibrium. He elaborated on this connection, stating, "While the severer symptoms of the same class, such as vomiting, and vertigo, &c, are to be associated with intra-auricular pressure (that is, pressure upon the labyrinth fluid, or on the auditory nerve-expansion itself), in a manner already explained." This comment from his "Lectures on Aural Catarrh" emphasizes the severity of

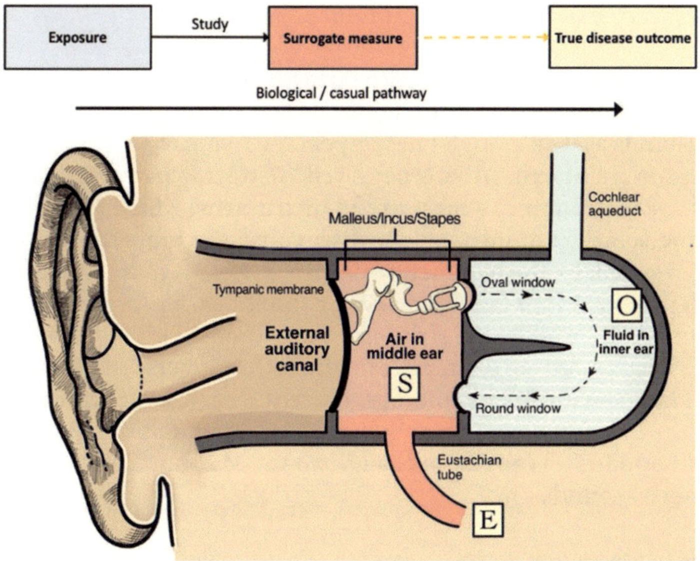


**Figure 3.**
*An anatomical illustration depicting the middle ear, vestibular systems, and Eustachian tube, illustrating the relationships between exposure, surrogate biomarker, and outcome in the context of Eustachian tube dysfunction [7] (Figure adapted from the cited study). Note: E, exposure; S, surrogate biomarker; O, outcome.*

symptoms caused by such pressure fluctuations. His work remains to be a cornerstone in the study of otolaryngological disease, particularly those that affect vestibular function. Furthermore, Allen noted the predominance of tinnitus in chronic aural disorders, attributing it to this phenomenon: "Increased intra-auricular pressure, of course, causes most troublesome tinnitus; so that the almost universal occurrence of this symptom in chronic catarrh may be expected." His findings link the common symptom of tinnitus to the mechanics of MEP management, further highlighting the importance of his contributions to understanding ear disorders (**Figure 3**) [7, 23].

### *5.2.2 Empirical validation of Allen's hypothesis*

Recent research confirms Peter Allen's idea that intralabyrinthine pressure influences vestibular symptoms [23, 25, 26]. These results validate Allen's theoretical paradigm by showing that changes in MEP have a direct impact on intralabyrinthine pressure. This confirmation is significant because it connects historical observations to current scientific studies, enhancing our understanding of the physiological basis for vestibular symptoms associated with ETD. Failure to equalize *via* the ET in the ME space results in a pressure discrepancy between the outer and inner ears. During descent, the TM retracts, and blood or fluid may leak into the ME due to the vacuum formed. Depending on the fragility of TM and the rate and depth of descent, the TM may rupture. If the pressure is high enough or the inner ear membranes are unstable, the oval or round windows may burst, with the round window being the most common. This could result from the rapid movement of the stapes footplate combined with quick TM positional changes, or from increasing pressure gradients between the inner and ME spaces generated by a Valsalva maneuver during descending. A Valsalva maneuver generates an increase in cerebrospinal fluid pressure and eventually raising inner ear pressure due to the connection between the two regions *via* the cochlear aqueduct [25].

### *5.2.3 Low-frequency hearing loss in ETD in Allen's insights*

The phenomenon of low-frequency hearing loss was also covered by Peter Allen in his publications. He noted that individuals with auditory catarrh often struggle to hear low sounds as well as high ones, especially in noisy environments. In "Lectures on Aural Catarrh," Allen's observed "In testing patients' hearing powers by means of the metronome (a most useful instrument, which I will show you after lecture), I find some are quite unable to distinguish the acute sound of the bell inside it when struck by the hammer, while others hear it more distinctly than I do myself. Such persons as the latter, however, cannot hear proportionately well the dull low sounds produced by the striking on the wood." This statement illustrates how diseases such as auditory catarrh can affect the perception of low-frequency sounds [22]. In line with Allen's findings, current research supports the idea that ETD may cause low-frequency hearing loss. These studies indicate that ETD can result in fluid buildup and pressure changes in the ME, impairing the transmission of low-frequency sounds [5].

### *5.2.4 Focus on symptom complexity*

Peter Allen's observations in "Lectures on Aural Catarrh" emphasize the systemic effects of ETD, notably on GI disorder. He stated, "A patient suffering from catarrh disease of the ear is commonly disordered in general health; especially are the digestive functions disturbed." This shows that ETD, which is commonly referred to as ear catarrh, can have an impact on overall health, including the digestive system. Allen's findings suggest that ETD can generate GI symptoms *via* common neuronal connections or systemic inflammatory responses that affect both the ear and digestive tract [23]. He referred to Yearsley's concept of "stomach deafness," emphasizing the relationship between GI issues and ear health [22]. Allen also stated that ETD can lead to GERD and vice versa, implying a complex bidirectional link. Allen argued for a treatment strategy that extends beyond local ear care, emphasizing the importance of using suitable medications to address both ear pathology and concomitant GI disorders. His thoughts highlight the need for a comprehensive management strategy that incorporates ENT and GI care to provide holistic treatment for ETD patients [22].

### *5.2.5 Merica's perspectives on ETD and GI disorders*

F. W. Merica's thorough study on vertigo caused by ET obstruction highlights the importance of identifying and treating this often-looked condition. His study, which included 135 cases, demonstrated the effectiveness of mechanical expansion of the ETs as a treatment for vertigo, nausea, and vomiting, underscoring the significant relationship between ear, nose, and throat diseases and GI symptoms. Merica particularly emphasized the risk of overlooking cases with an insidious onset, where "the gastrointestinal symptoms are predominant, the patients are likely to be subjected to various types of treatment over long periods for diseases of the digestive system." This insight stresses the need for a comprehensive diagnostic approach that considers both GI and auditory symptoms to avoid misdiagnosis and inappropriate treatment [9].

#### *5.2.6 John A. Rutka's insights into vestibular and GI interactions*

John A. Rutka has made substantial contributions to our understanding of the vestibular system, particularly how vestibular dysfunction can be mistaken for or contribute to GI symptoms. Rutka's thorough descriptions of vestibular circuits and their effects on balance and spatial orientation shed light on why abnormalities in this system can have far-reaching systemic consequences, including those affecting the digestive system. Rutka's insights support Allen's observations by highlighting the intricate link between vestibular dysfunction and GI disturbances, emphasizing the need for a comprehensive approach to diagnosis and treatment [23–26].

#### *5.2.7 Reciprocal causal relationship between GERD and ETD*

A recent study suggests a complex link between ETD and GERD, emphasizing the involvement of GI symptoms in the development of ETD and their impact on the vestibular system, as underlined by Rutka [7, 8, 26]. ETD frequently develops insidiously, with GI symptoms preceding and dominating the clinical presentation. This gradual onset allows the vestibular system to respond to different sensory inputs, lowering the severity of vertigo symptoms. Despite this adaptability, the vestibular system's connection with the brainstem's emetic areas remains delicate. Even slight abnormalities in vestibular function can result in nausea and vomiting, while compensatory adjustments may make vertigo less severe [26]. Understanding this connection is crucial to detecting and treating GERD and ETD. Clinicians should be aware that prolonged GI symptoms in ETD patients might indicate an underlying reflux disease that needs to be addressed. This comprehensive approach can help in accurately diagnosing and effectively treating the interconnected symptoms of both conditions.

#### *5.2.8 The role of muscles in swallowing and ET function*

Peter Allen highlighted the connection between the muscles involved in swallowing and the functioning of the ET. He stated, "There is a want of power over the muscles of deglutition, swallowing is therefore difficult, and accomplished with pain, which is aggravated by every motion of the throat; for it will be remembered that the muscles concerned in deglutition are also muscles of the Eustachian tube, and that their fibers interlace themselves among the glands and neighboring mucous surfaces of the soft palate." He observed that inflammation and uncomfortable conditions render these muscles unable to perform the function of separating the walls of the ET during swallowing, yawning, sneezing, and chewing, which is essential for maintaining balance in MEP and drainage [23].

#### *5.2.9 Legacy and modern relevance*

Peter Allen made important contributions to modern otolaryngology, notably in terms of understanding intralabyrinthine pressure and its implications on vestibular symptoms. His studies on ETD and vertigo elucidated the relationship between ear function and balance. Allen advocated for the use of ETC to treat ETD, highlighting out how inflammation and pain can impair the muscles involved in swallowing and

| Aspect/factor | James Yearsley | Peter Allen |
|---|---|---|
| Era | 1805–1869 | 1826–1874 |
| Main Contributions | Highlighted the role of swallowing mechanics in ENT health and systemic connections. | Furthered and applied Yearsley's pioneering concepts in modern otology. |
| Key Works | "Deafness Practically Illustrated: Being an Exposition of the Nature, Causes and Treatment of Diseases of the Ear" | "Lectures on Aural Catarrh: Or, the Commonest Forms of Deafness and Their Cure" |
| Focus Areas | Multisystemic effects of pharyngeal disorders on speech, hearing, swallowing, and breathing. | Intralabyrinthine pressure, vestibular function, and mechanical changes in the ME. |
| Treatment Innovations | Innovated in ETC; systemic treatment approaches involving GI and ENT care. | Supported ETC and comprehensive therapeutic approaches integrating medication for ear and GI disorders. |
| Impact on Modern Medicine | Influenced holistic approaches in diagnosing and treating ENT disorders with GI involvement. | Groundbreaking research on intralabyrinthine pressure, integrating historical ideas with current practice. |
| Legacy | Laid the groundwork for understanding the interconnectedness of physiological systems. | Enhanced and disseminated Yearsley's innovative approaches, ensuring their adoption and further development. |
| Causation Direction | GI and SD affecting auditory function. | Reinforced Yearsley's theories on ETD's influence on GI issues and vestibular symptoms. |
| Primary Condition | GI and swallowing issues leading to auditory issues. | Echoed and expanded on Yearsley's findings on auditory issues leading to GI and balance disorders. |
| Impact on Diagnosis | Considering GI and swallowing issues in diagnosing ETD. | Promoted considering ETD as a potential cause of vertigo and GI symptoms, building on Yearsley's work. |
| Swallowing Disorders | SD affecting ET function and leading to ear issues. | Supported the idea that ETD might contribute to or complicate SD, following Yearsley's theories. |
| Vertigo | GI issues leading to "giddiness of the stomach," but not linking vertigo specifically to ETD. | Identified vertigo as a symptom of ETD, possibly influencing GI function, as proposed by Yearsley. |
| Reciprocity Acknowledgment | Interdependence of swallowing, GI health, and auditory function. | Affirmed the bidirectional influence between ETD and conditions affecting swallowing and balance. |
| Low-Frequency Hearing Loss | ETD causing better hearing of high tones compared to low tones. | Observed similar patterns of low-frequency hearing loss, reinforcing Yearsley's findings. |
| Historical Significance | Crucial figure in the progress of ENT procedures and influential in the history of ETC. | Prominent figure in modern otology, renowned for integrating historical ideas with current practice. |

**Table 1.**
*Comparison between the legacy of James Yearsley and Peter Allen.*

ET function, both of which are necessary for maintaining MEP balance. His work bridges historical concepts with contemporary practice, aiding in the development of contemporary diagnosis and treatment procedures [23].

### 5.3 Comparison of James Yearsley and Peter Allen

#### *5.3.1 Comparison of legacy*

**Table 1** provides a comprehensive comparison of the contributions made by James Yearsley and Peter Allen in the field of otolaryngology. It highlights their main contributions, key works, areas of focus, innovations in treatment, impact on modern medicine, legacy, primary conditions they focused on, impact on diagnosis, perspectives on SD and vertigo, acknowledgment of reciprocal influences, and notes on low-frequency hearing loss. Yearsley is recognized as a crucial figure in advancing ENT procedures and is considered the most influential person in the history of ETC. On the other hand, Allen is highly regarded as a prominent figure in modern otology. He is renowned for his groundbreaking research on intralabyrinthine pressure and for integrating historical ideas with current medical practice [22–24].

#### *5.3.2 Common ground*

They underlined the link between swallowing mechanics, ET function, and ENT health, highlighting the importance of holistic care. They concluded that SD may compromise ET function, compromising swallowing and digestion. Both acknowledged the impact of ETD in contributing to these disorders and proposed ETC as a treatment to restore MEP balance and minimize symptoms. Their combined findings emphasized the importance of an MDA that includes otolaryngology, gastroenterology, and neurovestibular sciences, and which continues to influence modern otolaryngology [22–24].

## 6. Clinical management and interdisciplinary treatment approaches

### 6.1 Management strategies

Treatment of ETD, associated SD, and reflux-related diseases such as GERD, LPRD, and NPR requires an MDA [1, 2, 17–20]:

*Medical management.* Use of proton pump inhibitors or H2 blockers to reduce acid production and alleviate reflux, along with corticosteroid nasal sprays and other decongestants to reduce inflammation and enhance ET function. Systemic pseudoephedrine did not improve gas bolus transfer through the ET during swallows [1–5, 17–20].

*Dietary and lifestyle modifications.* Recommendations include avoiding reflux-causing foods, eating smaller meals, avoiding recumbency after consuming water, medication, or meals, managing weight, and quitting smoking [1, 17–20].

*Speech and swallowing therapy.* Conducted by speech-language pathologists to improve swallowing mechanics and reduce aspiration risk [1].

*Surgical and procedural interventions.* Include anti-reflux surgery for severe cases [17, 18]. Adenoidectomy removes hypertrophied adenoids that block the ET, making it advantageous for ETD, especially in children [2]. Radiation and chemotherapy can shrink tumors and improve ETD caused by tumor blockage or inflammation. However, these treatments can also produce mucositis and other inflammatory responses in the nasopharyngeal region, which can harm the ET and exacerbate ETD symptoms. The well-documented side effects of head and neck cancer treatments, such as mucositis, esophagitis, and xerostomia, can cause substantial discomfort and SD. To manage these challenges, supportive care measures, dietary modifications, and swallowing exercises are recommended [27]. Turbinectomy, which reduces the size of nasal turbinates to enhance airflow and reduce inflammation, can help relieve ETD [14].

*Eustachian tube catheterization (ETC)*. Used for both the diagnosis and treatment of ETD, ETC addresses blockages or ETD to stabilize MEP. It is particularly useful in cases of chronic ETD, persistent ear fullness, negative MEP, and when other treatments have failed [3, 7–10, 12, 13, 15, 21–24].

### 6.2 Role of interdisciplinary teams

Collaboration among various specialists ensures comprehensive treatment for ETD and related conditions [1, 2]. Interdisciplinary teams should incorporate a specialist for ETD to optimize patient outcomes [14]:

*Otolaryngologists.* Diagnose and treat ENT disorders, including ETD.

*Gastroenterologists.* Manage GERD, LPRD, and NPR, which can worsen ETD and impair swallowing.

*Neurologists.* Address neurological problems that impact swallowing and balance.

*Speech-language pathologists.* Improve swallowing mechanics and treat speech disorders.

*Audiologists.* Assess hearing and balance to determine the impact of ETD.

*Neuro-vestibular specialists.* Treat balance and vestibular function.

*Pulmonologists.* Manage respiratory problems that influence or are influenced by ETD.

*Cardiologists.* Address cardiovascular symptoms like bradycardia caused by ETD.

*Ophthalmologists.* Treat visual disturbances such as oscillopsia and nystagmus.

*Dietitians/nutritionists.* Offer dietary guidance to manage reflux disorders and enhance general health.

*Physical therapists.* Enhance muscle function related to swallowing and balance.

*Occupational therapists.* Assist with daily tasks affected by SD.

*Psychologists.* Support patients in managing anxiety and stress associated with chronic ETD and SD [1].

### 6.3 Coordinated care approach

A coordinated care approach, involving the collaboration of these specialists, is essential for effectively addressing complex symptoms of ETD and related conditions. This approach improves treatment outcomes but ensures a comprehensive evaluation of all patient health issues, enhancing patient satisfaction and quality of life [1, 2, 7, 13].

## 7. Case studies and practical applications

### 7.1 Presentation of case studies

#### *7.1.1 Case study 1: treatment of chronic ETD with asymmetric ME pressures*

- Patient background: A 45-year-old male with chronic sinusitis, recurrent ear fullness, occasional hearing loss, SD, and tinnitus. Whenever he experienced a sensation of fullness in his ears, it felt as though there was a constriction in the laryngeal area of his neck. Nasal obstruction led to frequent sniffing, worsening his symptoms.

- Diagnostic findings: Irritated nasal mucosa, retracted TM, mild-to-moderate low-frequency hearing loss, asymmetrical MEP, and indications of LPRD including laryngoscopic findings such as erythema, edema of the laryngeal mucosa, and interarytenoid hypertrophy.

- Treatment strategy: Corticosteroid nasal sprays, nasal decongestants, LPR management, and ETC. Behavioral advice to reduce sniffing.

- Outcome: Significant reduction in ear fullness and improved hearing within 3 weeks. Long-term improvement with adherence to behavioral changes.

#### *7.1.2 Case study 2: complex GERD, NPR, and ETD*

- Patient background: A 55-year-old female with long-standing GERD, persistent SD, dizziness, sudden tinnitus, and vertigo. Symptoms worsened by taking medication with water before bed.

- Diagnostic findings: LPRD and NPR interfering with ET function, confirmed by nasopharyngoscopy showing refluxed gastric contents in the nasopharynx, erythema, and edema, and aggravated by bedtime medication habits.

- Treatment strategy: PPI therapy, dietary changes, altering medication habits, and ETC.

- Outcome: Notable improvement in GERD, LPRD, NPR, and auditory symptoms. Ceased vertigo bouts and significantly improved tinnitus.

### 7.2 Multidisciplinary approach (MDA) in clinical practice

#### *7.2.1 Advantages of a solo MDA*

Managing complex problems alone necessitates a solid consciousness of numerous specializations, allowing for faster decision-making and personalized treatment strategies without extensive coordination among multiple specialists.

#### *7.2.2 Conclusion*

These case studies demonstrate the significance of using an interdisciplinary approach, even in solo practice, to provide comprehensive treatment by considering all potential factors on a patient's health for optimal management and satisfaction.

## 8. Future directions

### 8.1 Emerging research areas

Ongoing advances in otolaryngology, gastroenterology, and neuro-vestibular sciences promise to enhance the diagnosis and treatment of SD and ETD. Future studies should focus on these crucial areas.

### *8.1.1 Functional restoration and maintenance*

The focus is shifting to therapies that restore and maintain ET function, crucial for balancing MEP and promoting drainage. Treating SD, which frequently coexists with or worsens ETD, is critical. Researchers are exploring the relationship between swallowing mechanics and ET function to develop integrated treatments for both disorders [12].

### *8.1.2 Advanced diagnostic tools*

*Biomarker identification.* Biomarkers like MEP help in the early detection and monitoring of ETD and SD [7]. Salivary pepsin, detectable with non-invasive instruments, is a reliable biomarker for airway reflux and LPR [28], providing quick and accurate measurements of LPR severity.

*Enhanced imaging techniques.* High-resolution imaging and 3D CT scans produce exact images of the ET and surrounding structures, which are necessary for accurate diagnosis and simulation [5, 6, 29].

*Wideband acoustic immittance.* This emerging technology provides a comprehensive evaluation of ME function over a wide frequency range, enabling more accurate identification of ME disorders [30, 31].

### *8.1.3 Multidisciplinary approach (MDA)*

Encouraging MDA involves gathering a variety of professionals to focus on interrelated systems, utilizing shared databases, and obtaining funding [1, 2]. Creating integrated care models enhances patient outcomes by incorporating multidisciplinary teams, central care coordinators, shared EHRs, complete care plans, and regular treatment planning and outcome monitoring.

### *8.1.4 Innovative therapeutic approaches*

Research into new minimally invasive procedures, such as Balloon Eustachian Tuboplasty, and Laser Eustachian Tuboplasty, as well as renewed interest in established ones, is advancing the field of ETD treatment [2, 3, 7–10, 12, 13, 15, 21–24].

### *8.1.5 Rehabilitation and therapy*

Development of advanced therapeutic techniques and devices to improve swallowing function and reduce the risk of aspiration in patients with SD is ongoing [1]. Examples include neuromuscular electrical stimulation (NMES) to stimulate swallowing muscles, customized swallowing exercises and maneuvers, adapted equipment such as specialized utensils and cups, and biofeedback therapy to improve swallowing techniques [1].

## 8.2 Addressing current gaps

Future research should focus on these key areas to address current gaps:

*Early detection.* Improved diagnostic tools and biomarkers can lead to earlier detection of ETD and SD, allowing for timely intervention [7, 28].

*Personalized care.* Precision medicine approaches for more personalized and effective treatment plans, reducing trial-and-error in therapy [13].

*Patient-centered care.* Telemedicine and digital health tools to empower patients improving adherence and outcomes [7, 31].

*Comprehensive management.* Interdisciplinary research and integrated care models to address all aspects of complex conditions, leading to better overall management and patient satisfaction [1, 2].

## 9. Contribution

### 9.1 Summary of key findings

This chapter investigates the intricate links between SD and ETD from a multidisciplinary perspective. The key findings include:

*Interplay of swallowing and ET* SD have an impact on ET function, and SD can exacerbate ETD.

*Comprehensive management strategy.* Highlights the need of integrating otolaryngology, gastroenterology, and speech-language pathology for a complete diagnosis. Treatment options include ETC and medication adjustments.

*Effectiveness of interdisciplinary teams.* Emphasizes the significance of professional collaboration in developing comprehensive treatment programs for both swallowing and auditory issues.

### 9.2 Key contributions

Ongoing research and interdisciplinary collaboration are essential for advancing our understanding and treatment of SD and ETD. Research enhances diagnostic tools and treatment options, and interdisciplinary collaboration promotes holistic care and innovation. This chapter addresses the relationship between SD and ETD, emphasizing the value of MDA, advanced diagnostics, telemedicine, digital health, and innovative treatments. Continued research and collaboration will lead to improved patient outcomes and quality of life.

## Conflict of interest

The author declares no conflict of interest.

## Author details

Hee-Young Kim
Center for Executive and Continuing Professional Education, Harvard T.H. Chan School of Public Health, Boston, MA, USA

*Address all correspondence to: hee-young.kim-2022@ppcr.org

## References

[1] Azer SA. Dysphagia. In: StatPearls [Internet]. Treasure Island (FL): StatPearls Publishing; 2023. Available from: https://www.ncbi.nlm.nih.gov/books/NBK559174/

[2] Hamrang-Yousefi S, Ng J, Andaloro C. Eustachian tube dysfunction. In: StatPearls [Internet]. Treasure Island (FL): StatPearls Publishing; 2021. Available from: https://www.ncbi.nlm.nih.gov/books/NBK555908/

[3] Bluestone CD. Eustachian Tube: Structure, Function, and Role in Middle Ear Disease. 2nd ed. Raleigh, North Carolina: People Medical Publishing House USA; 2018

[4] Llewellyn A, Norman G, Harden M, Coatesworth A, Kimberling D, Schilder A, et al. Interventions for adult Eustachian tube dysfunction: A systematic review. Health Technology Assessment. 2014;**18**(46):1-180

[5] Alper CM, Luntz M, Takahashi H, Ghadiali SN, Swarts JD, Teixeira MS, et al. Panel 2: Anatomy (Eustachian tube, middle ear, and mastoid—Anatomy, physiology, pathophysiology, and pathogenesis). Otolaryngology–Head and Neck Surgery. 2017;**156**(4_suppl):S22-S40

[6] Alper CM, Teixeira MS, Mandel EM, Swarts JD. Dissecting Eustachian tube dysfunction: From phenotypes to endotypes. PLoS ONE. 2023;**18**(4). DOI: 10.1371/journal.pone.0283885

[7] Kim HY. Validation of biomarkers and patient-reported outcome measures to improve the diagnosis and treatment of Eustachian tube dysfunction. Principles and Practice of Clinical Research Journal. 2024;**10**(1):27-38

[8] Kim HY. Reciprocal causal relationship between nasopharyngeal reflux and Eustachian tube dysfunction. Journal of Otolaryngology-ENT Research. 2021;**13**(3):46-47

[9] Merica FW. Vertigo due to obstruction of the Eustachian tubes. Journal of American Medical Association. 1942;**118**(15):1282-1284

[10] Kim HY. Alternobaric vertigo: Asymmetrical vestibular function due to asymmetrical middle ear pressures (iron man's archenemy). ENT and Audiology News. 2021. Available from: https://cloud.3dissue.net/30176/30070/30342/63730/index.html?page=42

[11] Heidsieck DSP, Smarius BJA, Oomen KPQ, Breugem CC. The role of the tensor veli palatini muscle in the development of cleft palate-associated middle ear problems. Clinical Oral Investigations. 2016;**20**(7):1389-1401. Available from: https://pubmed.ncbi.nlm.nih.gov/27153847/

[12] Teixeira MS. Understanding Eustachian tube function. Brazilian Journal of Otorhinolaryngology. 2020;**86**(5):523-524

[13] Kim HY. Ground-level alternobaric vertigo: A contemporary perspective on Eustachian tube. In: Giourgos G, editor. Studies in Otorhinolaryngology. London, UK: IntechOpen; 2025. pp. 1-21. DOI: 10.5772/intechopen.1004951

[14] Bluestone CD, Swarts JD, Forman JM, Yellon RF. Persistent alternobaric vertigo at ground level. The Laryngoscope. 2012;**122**:868-872. DOI: 10.1002/lary.22182

[15] Kim HY. A case report on ground-level alternobaric vertigo due to Eustachian tube dysfunction with the assistance of conversational generative pre-trained transformer (ChatGPT). Cureus. 28 Mar 2023;**15**(3). DOI: 10.7759/cureus.36830

[16] Kim HY. Reevaluating "within normal limits" in tympanometry: Implications for alternobaric vertigo. Journal of Otolaryngology-ENT Research. 2024;**16**(2):41-42. DOI: 10.15406/joentr.2024.16.00546

[17] American Academy of Otolaryngology-Head and Neck Surgery Foundation. GERD and LPR. ENT Health [Internet]. Alexandria (VA): American Academy of Otolaryngology-Head and Neck Surgery Foundation; 2018. Available from: https://www.enthealth.org/conditions/gerd-and-lpr/

[18] Antunes C. Gastroesophageal reflux disease. In: StatPearls [Internet]. Treasure Island (FL): StatPearls Publishing; 2023. Available from: https://www.ncbi.nlm.nih.gov/books/NBK441938/

[19] Joshi AA, Chiplunkar B. Laryngopharyngeal reflux. International Journal of Head and Neck Surgery. 2022;**13**(1):8-17

[20] Brunworth JD, Mahboubi H, Garg R, Johnson B, Brandon B, Djalilian HR. Nasopharyngeal acid reflux and Eustachian tube dysfunction in adults. Annals of Otology, Rhinology and Laryngology. 2014;**123**(6):415-419

[21] Kim HY. Eustachian tube catheterization: Fundamental skill for competent otolaryngologists. Journal of Otolaryngology-ENT Research. 2019;**4**:11. DOI: 10.15406/joentr.2019.11.00401

[22] Yearsley J. Deafness Practically Illustrated: Being an Exposition of the Nature, Causes and Treatment of Diseases of the Ear. London: John Churchill; 1863

[23] Allen P. Lectures on Aural Catarrh: Or, the Commonest Forms of Deafness and their Cure. London: Churchill; 1871

[24] Kim HY. From pioneers to modern medicine: Tracing the evolution of our understanding of the relationship between Eustachian tube dysfunction, alternobaric vertigo, and laryngopharyngeal reflux. Journal of Otolaryngology-ENT Research. 2023;**12**:23-24. DOI: 10.15406/joentr.2023.15.00521

[25] Mallen JR, Roberts DS. SCUBA medicine for otolaryngologists: Part I. Diving into SCUBA physiology and injury prevention. The Laryngoscope. 2019;**130**(1):1-7

[26] Roland PS, Rutka JA. Physiology of the vestibular system. In: Rutka JA, editor. Ototoxicity. Hamilton, Ontario, Canada: BC Decker Inc.; 2004. pp. 24-25

[27] Blanchard P, Lee AW, Carmel A, Ng WT, Ma J, Chan ATC, et al. Meta-analysis of chemotherapy in nasopharynx carcinoma (MAC-NPC): An update on 26 trials and 7080 patients. Clinical and Translational Radiation Oncology. 2022;**32**:59-68

[28] Dettmar PW, Watson M, McGlashan J, et al. A multicentre study in UK voice clinics evaluating the non-invasive reflux diagnostic peptest in LPR patients. SN Comprehensive Clinical Medicine. 2020;**2**:57-65. DOI: 10.1007/s42399-019-00184-0

[29] Schuon R, Schwarzensteiner J, Paasche G, Lenarz T, John S. Functional aspects of the Eustachian tube by means of 3D-modeling. PLoS ONE. 2021;**16**(8). DOI: 10.1371/journal.pone.0244909

[30] Shahnaz N, AlMakadma H, Sanford CA. The rise and fall of aural acoustic immittance assessment tools. Seminars in Hearing. 2023;**44**(01):005-016

[31] Chan J, Najafi A, Baker M, Kinsman J, Mancl LR, Norton S, et al. Performing tympanometry using smartphones. Communications Medicine. 2022;**2**(1):1-11. Available from: https://www.nature.com/articles/s43856-022-00120-9

Chapter 8

# Perspective Chapter: Spinal Etiologies of Swallowing Dysfunction

*Samir Alsalek, Nghiem H. Nguyen and Shayan U. Rahman*

## Abstract

Swallowing dysfunction, or dysphagia, presents a persistent and common challenge in many patients, with consequences on quality of life and life expectancy. Dysphagia results from a variety of structural and functional causes that affect the deglutition process, including central and peripheral nervous system disease, stroke, neoplasms and their treatment, and psychogenic disturbances. Spinal etiologies of dysphagia are of particular concern for combining both structural and functional processes. Dysphagia is a common concern following anterior cervical spine surgery such as fusion, due to spinal cord manipulation and traction on surrounding soft tissue. Furthermore, dysphagia observed in patients with spinal injury due to direct and indirect causes. Spinal deformities (e.g., kyphosis) and degenerative processes affecting the cervical spine (e.g., osteophytes) can also result in compression on the esophagus or adjacent neural structures with subsequent swallowing dysfunction. Management of dysphagia consists of conservative therapy by multi-disciplinary teams in most cases, involving speech therapists, nutritional specialists, and surgeons, among other providers. In rare instances, surgical treatment may be necessary for severe spinal deformities and compressive lesions.

**Keywords:** spinal, swallowing, dysfunction, dysphagia, ACDF, osteophytes

## 1. Introduction

Swallowing dysfunction, or dysphagia, is a debilitating condition that can substantially affect a person's quality of life, in some cases leading to significant morbidity and even death. Dysphagia manifests as difficulty initiating and completing swallowing, retention and regurgitation of food in the pharynx or esophagus, pain with eating, or more serious complications such as aspiration and respiratory infections. These complications are particularly concerning in vulnerable populations, such as older adults or individuals with pre-existing conditions, where aspiration can rapidly progress to pneumonia. Even in the absence of severe complications, acute dysphagia may lead to prolonged hospitalization, malnutrition, and respiratory compromise, contributing to increased healthcare costs and patient burden. Chronic dysphagia can also result in psychological distress, social isolation, and reduced overall quality of life.

Dysphagia can arise due to a variety of causes, including neurological, structural, and iatrogenic factors. Disorders of the spinal cord and spinal column are particularly important contributors to swallowing dysfunction, due to the diverse etiologies encompassing degenerative, inflammatory, traumatic, and iatrogenic processes. Cervical spine injuries and surgeries, for example, can disrupt neural pathways or compress anatomical structures critical to swallowing, often leading to significant functional impairments.

Given the complexity of the swallowing process, dysphagia associated with spinal conditions demands a nuanced understanding of both anatomy and pathology. Understanding the multifactorial nature of dysphagia in these contexts is essential for developing effective diagnostic and therapeutic strategies to enhance patient outcomes. This chapter seeks to explore the multifactorial etiologies, mechanisms, and management strategies for swallowing dysfunction linked to spinal disorders. It aims to provide a holistic perspective, integrating insights from recent studies to offer clinicians a framework for understanding and addressing dysphagia in the context of spinal pathology. This approach emphasizes the importance of early detection, targeted treatment, and interdisciplinary care to mitigate the potentially severe impacts of dysphagia on patient health and quality of life.

## 2. Mechanism and physiology of swallowing

Swallowing, or deglutition, occurs through a complex, multi-phasic process that involves voluntary and involuntary muscle actions coordinated by the central and peripheral nervous systems, with input from cranial and cervical nerves. The swallowing reflex is initiated voluntarily and can be divided into four distinct phases: oral preparatory, oral, pharyngeal, and esophageal. During these phases, the food bolus is sequentially manipulated, processed, and broken down, then propelled into the pharynx and through the esophagus by a series of well-executed steps. An essential component in the swallowing reflex includes closure of the larynx and inhibition of respiration to prevent aspiration [1].

Each phase in the deglutition process requires the precise coordination of muscles in the oral cavity, pharynx, and esophagus, as well as input from six cranial nerves: the trigeminal (CN V), facial (CN VII), glossopharyngeal (CN IX), vagus (X), accessory (XI), and hypoglossal (XII). Cervical spinal nerves, particularly C1-C5, also play a supportive role in swallowing by contributing to the movement and stabilization of key muscles involved in the process (**Figure 1**). The C1 nerve innervates the geniohyoid and thyrohyoid muscles, which assist in elevating the hyoid bone and larynx. Additionally, C2 and C3 innervate the infrahyoid muscles responsible for stabilizing the hyoid bone, facilitating smooth bolus transfer from the mouth to the esophagus. Lastly, the C3-C5 nerves collectively form the phrenic nerve, which controls the diaphragm, ensuring proper coordination between respiration and swallowing to prevent aspiration. Together, these cervical nerves complement the role of cranial nerves and help maintain the integrity of the swallowing mechanism [1, 2].

Dysphagia can result from interruption or dysfunction at any point along this pathway, from neural damage to structural impingement. In particular, cervical spine pathology can compromise the neuromuscular control required for smooth swallowing, leading to difficulty in bolus propulsion or airway protection. The structural integrity of the cervical vertebrae also plays a crucial role, as any deformation,

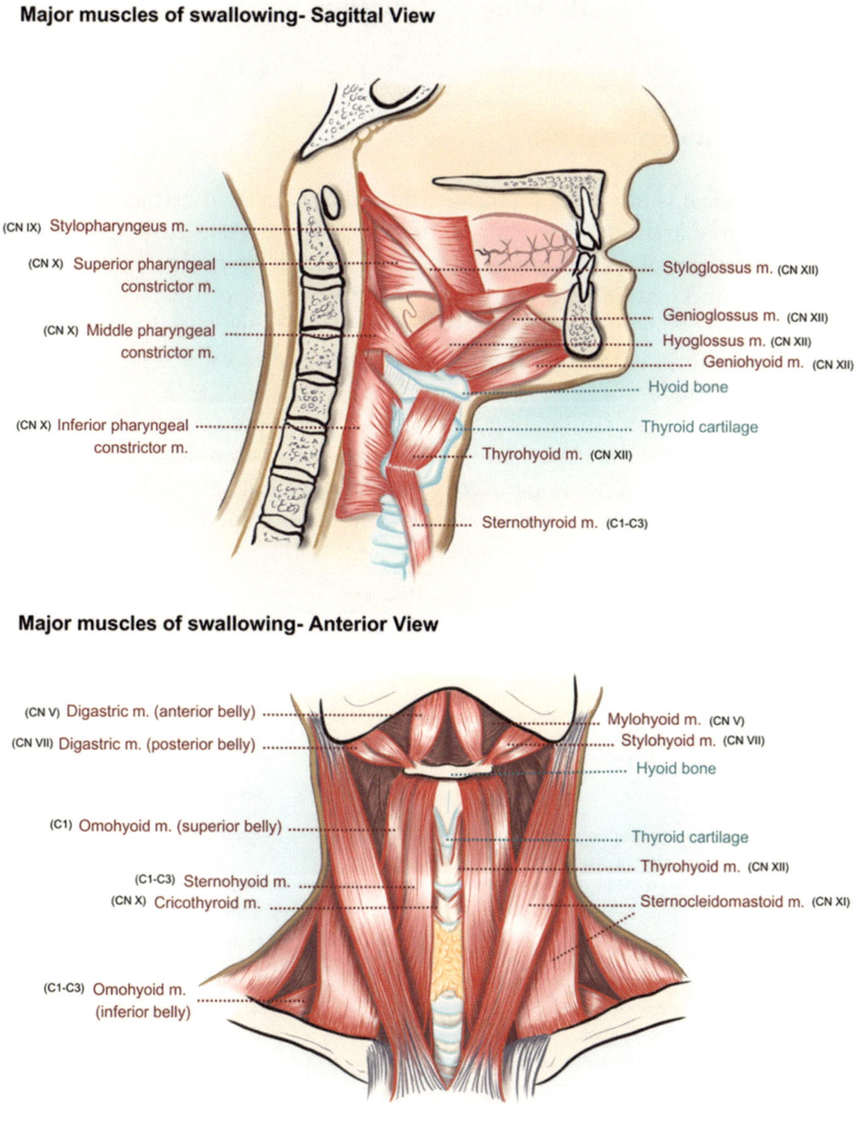


**Figure 1.**
*Sagittal and anterior views of the neck illustrating the primary muscles and anatomical structures involved in the swallowing process, including their innervation by cranial and cervical spinal nerves. These muscles work in coordination to facilitate the complex phases of swallowing, including bolus propulsion, airway protection, and esophageal clearance.*

degeneration, or compression can lead to mechanical obstruction of the passage of food or disrupt the nerve signaling needed for coordinated swallowing. Additionally, inflammatory responses around compressed tissues may cause fibrosis and scarring, further narrowing the esophageal lumen and exacerbating swallowing difficulties. Over time, these disruptions can reduce the efficiency of both voluntary and reflexive swallowing phases, increasing the risk of aspiration and subsequent respiratory complications.

## 3. Spinal etiologies of swallowing dysfunction

See **Table 1.**

### 3.1 Anterior cervical spine surgery

Anterior cervical spine procedures, such as anterior cervical discectomy and fusion (ACDF) and artificial disc replacement (ADR), are frequently performed to alleviate conditions such as cervical spondylotic myelopathy, radiculopathy due to disc herniation, and instability due to trauma. However, one of the most feared complications of these procedures is the development of postoperative dysphagia, which may lead to short-term patient morbidity, and in some cases rapid deterioration and surgical intervention.

Swallowing dysfunction following anterior cervical spine approaches is attributed to a variety of mechanical and physiological factors such as esophageal and tracheal retraction during surgery, post-operative soft tissue swelling, and injury to the neural and vascular structures in the anterior neck. The incidence of dysphagia after

| Etiology | Mechanism | Diagnosis | Management | Risk factors |
|---|---|---|---|---|
| Postoperative | Nerve traction, soft tissue swelling, esophageal motility changes, nerve injury | Bedside swallow, VFSS, endoscopy, laryngoscopy | Corticosteroids, swallowing therapy, dietary modification, surgical re-exploration if severe | Older age, multi-level ACDF, Parkinson's disease |
| Osteodegenerative | Osteophyte formation and protrusion into the esophagus, inflammation and fibrosis | CT scan, X-ray | Speech and swallowing therapy, osteophyte resection | Older age, male sex, diabetes, hyperlipidemia |
| Deformities | Abnormal spinal curvature with compression of soft tissues and pharyngeal/esophageal narrowing | MRI, FEES, VFSS | Postural adjustments, corrective surgery | Severe scoliosis, trauma, congenital abnormalities |
| Spinal Cord Injury | Direct spinal cord and nerve damage, respiratory muscle weakness impair airway protection, especially with tracheostomy, impaired cranial nerves (IX, X) | Bedside swallow, neurological exam, FEES, VFSS | Swallowing exercises, tracheostomy care | High cervical injury (C1-C2), prolonged intubation |
| Neurodegenerative | Neuromuscular degeneration disrupts coordination of swallowing muscles | Neurological exam, VFSS, FEES | Dietary modifications, swallowing maneuvers | Older age (>60), advanced disease stage |

*Abbreviations: VFSS: Videofluoroscopic Swallowing Study, ACDF: Anterior Cervical Discectomy and Fusion, FEES: Functional Endoscopic Evaluation of Swallowing, CT: Computed Tomography, MRI: Magnetic Resonance Imaging.*

**Table 1.**
*Overview of spinal etiologies of swallowing dysfunction.*

cervical spine surgery varies widely in the current literature, partly due to the lack of a conventional definition, with some reports suggesting rates of up to 70%. [3] While the majority of cases resolve within the first few months after surgery, a subset of patients may experience persistent dysphagia for up to a year or longer. One systematic review reported the prevalence of dysphagia was 33.1% within the first week following surgery, and this decreased to 19.8% at 6 months and 12.9% at 24 months. [3] However, some patients continue to experience significant swallowing difficulties up to 2 years postoperatively, indicating that long-term management may be required for certain individuals. A particular and enduring challenge in studying etiologies of postoperative dysphagia has been the lack of consensus on the definition, risk factors, and best practices to prevent this complication.

Nonetheless, it is clear that the pathophysiology of postoperative dysphagia is multifactorial, incorporating mechanical, neurological, and inflammatory causes. For example, direct esophageal injury is a serious intraoperative complication that can result in severe dysphagia, particularly if left unrecognized intraoperatively. This complication is quite rare, however, with a reported incidence of less than 0.5%. [4] More commonly, intraoperative esophageal retraction is thought to cause local ischemia through prolonged pressure exerted by the retractor blades, which impairs blood perfusion to the esophageal musculature and produces subsequent swelling with reperfusion. [5] Combined with the expected postoperative edema in the surrounding soft tissues, these changes can cause significant compression on the esophagus. Despite this, the strength of association between intraoperative retraction and the severity of postoperative dysphagia remains unclear, with some studies reporting no correlation between the degree of intraoperative esophageal pressure and the incidence of postoperative dysphagia [5]. This suggests that other factors, such as individual patient anatomy, duration of surgery, and specific hardware used, may also play a role in the development of dysphagia.

Another serious cause of postoperative swallowing dysfunction is the development of postoperative soft tissue swelling, such as wound hematomas, often due to the accumulation of postoperative blood and edema within the surgical site, or rarely, due to direct vascular injury. This complication presents early in the postoperative period as a rapidly-enlarging anterior neck lesion constricting the esophageal lumen and compressing the airways. In addition to causing swallowing dysfunction, these lesions can cause acute deterioration and respiratory compromise, requiring emergent surgical decompression. Incidence of post-operative wound hematomas also varies in the literature, with studies reporting estimates of up to 5% [6]. Strategies to mitigate the risk of this complication include meticulous hemostasis, minimizing soft tissue retraction, and the use of surgical wound drains.

A well-known precursor to speech and swallowing dysfunction following anterior neck surgery is injury to the pharyngeal plexus or the hypoglossal, superior laryngeal, and recurrent laryngeal nerves. These nerves can be damaged directly or indirectly via retraction due to their close proximity to the operating field. Injury to the recurrent laryngeal nerve, for example, can result in vocal cord paralysis, which compromises airway protection during swallowing and increases the risk of aspiration. This complication presents through postoperative hoarseness, cough, dysphagia, and aspiration.

With regard to risk factors influencing the development of postoperative dysphagia following anterior cervical spine surgery, a combination of patient characteristics and intraoperative techniques have been associated with this complication. For example, multilevel surgery, female sex, and the use of recombinant human bone morphogenetic protein 2 (rhBMP-2) have all been identified as significant risk factors for postoperative dysphagia. Multilevel fusions are more likely to develop dysphagia, likely due to the greater amount of tissue retraction and longer operative times associated with these procedures. A possible explanation for why female patients are at higher risk of developing dysphagia may be due to anatomical differences or heightened sensitivity to retraction pressure. The use of rhBMP-2, particularly in multilevel procedures, has also been associated with higher rates of dysphagia due to its pro-inflammatory properties, which can exacerbate tissue swelling and edema postoperatively.

### 3.2 Degenerative disease of the spine and diffuse idiopathic skeletal hyperostosis

In addition to cervical spine procedures, degenerative conditions of the spine, including both age-related and pathologic processes, also contribute swallowing dysfunction. For example, diffuse idiopathic skeletal hyperostosis (DISH) is a rare, non-inflammatory ankylosing condition characterized by calcification and ossification of the spinal ligaments, particularly the anterior longitudinal ligament. This process leads to the formation of extensive, flowing osteophytes, especially in the cervical spine, which can encroach upon the esophageal space and produce mechanical compression on the esophagus (**Figure 2**). The condition predominantly affects older adults, particularly men, and is frequently associated with metabolic comorbidities such as diabetes and hyperlipidemia. The mechanical effects of DISH are often exacerbated when the neck is extended, as osteophytes protrude further into the esophageal space, worsening dysphagia symptoms [8, 9]. In addition to direct mechanical compression, soft tissue inflammation around the osteophytes can lead to fibrosis and formation of adhesions, further narrowing the esophagus and intensifying dysphagia. In more severe cases, impingement by cervical osteophytes may affect nearby nerves. For instance, recurrent laryngeal nerve palsy can occur due to direct compression by such osteophytes, leading to vocal fold dysfunction, which further contributes to dysphagia and may cause hoarseness, vocal fatigue, or choking [9].

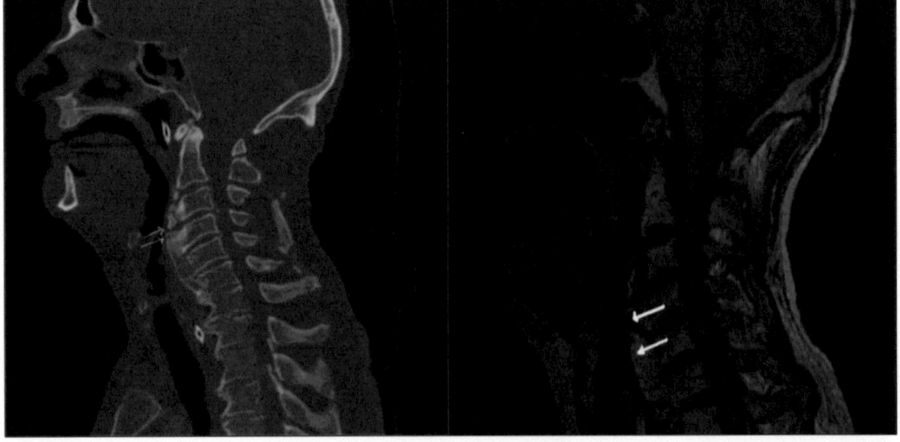

**Figure 2.**
*Sagittal CT (left) and MRI (right) of the neck demonstrating radiographic features of Diffuse Idiopathic Skeletal Hyperostosis (DISH). Bridging osteophytes (arrows) from C3 to C6 contributing to mechanical compression of the esophagus and subsequent dysphagia. Adapted from: Ref. [7].*

More prevalent and common than DISH, however, is the formation of anterior cervical osteophytes due to natural, age-related degenerative processes. These form along the edges of cervical vertebrae and, although generally smaller than the osteophytes seen in DISH, can exert significant mechanical pressure on the esophagus. As with DISH, the dysphagia caused by these osteophytes is primarily mechanical, as the bony protrusions obstruct the esophageal passage or interfere with the normal function of the upper esophageal sphincter. The severity of dysphagia often correlates with the size and precise location of these growths. Large osteophytes, especially those at the C3-C4 level, can affect the normal tilt of the epiglottis, reducing its ability to seal the airway during swallowing. This can result in choking, regurgitation, or even aspiration, particularly in older patients who may already have compromised muscle strength and reflexes.

When conservative measures—such as dietary modifications and swallowing therapy—prove ineffective in managing dysphagia, surgical resection of the osteophytes may be necessary in age-related degeneration and DISH. Surgical intervention is typically reserved for severe cases, where the mechanical obstruction severely limits esophageal function, causing significant risk of aspiration or nutritional deficiency. In these cases, an anterior approach may be used to resect the obstructive osteophytes, often resulting in marked improvement in swallowing function. However, surgery carries its own risks, including potential recurrence of osteophyte formation and post-operative dysphagia as previously outlined, which underscores the need for thorough assessment before proceeding with invasive treatment.

### 3.3 Deformities and postural disorders

Cervical spinal deformities, such as kyphosis, scoliosis, and hyperlordosis, can significantly impact swallowing by altering the anatomical alignment of the esophagus and pharynx. These changes can compress the esophagus and surrounding soft tissues, creating mechanical barriers that interfere with the normal passage of food. For instance, severe scoliosis can displace the pharynx and esophagus laterally, leading to increased pharyngeal residue. As a result, patients with pronounced cervical deformities often experience difficulty coordinating the swallowing process, which can exacerbate dysphagia and increase the likelihood of aspiration pneumonia [2].

Hyperlordosis, characterized by an exaggerated inward curvature of the cervical spine, contributes to swallowing dysfunction by causing posterior bulging of the pharyngeal wall. This reduces the space available for food passage, affecting the efficiency of pharyngeal squeeze and laryngeal elevation. As a result, patients may experience increased difficulty in propelling food through the pharynx, leading to choking or incomplete swallowing. In contrast, severe cervical kyphosis, which involves a reversal of the natural cervical curve, can create a forward-leaning posture that compresses the airway and esophagus, contributing to both swallowing and breathing difficulties. This condition often necessitates surgical correction, especially when associated with significant dysphagia and airway obstruction.

While helpful and deliver relief in many cases, surgical interventions to address spinal deformities, such as occipitocervical fusion can inadvertently worsen dysphagia by creating oropharyngeal stenosis. Malalignment during such surgeries, especially if performed in an excessively flexed position, can lead to airway compression, resulting in postoperative swallowing difficulties.

In addition to acquired deformities, certain congenital conditions are associated with cervical spinal malalignment and dysphagia. For example, Klippel-Feil syndrome (KFS), characterized by congenital fusion of cervical vertebrae, frequently results in a shortened neck and restricted range of motion, complicating the swallowing process due to altered pharyngeal mechanics. The abnormal alignment can compress the esophagus or distort the airway, making both swallowing and breathing more difficult. Similarly, children with Chiari I malformation or craniocervical junction abnormalities often present with coexisting scoliosis and dysphagia, wherein structural compression at the cervicomedullary junction leads to impaired swallowing coordination. These congenital anomalies not only affect the neuromuscular control of the upper digestive tract but can also exacerbate symptoms over time, requiring close monitoring and, in some cases, surgical intervention to prevent severe complications like aspiration and malnutrition [2].

### 3.4 Cervical spine injuries

Cervical spine injuries, especially at the higher vertebral levels (C1-C2) also present a multi-factorial etiology for swallowing dysfunction. These injuries may be due to traumatic (e.g., falls, accidents) or non-traumatic (e.g., tumors, infections) causes. Regardless, the prevalence of dysphagia in cervical spine injury patients has been shown to be significant, present in up to 80% of patients by some estimates [10, 11]. Dysphagia in this group can be attributed to a variety of mechanisms including direct neural injury to the spinal cord and adjacent nerves, surgical treatment, and other associated interventions, such as tracheostomy [12].

Compressive injury to the glossopharyngeal, vagus, and hypoglossal nerves, leads to impaired control over muscles of the neck involved in swallowing, including the sternohyoid, sternothyroid, and thyrohyoid muscles. Damage to the spinal nerves, particularly the phrenic nerve (C3-C5), further complicates swallowing as it impacts the function of the diaphragm and coordination of the respiration-swallowing response, compromising airway protection during swallowing.

In addition to direct neural injury, the management of cervical spine injuries involves interventions that can further complicate swallowing. Surgical procedures for spinal stabilization, particularly those involving the anterior approach, increase the risk of soft tissue trauma, swelling, and scarring, which as discussed previously, can collectively constrict the airways, compress the esophagus, and interfere with normal swallowing mechanics. The use of cervical collars and braces to immobilize the spine can also restrict head and neck movement, causing difficulty in the swallowing phases, particularly the oral and pharyngeal stages. Lastly, tracheostomy, commonly used to support breathing in patients with spinal injuries, hinders normal swallowing mechanics by limiting vocal fold mobility and reducing subglottic pressure, thus preventing bolus propulsion and increasing the risk of dysphagia [10, 13].

### 3.5 Other causes

In addition to direct spinal pathologies, several related neurological and systemic conditions contribute to swallowing dysfunction. Notably, neurodegenerative disorders that do not directly impact the spinal cord can nonetheless affect the nerves and muscles involved in the deglutition process.

Parkinson's disease (PD) is a prime example of such disorders, as it predisposes patients to dysphagia due to progressive neuromuscular impairment. The motor symptoms of PD, including bradykinesia, muscle rigidity, and impaired reflexes, disrupt the precise coordination required for effective swallowing. These impairments commonly affect both the pharyngeal and esophageal phases of swallowing, leading to a heightened risk of aspiration, prolonged swallowing times, and difficulty in managing solid foods. Dysphagia in PD patients is a significant contributor to morbidity, resulting in malnutrition, dehydration, and aspiration pneumonia, which is one of the leading causes of mortality in this patient group [14, 15].

Furthermore, when PD patients undergo cervical spine surgery, such as anterior cervical discectomy and fusion, their risk of postoperative dysphagia increases significantly compared to non-PD patients. Studies indicate that PD patients are approximately three times more likely to require nasogastric tube placement following cervical spine surgery due to severe dysphagia. The preexisting neuromotor deficits inherent to PD complicate the recovery process, as these patients often struggle to regain adequate swallowing function after surgery. This can lead to longer hospital stays, increased reliance on assisted feeding, and a higher incidence of postoperative complications, particularly aspiration pneumonia [14].

Other neurological conditions, such as amyotrophic lateral sclerosis (ALS) and multiple sclerosis (MS), also contribute to dysphagia due to progressive neuromuscular degeneration. The pathophysiology of dysphagia in ALS is multifactorial, including tongue atrophy, impaired closure of the soft palate, and degeneration of the glossopharyngeal, vagus, and hypoglossal nerves. Additionally, neuromuscular degeneration affects the diaphragm and compromises the coordination of swallowing and breathing. These impairments lead to a high incidence of aspiration pneumonia, malnutrition, and dehydration, which are common causes of death in ALS patients [16, 17].

Multiple sclerosis, characterized by demyelination of the central nervous system, can affect the cranial nerves involved in swallowing, leading to coordination deficits in the oral, pharyngeal, and esophageal phases. Both ALS and MS patients are at risk for progressive dysphagia that worsens over time, necessitating regular swallowing assessments and, in advanced stages, the use of feeding tubes to maintain adequate nutrition.

## 4. Prevention, management, and treatment

Addressing the risk of dysphagia due to spinal etiologies requires a comprehensive approach aimed at preventing, detecting, and managing swallowing dysfunction. Preventative measures are particularly important for reducing the risk of postoperative dysphagia. Prevention involves meticulous surgical planning and execution, especially in procedures involving the anterior cervical spine. For example, the use of smaller endotracheal tubes and ensuring proper alignment during intubation can help reduce prevertebral soft tissue swelling in the postoperative period.

During surgery, optimizing techniques, such as sharp dissection rather than blunt methods, is critical for minimizing tissue trauma and inflammation. Furthermore, reducing excessive retraction pressure on the esophagus can help prevent mechanical trauma, edema, or scarring. Gentle, short-duration retraction significantly lowers the risk of direct injury to the esophageal wall. Special care should also be taken to protect critical nerves involved in swallowing, particularly the recurrent laryngeal nerve, which is highly susceptible to traction injury at the C5–C6 level. Awareness of anatomic variations and the use of intraoperative nerve monitoring are key strategies to avoid inadvertent damage. Proper placement of anterior plates and screws is also essential to prevent impingement on the esophagus or displacement into adjacent structures [18].

In addition, pharmacological interventions, such as intraoperative administration of corticosteroids, have demonstrated effectiveness in reducing postoperative swelling and improving early swallowing outcomes [2, 3, 18]. Finally, for multilevel surgeries, selecting less invasive options where possible may decrease esophageal pressure and reduce the risk of postoperative dysphagia compared to techniques with extensive anterior plating.

The management of dysphagia in patients with spinal etiologies varies depending on the underlying cause, severity of dysfunction, and the specific swallowing physiology, and involves both conservative and surgical approaches. Treatment frequently requires multi-disciplinary care by various providers, including speech pathologists, occupational therapists, nutritionists, otolaryngologists, neurologists, and surgeons. Postural adjustments, such as chin-tucking, head lifting, rotating or tilting the head, or lying down, can assist in improving the flow of food and modifying the relationship between the oropharyngeal structures during swallowing. Dietary modifications, such as gradually increasing the viscosity of liquids or using pureed foods, can help in cases where patients cannot follow directions. Exercise programs are another treatment option, aimed at improving structural movement during swallowing, increasing airway closure, and strengthening the tongue.

For dysphagia following anterior cervical spine injuries and procedures, conservative treatments such as swallowing therapy, dietary modifications, and speech therapy are often the first line of treatment. However, immediate surgical intervention may sometimes be necessary in cases of compressive soft tissue hematomas, which in addition to causing severe swallowing dysfunction can expand rapidly and cause progressive compression of the airways and respiratory failure. In cases where dysphagia persists, endoscopic evaluation of swallowing or videofluoroscopy can help identify the underlying issues and guide further treatment.

Management of dysphagia in DISH ranges from conservative to surgical interventions, depending on the severity of symptoms. For mild cases, conservative treatment with nonsteroidal anti-inflammatory drugs (NSAIDs) and muscle relaxants can help reduce inflammation and relieve symptoms. In more severe cases, where significant mechanical obstruction occurs, surgical resection of the osteophytes may be necessary to restore esophageal patency and alleviate symptoms, commonly through the anterior neck approach. However, the risk of esophageal injury and nerve damage during surgery must be considered and balanced against the benefits. Recurrence of osteophytes remains common even after surgical resection.

In patients with neurodegenerative disorders, the management of dysphagia is more complex due to the progressive nature of these diseases. Intensive speech therapy and close monitoring of swallowing function are crucial. When dysphagia becomes severe, interventions such as feeding tube placement may be required to prevent malnutrition and aspiration pneumonia.

## 5. Conclusions

Swallowing dysfunctions resulting from spinal disorders pose significant challenges for both patients and clinicians. The interplay between structural abnormalities, postoperative complications, and underlying neurological conditions necessitates a comprehensive approach to diagnosis and treatment. Early detection and intervention are critical for improving patient outcomes, as delays in addressing dysphagia can lead to severe complications like malnutrition, aspiration pneumonia, and reduced quality of life. In cases of mechanical obstruction, surgical intervention may be required to restore esophageal patency. By thoroughly understanding the multifactorial causes of dysphagia and customizing treatment plans, clinicians can not only mitigate symptoms but also enhance long-term functional recovery. Continued research into less invasive surgical techniques and multidisciplinary rehabilitation strategies will be essential to advance patient care.

## Conflict of interest

The authors declare no conflict of interest or financial interests.

## Author details

Samir Alsalek[1], Nghiem H. Nguyen[1] and Shayan U. Rahman[2*]

1 Kaiser Permanente Bernard J. Tyson School of Medicine, Pasadena, CA, United States

2 Department of Neurological Surgery, Kaiser Permanente Los Angeles Medical Center, Los Angeles, CA, United States

*Address all correspondence to: shayan.x.rahman@kp.org

## References

[1] Logemann JA, Larsen K. Oropharyngeal dysphagia: Pathophysiology and diagnosis for the anniversary issue of diseases of the esophagus. Diseases of the Esophagus. 2012;**25**(4):299-304. DOI: 10.1111/j.1442-2050.2011.01210.x

[2] Papadopoulou S, Exarchakos G, Beris A, Ploumis A. Dysphagia associated with cervical spine and postural disorders. Dysphagia. 2013;**28**(4):469-480. DOI: 10.1007/s00455-013-9484-7

[3] Riley LH 3rd, Vaccaro AR, Dettori JR, Hashimoto R. Postoperative dysphagia in anterior cervical spine surgery. Spine (Phila Pa 1976). 2010;**35**(9 Suppl):S76-S85. DOI: 10.1097/BRS.0b013e3181d81a96

[4] Daniels AH, Riew KD, Yoo JU, et al. Adverse events associated with anterior cervical spine surgery. The Journal of the American Academy of Orthopaedic Surgeons. 2008;**16**(12):729-738. DOI: 10.5435/00124635-200812000-00005

[5] Papavero L, Heese O, Klotz-Regener V, Buchalla R, Schröder F, Westphal M. The impact of esophagus retraction on early dysphagia after anterior cervical surgery: Does a correlation exist? Spine (Phila Pa 1976). 2007;**32**(10):1089-1093. DOI: 10.1097/01.brs.0000261627.04944.cf

[6] Fountas KN, Kapsalaki EZ, Nikolakakos LG, et al. Anterior cervical discectomy and fusion associated complications. Spine (Phila Pa 1976). 2007;**32**(21):2310-2317. DOI: 10.1097/BRS.0b013e318154c57e

[7] Krishnarasa B, Vivekanandarajah A, Ripoll L, Chang E, Wetz R. Diffuse idiopathic skeletal hyperostosis (DISH)—A rare etiology of dysphagia. Clinical Medicine Insights: Arthritis and Musculoskeletal Disorders. 2011;**4**:71-75

[8] Le HV, Wick JB, Van BW, Klineberg EO. Diffuse idiopathic skeletal hyperostosis of the spine: Pathophysiology, diagnosis, and management. The Journal of the American Academy of Orthopaedic Surgeons. 2021;**29**(24):1044-1051. DOI: 10.5435/JAAOS-D-20-01344

[9] Lee JH, Paeng SH, Pyo SY, Kim ST, Lee WH. Swallowing difficulty in diffuse idiopathic skeletal hyperostosis with metabolic syndrome. Korean Journal of Neurotrauma. 2020;**16**(1):90-98. Published 2020 Apr 1. DOI: 10.13004/kjnt.2020.16.e4

[10] Choi JW, Kim DY, Joo SY, Park D, Chang MC. Evaluation of clinical factors predicting dysphagia in patients with traumatic and non-traumatic cervical spinal cord injury: A retrospective study. Frontiers in Neurology. 2024;**15**:1376171. Published 2024 May 15. DOI: 10.3389/fneur.2024.1376171

[11] McRae J, Morgan S, Wallace E, Miles A. Oropharyngeal dysphagia in acute cervical spinal cord injury: A literature review. Dysphagia. 2023;**38**(4):1025-1038. DOI: 10.1007/s00455-022-10535-0

[12] Hayashi T, Fujiwara Y, Sakai H, Maeda T, Ueta T, Shiba K. Risk factors for severe dysphagia in acute cervical spinal cord injury. Spinal Cord. 2017;**55**(10):940-943. DOI: 10.1038/sc.2017.63

[13] Wolf C, Meiners TH. Dysphagia in patients with acute cervical spinal cord

injury. Spinal Cord. 2003;**41**(6):347-353. DOI: 10.1038/sj.sc.3101440

[14] Avila MJ, Aguilar-Salinas P, Burket AR, Dumont TM. Parkinson disease, dysphagia, and cervical spine surgery. Clinical Spine Surgery. 2022;**35**(1):E26-E30. DOI: 10.1097/BSD.0000000000001197

[15] Suttrup I, Warnecke T. Dysphagia in Parkinson's disease. Dysphagia. 2016;**31**(1):24-32. DOI: 10.1007/s00455-015-9671-9

[16] Onesti E, Schettino I, Gori MC, et al. Dysphagia in amyotrophic lateral sclerosis: Impact on patient behavior, diet adaptation, and Riluzole management. Frontiers in Neurology. 2017;**8**:94. Published 2017 Mar 21. DOI: 10.3389/fneur.2017.00094

[17] Mariani L, Ruoppolo G, Cilfone A, et al. Progression of oropharyngeal dysphagia in amyotrophic lateral sclerosis: A retrospective cohort study. Dysphagia. 2022;**37**(4):868-878. DOI: 10.1007/s00455-021-10346-9

[18] Alentado VJ, Bisson EF, Potts EA. Dysphagia after cervical spine surgery: A review of risk factors and preventative measures. Journal of Neurosurgery. Spine. 2022;**38**(3):382-388. Published 2022 Dec 16. DOI: 10.3171/2022.11.SPINE221247

Chapter 9

# Dysphagia Caused by Esophageal Neoplasms: Approach and Management

*Lilamani Rajthala*


## Abstract

Esophageal carcinoma has been one of the leading causes of cancer deaths worldwide due to its higher stage at the time of diagnosis and poor prognosis. The incidence of esophageal adenocarcinoma (EAC) is increasing even though the incidence of esophageal squamous cell carcinoma (ESCC) has declined. Tobacco and smoking are the prominent risk factors for ESCC while Barrett's esophagus (BE) is a known precursor lesion for EAC. Dysphasia is the most common presentation while patients may also present with fatigue, retrosternal pain, anemia, weight loss, and even hoarseness. An endoscopic biopsy is required for definitive diagnosis. BE with suspicious morphology is evaluated with multiple biopsies. High-grade dysplasia and intramucosal carcinoma associated with BE are treated with endoscopic resection followed by ablative therapies. For staging of esophageal carcinoma, endoscopic ultrasound, computed tomography (CT), and positron emission tomography (PET)/CT have crucial roles. Early-stage lesions limited to mucosa and submucosa can be cured with endoscopic resection while nodal metastasis and deeper lesions mandate esophagectomy. Trimodal therapy including chemoradiation followed by surgery has increased the overall survival. The unresectable disease is treated with multimodal therapy with systemic therapy. The addition of novel agents like trastuzumab, nivolumab, and pembrolizumab to conventional chemotherapy has encouraging outcomes.


**Keywords:** dysphagia, Barrett's esophagus, esophageal carcinoma, esophagectomy, trimodal therapy

## 1. Introduction

Esophageal cancer (EC) is one of the most aggressive gastrointestinal cancers characterized by its high mortality rate, poor prognosis, and higher stage at the time of diagnosis [1]. Squamous cell carcinoma and adenocarcinoma comprise the vast majority of esophageal cancers [2]. The incidence of esophageal adenocarcinoma (EAC) has rapidly increased in the Western world, surpassing esophageal squamous cell carcinoma (ESCC) as the most prevalent type of esophageal malignancy.

Esophageal cancer is the eighth most common type of cancer worldwide and presents as the sixth leading cause of cancer deaths [3]. Efforts have targeted prevention and early identification, screening, surveying, and treating Barrett's esophagus (BE), the only established precursor of EAC [4]. Advances in endoscopic eradication therapy, and management of Barrett's-related dysplasia and early EAC have obviated the need for esophagectomy in many patients presenting with localized lesions. Other rare types of esophageal tumors include mesenchymal tumors, neuroendocrine cancers, and benign tumors [5].

The objective of the chapter highlights the clinical presentation, approach, and investigation of patients presenting with dysphasia secondary to BE and EC. Recent guidelines for the management of early, advanced and metastatic esophageal carcinoma along with palliative therapy for dysphagia are discussed in this chapter.

## 2. Epidemiology

The incidence and mortality of EC have wide geographical variations [6]. In 2019, 17,650 new cases of EC were detected in the United States, with a total of 16,080 deaths due to EC [7]. The most common type of EC is ESCC. However, the incidence of ESCC is declining and the incidence of EAC has peaked sharply during the past four decades and has become the major type of EC in Western countries [8]. The age-standardized death rates of EC decreased from 23.19/100,000 in 1973–1975 to 13.73/100,000 in 2004–2005, showing a decline of 59%, in China [8]. Similarly, in the United States, the incidence rate of ESCC in African Americans is much higher than in European Americans, but the overall incidence has declined during the past decades. A similar decline is also noticed in Asian/Pacific Islander and Hispanic groups. In males, the incidence rates for both types of carcinomas are 2- to 3-fold higher than in females; however, the trend of decreasing ESCC and increasing EAC are similar [9]. However, the National Cancer Report 2010 issued by the Robert Koch Institute showed an incidence of 5200 for EC in Germany—with a 4:1 preponderance in male patients [10]. The gradual decrease in the incidence of ESCC in the past decades has been attributed to the improvement in diet and nutrition in many populations [11].

## 3. Etiology

### 3.1 ESCC

Tobacco smoking and alcohol consumption have been the established major risk factors for ESCC. The risk of ESCC increases linearly with increasing consumption when alcohol ingestion exceeds 170 g/week [12]. Smoking increases the risk by nine-fold compared to nonsmokers (hazard ratio 9.3; 95% CI: 4.0–21.3) [13]. Other risk factors included low intake of fruits and vegetables with deficiencies of vitamin and trace elements. Nitrosamines and polyaromatic hydrocarbons play a role as carcinogens. Consumption of hot beverages, chewing betel quid, and extremely high intake of salt are associated with increased risk of ESCC. The association between HPV 16 and 18 with ESCC has been inconsistent [8]. Worldwide, parts of the Middle East, Central Asia, and China have the highest rates of SCC, after adjusting for tobacco and alcohol use, indicating genetic predisposition or other environmental factors behind the pathogenesis of ESCC [5]. ESCC is associated with certain intrinsic disorders of the esophagus, such as Plummer-Vinson syndrome and achalasia. Tylosis and Fanconi anemia are the hereditary cancer syndromes associated with esophageal SCC. Patients with a history of caustic ingestion have a significantly increased risk for ESCC [5].

### 3.2 EAC

Regarding EAC, it is now the most common histologic type in the United States even though it is relatively rare among African Americans and Asian Americans [5]. BE and gastroesophageal reflux disease (GERD) have been the major risk factors. Other etiology includes obesity, cigarette smoking, low intake of fiber, alcohol consumption, and genetic susceptibility [8]. The development of BE is strongly associated with GERD and obesity. Metaplastic BE is characterized by increased cellular proliferation and turnover with an increased risk of progression to neoplasia. Reports suggest a 30- to 40-fold increased risk of the development of EAC with metaplastic BE [14].

Normal esophageal lining comprises squamous epithelium. The chronic insult by gastric acid reflux results in the metaplastic transformation of the squamous epithelial lining into columnar epithelium. This condition is known as BE. The estimated prevalence of BE is 1.6% in the general population, but the incidence increases in patients with GERD [15]. Increasing age, male gender, chronic GERD, tobacco usage, family history of BE, Caucasian race, and central obesity are the risk factors associated with BE. The risk of malignant transformation of metaplastic columnar epithelium of BE into adenocarcinoma is minimal which is less than 0.5% per year. However, the incidence of EAC is increasing and the prognosis is poor with 5-year overall survival rate of <20%. The epidemiological trend and unfavorable prognosis advocate the need for well-designed screening and surveillance methods [16].

## 4. Clinical presentation

The majority of cases are diagnosed during the evaluation of symptoms related to EC. Only few patients (<1%) are diagnosed during BE surveillance without any symptoms. Dysphagia is the most common presentation. Approximately, 74 to 83% of patients diagnosed with esophageal carcinoma present initially with difficulty in swallowing [17]. It is characterized by progressive dysphagia, initially with solid food and later progressing to liquid as well. Adaptive behaviors like chewing more thoroughly, avoiding hard foods, or drinking liquids with swallows temporarily ease the patients. Thus, patients seek medical attention only when the dysphagia has become problematic and the majority have weight loss. Many patients with EAC recall a long history of reflux symptoms including heartburn and regurgitation. Fatigue, retrosternal pain, and anemia are the associated presenting symptoms. Locally advanced tumors may manifest with laryngeal nerve involvement causing hoarseness or even with tracheoesophageal fistula. Cervical and supraclavicular lymphadenopathy might be present in the examination. Early-stage tumors are often asymptomatic and are occasionally discovered during endoscopy performed for BE [5]. The clinical presentation of patients with esophageal carcinoma is summarized in **Table 1**.

| Barrett's esophagus | Esophageal carcinoma |
|---|---|
| Most commonly gastroesophageal reflux | Dysphagia |
| Retrosternal burning sensation | Weight loss |
| Dysphagia | Pain abdomen |
| Globus | Chest pain |
| Cough | Upper GI bleed |
| Chest pain | Gastroesophageal reflux |
| Laryngitis | Nausea and vomiting |
| Rarely asymptomatic | Fatigue |

**Table 1.**
*Presenting symptoms of Barrett's esophagus and esophageal carcinoma.*

## 5. Diagnosis and staging

Irregular filling defects and ulcerations may be prominent features in the barium esophagogram. A symmetrical and circumferential narrowing would create a classical 'apple core' filling defect. Endoscopic biopsy establishes the definitive diagnosis of esophageal cancer. Early tumors may be visualized as small nodules or ulcerations while advanced tumors are more friable, ulcerated, and necrotic masses associated with stricture formation (**Figure 1**). Multiple biopsies may be required for suspicious lesions as there is a high probability of false negative results [5]. Four quadrant biopsies at the interval of 1 cm along the length of BE and additional targeted biopsy from the suspicious area enhance the diagnostic yield. Chromoendoscopy and narrow-band imaging enable better visualization of the lesions.

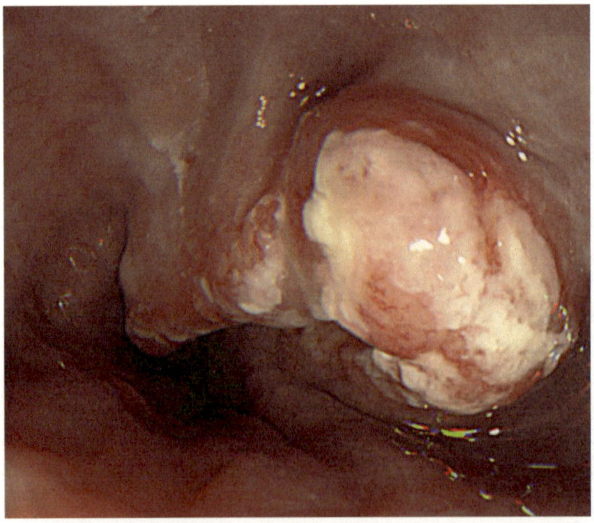

**Figure 1.**
*Endoscopic image of esophageal squamous cell carcinoma showing nodular lesion with ulceration and necrosis (Source: Brooks et al. [18]. License: CC BY 2.5).*

After the definite diagnosis of EC, accurate staging is mandatory to guide the appropriate therapy and prediction of prognosis. The 8th edition of the American Joint Committee on Cancer (AJCC) staging of epithelial cancers (**Tables 2** and **3**, **Figure 2**) of the esophagus and esophagogastric junction (EGJ) has acknowledged

| Category | Criteria |
|---|---|
| T category | |
| TX | Tumor cannot be assessed |
| T0 | No evidence of primary tumor |
| Tis | High-grade dysplasia, defined as malignant cells confined by the basement membrane |
| T1 | Tumor invades the lamina propria, muscularis mucosae, or submucosa |
| T1a | Tumor invades the lamina propria or muscularis mucosae |
| T1b | Tumor invades the submucosa |
| T2 | Tumor invades the muscularis propria |
| T3 | Tumor invades adventitia |
| T4 | Tumor invades adjacent structures |
| T4a | Tumor invades the pleura, pericardium, azygos vein, diaphragm, or peritoneum |
| T4b | Tumor invades other adjacent structures, such as aorta, vertebral body, or trachea |
| N category | |
| NX | Regional lymph nodes cannot be assessed |
| N0 | No regional lymph node metastasis |
| N1 | Metastasis in 1–2 regional lymph nodes |
| N2 | Metastasis in 3–6 regional lymph nodes |
| N3 | Metastasis in 7 or more regional lymph nodes |
| M category | |
| M0 | No distant metastasis |
| M1 | Distant metastasis |
| Adenocarcinoma G category | |
| GX | Differentiation cannot be assessed |
| G1 | Well-differentiated, >95% of tumor is composed of well-formed glands |
| G2 | Moderately differentiated. 50–95% of tumor shows gland formation |
| G3 | Poorly differentiated. Tumors composed of nest and sheets of cells with <50% of tumor demonstrating glandular formation |
| Squamous cell carcinoma G category | |
| GX | Differentiation cannot be assessed |
| G1 | Well-differentiated. Prominent keratinization with pearl formation and a minor component of nonkeratinizing basal-like cells. Tumor cells are arranged in sheets, and mitotic counts are low. |
| G2 | Moderately differentiated. Variable histologic features, ranging from parakeratotic to poorly keratinizing lesions. Generally, pearl formation is absent. |
| G3 | Poorly differentiated. Consists predominantly of basal-like cells forming large and small nests with frequent central necrosis. The nests consist of sheets or pavement-like arrangements of tumor cells, and occasionally are punctuated by small numbers of parakeratotic or keratinizing cells. |

| Category | Criteria |
|---|---|
| Squamous cell carcinoma L category (defined by epicenter of esophageal tumor) | |
| LX | Location unknown |
| Upper | Cervical esophagus to lower border of azygos vein |
| Middle | Lower border of azygos vein to lower border of inferior pulmonary vein |
| Lower | Lower border of inferior pulmonary vein to stomach, including esophagogastric junction |

**Table 2.**
*AJCC 8th edition TNM staging for esophageal and gastroesophageal junction carcinoma.*

| Clinical stage | cT | cN | cM |
|---|---|---|---|
| Squamous cell carcinoma | | | |
| 0 | Tis | N0 | M0 |
| I | T1 | N0–1 | M0 |
| II | T2 | N0–1 | M0 |
| | T3 | N0 | M0 |
| III | T3 | N1 | M0 |
| | T1–3 | N2 | M0 |
| IVA | T4 | N0–2 | M0 |
| | T1–4 | N3 | M0 |
| IVB | T1–4 | N0–3 | M1 |
| Adenocarcinoma | | | |
| 0 | Tis | N0 | M0 |
| I | T1 | N0 | M0 |
| IIA | T1 | N1 | M0 |
| IIB | T2 | N0 | M0 |
| III | T2 | N1 | M0 |
| | T3–4a | N0–1 | M0 |
| IVA | T1–4a | N2 | M0 |
| | T4b | N0–2 | M0 |
| | T1–4 | N3 | M0 |
| IVB | T1–4 | N0–3 | M1 |

**Table 3.**
*Clinical staging (cTNM) of esophageal carcinoma.*

separate classifications for clinical (cTNM), pathologic (pTNM), and post-neoadjuvant (ypTNM) stage groups [19]. Adenocarcinomas with epicenters no more than 2 cm into the gastric cardia are staged as EACs. The extensions beyond that are staged as gastric cancers [20]. The genetic analysis of cancer cells may more accurately identify the cellular origin of cancer rather than its gross location [19]. Although clinical staging facilitates decision-making, it may not reflect the pathologic stage.

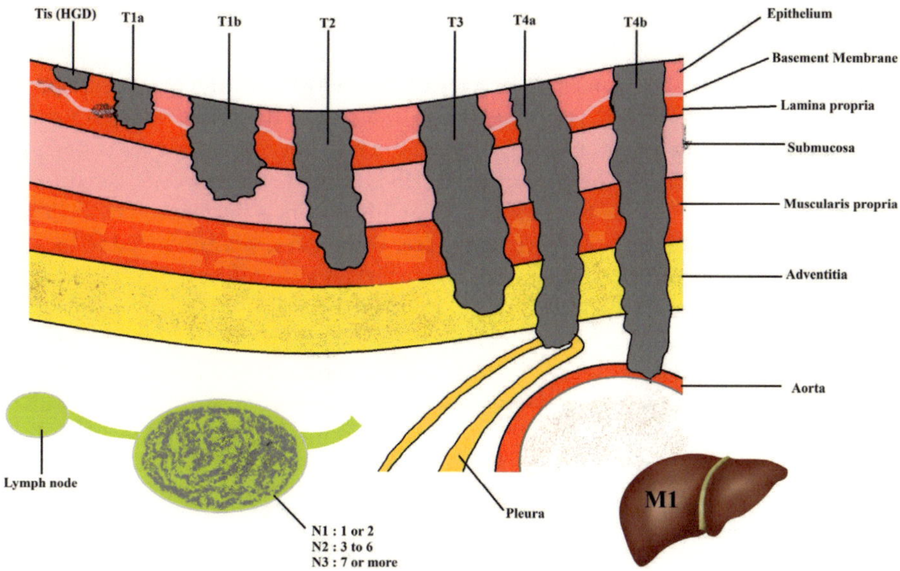


**Figure 2.**
*Schematic diagram showing TNM staging of esophageal carcinoma.*

## 5.1 Diagnostic workup

National Comprehensive Cancer Network (NCCN) guidelines, 2024 for esophageal carcinoma highlights the following diagnostic workup in the evaluation of the patients:

- History and physical examination,
- Upper gastrointestinal endoscopy and biopsy,
- Contrast-enhanced chest and abdominal CT,
- FDG-PET/CT if there is no evidence of metastasis in CECT,
- Endoscopic ultrasound,
- Endoscopic resection for T1a and T1b,
- Testing for microsatellite instability (MSI) and Mismatch gene repair (MMR),
- Programmed cell death ligand 1 (PD-L1) and HER2 testing for metastatic disease,
- Bronchoscopy for esophageal lesions above carina,
- Nutritional assessment and rehabilitation, and
- Screening for family history and syndromic association.

### 5.2 Endoscopic biopsy

Superficial and small lesions may be excised by endoscopic mucosal resection (EMR) and evaluated for depth of penetration and risk of nodal metastasis. For T1a lesions, further staging may not be required as the risk of lymph node metastasis is very low. For earlier lesions, the accuracy of EUS is lower [21]. However, the differentiation between T1 or T2 tumors and T3 or T4 tumors is performed by EUS with high efficiency and accuracy [22]. Furthermore, the accuracy is enhanced in locally advanced EC than in comparison with early cancers. A systemic review demonstrated the sensitivity and specificity of EUS increased from 81.6 and 99.4% in T1 tumors to 81.4 and 96.3% in T2 tumors, respectively in cancer staging. In addition, the sensitivity and specificity further increase as the tumor stage increases from 91.4 and 94.4% in T3 tumors to 92.4 and 97.4% in T4 tumors [23]. In the contrary, the accuracy of EUS restaging after chemoradiation is poor, due to architectural distortion and post-treatment inflammation and fibrosis [24].

### 5.3 Imaging and metastatic workup

Contrast-enhanced computed tomography (CECT) of chest and abdomen, and positron emission tomography (PET)/CT are recommended for evaluation of distant metastatic disease. The CT cannot delineate different layers of esophageal wall. Hence, accurate radiological differentiation of lesion into cT1, cT2 and cT3 preoperatively is difficult. However, the infiltration of lesion across the fat plane adjacent to serosa into surrounding structures determines the clinical stage to be cT4 [25]. Local invasion can be identified with indentation or displacement of the surrounding structures in addition to the loss of adjacent fat planes [26]. The sensitivity and specificity of CT for detection of involvement of mediastinal structures ranges from 85 to 100%. For larger lesions, EUS is superior for the assessment of T and N stages in comparison to PET or CT. In addition, bronchoscopy should also be performed for tumors above the carina to rule out direct tracheal invasion. Appropriate decision-making is guided by the accurate staging of the cancer. T1a lesions can be treated by endoscopic resection while locally advanced lesions (T2 with nodal metastasis or T3) may require definite surgery with chemotherapy and radiation. Metastatic cancer requires palliative or systemic therapy [5].

## 6. Management of esophageal carcinoma

### 6.1 Management of Barrett's esophagus (BE)

BE is the only known precursor lesion of EAC. Currently, there are evidences of decrease in mortality from EAC with a screening program for BE [27]. Although screening in the general population is not routinely recommended, it may be considered in individuals with high risk. Men with chronic (>5 years) and/or frequent (weekly or more) symptoms of gastroesophageal reflux not responding to medical therapy can be possible candidates for screening [28]. The American College of Gastroenterology (ACG) recommends the diagnosis, screening, surveillance, and endoscopic and medical therapy of BE. Routine endoscopic biopsies are not recommended in the absence of visible lesions. At least 8 endoscopic biopsies should be obtained with the Seattle protocol for segments of longer than 4 cm if the endoscopic findings suggest BE [29]. Both white light endoscopy and chromoendoscopy are recommended in endoscopic surveillance of BE. Endoscopic eradication therapy is required if the biopsy shows high-grade dysplasia (HGD) or intramucosal carcinoma (IMC) [29]. Endoscopic eradication therapy is also recommended in patients with low-grade dysplasia (LGD) as it reduces the risk of progression to HGD or EAC. However, close endoscopic surveillance in every 3–5 years is also an alternative [27].

#### *6.1.1 Ablative therapies for BE*

##### *6.1.1.1 Radiofrequency ablation*

Endoscopic resection (ER) of any visible lesion followed by ablative techniques such as radiofrequency ablation (RFA) and cryotherapy are practiced for complete eradication. RFA has demonstrated the highest efficacy and effectiveness along with minimal complications [30]. In RFA, thermal energy is delivered to the esophageal mucosa via an endoscope which results in tissue necrosis. The overall safety data is encouraging. The pooled rate of adverse events from RFA was reported up to 8.8% which included esophageal strictures (5.6%), bleeding (1%), and perforation (0.6%) [30]. The AIM-Dysplasia trial was the landmark trial that demonstrated high efficacy of RFA in BE. This was a multicenter, sham-controlled study, in which 127 patients with dysplastic BE were enrolled in this study. The patients were assigned to RFA or a sham procedure group randomly. Ninety one percent of patients with LGD and 81% with HGD in the ablation group, compared with 23 and 19% in the control group ($P < 0.001$) respectively, achieved complete eradication at follow-up after 12 months [31].

##### *6.1.1.2 Cryotherapy*

Cryotherapy is another emerging technique designed for endoscopic management of BE, and related dysplasia and neoplasia. Various modalities of cryotherapy have been introduced. The spray catheter can use carbon dioxide or liquid nitrogen as a cryogen. Liquid nitrogen is the most widely utilized and studied method of cryotherapy [16]. A meta-analysis incorporated nine studies and 386 patients who were treated with cryotherapy. The complete eradication rate of HGD and IMC was 86.5 and 56.5% respectively. Furthermore, in subgroup patients who failed RFA, the eradication rate of IMC was 58.4% and HGD was 81.9% [32].

##### *6.1.1.3 Image enhanced endoscopy*

Novel image-enhanced endoscopies with surface enhancement, tone enhancement, and contrast enhancement can allow detailed observation of a mucosal surface structure [33]. A study indicated that the sensitivity, specificity, positive predictive value (PPV), and negative predictive value (NPV) for the prediction of dysplasia/early cancer using Narrow Band Imaging (NBI) overview and narrow band imaging-dual focus were 100, 93.8, 68.6, 100% and 100, 86.2, 73.3, 100%, respectively. The study also demonstrated an overall reduction in the number of biopsies with NBI endoscopy compared to white light, also detecting the dysplastic or neoplastic lesions with a high success rate [34]. Virtual chromoendoscopy adds no cost, additional time, or risk to the patient while adding accuracy to the diagnosis in routine endoscopy [27]. It is difficult to differentiate between microscopic tumor invasion and peritumoral inflammatory changes with EUS. Hence, EUS may overclassify dysplasia. EUS remains an appropriate technique to assess nodal status before performing endoscopic treatment.

#### *6.1.1.4 Endoscopic resection of BE*

Endoscopic mucosal resection (EMR) is an endoscopic technique adapted for possible curative resection of earlier esophageal lesions. This involves the dissection of submucosal layer via injection of saline or a solution mixed with a dye such as methylene blue resulting in formation of "submucosal cushion". The mucosa is then resected by snare [35]. Endoscopic submucosal dissection (ESD) is a more complex technique that creates a submucosal tract to dissect lesions restricted to the mucosa. HGD associated with BE should be treated with EMR and/or ablation therapy. Endoscopic eradication has an admirable success rate up to 83.7% while untreated patients have a high probability of progression to EAC [36]. ESD is more appropriate for larger lesions. In a study by O Pech et al., that included 1000 patients with T1a Barrett's mucosal adenocarcinoma undergoing EMR, the complete response rate was 96.3%. Surgery was necessary in 3.7% of the patients during the follow-up period of 5 years. Metachronous neoplasia was detected in 14.5% and could be re-treated, yielding a long-term complete remission rate of 93.8% and a calculated 10-year survival rate of patients of 75% [37].

The success rate of EMR for curative resection of lesions larger than 20 mm is not satisfactory. The lesions are excised in a piecemeal fashion and hence, the margins cannot be assessed for complete resection. This may result in residual disease and local recurrence [38]. This risk of inadequate resection margins can be avoided by ESD. It offers en bloc dissection regardless of lesion sizes and locations, along with the lateral and deep margins [39]. ESD has higher en bloc rates (96 vs. 50%) and R0 resection rates (82 vs. 40%) with fewer recurrences (2.5 vs. 12.4%) in comparison to EMR. Complication rates of endoscopic resection are low for both techniques. They include perforation, bleeding, and strictures. Stricture is more common after mucosal resection of more than 70–80% of the circumference [40]. EMR is preferable for lesions ≤10 mm, with similar en bloc resection, curative resection, and local recurrence rates in comparison to ESD with an advantage of shorter procedure time. For patients with lesions between 11 and 20 mm, both EMR and ESD are equivocal in terms of recurrence rate. ESD is the most appropriate choice for lesions >20 mm. The techniques of ESD need to be refined to shorten the procedure time avoiding procedure-related complications [38].

### 6.2 Management of early-stage esophageal cancer (T1a and T1b)

Endoscopic resection has been the mainstay of therapy for smaller lesions (Tis and T1a, ≤2 cm, and well or moderately differentiated carcinoma) because the risk of nodal involvement, local or distant recurrence, and mortality following esophageal cancer are low following endoscopic therapy. Larger lesions may be amenable to endoscopic intervention depending on the availability of advanced expertise. The goal of EMR, ESD, and/or ablation is the complete removal or eradication of early-stage disease and pre-neoplastic tissue associated with BE. Complete evaluation for the presence of nodularity, and lateral spread, and ruling out multifocal disease and lymph node metastases by EUS is of immense value. Areas of nodularity or ulceration and flat, small lesions (≤2 cm) of squamous cell HGD/Tis (carcinoma in situ) should be treated by ER as it provides more accurate histologic assessment. Larger flat lesions (>2 cm) are associated with a greater risk of complications. The successful curative resection rate is governed by various anatomical factors like size of the lesion less than 20 mm, presentation at an earlier clinical stage (T1a) and location of lesions in middle or distal esophagus [41]. The level of evidence for ablation of ESCC after ER is low.

In cases of early adenocarcinoma, the criteria for curative resection include complete (R0) resection with clear lateral and vertical margins, no lymphovascular invasion, and tumor grading G1/2. Infiltration depth of <500 μm into submucosal is acceptable [42]. Complete ablation of the remaining Barrett's epithelium starting from 5 to 10 mm above the squamocolumnar junction to 5–10 mm distal to the "neo Z-line" is recommended. The neo-z-line is the area at the gastroesophageal junction (GEJ) immediately above the top of the gastric fold. Alternatives to RFA are argon plasma coagulation, cryo-ablation, or photodynamic therapy [43].

### 6.3 Management of locally advanced esophageal carcinoma

Trimodal therapy with a combination of neoadjuvant chemoradiation therapy followed by esophagectomy has been established as the treatment option for locally advanced tumors (T2 or with nodal involvement) while for metastatic disease (Stage IV), systemic therapy with chemoradiation to sites of disease involvement would be appropriate [44]. Esophagectomy for operable non-metastatic patients with T1b or greater primary lesions and/or any nodal disease are performed with transhiatal, transthoracic, three field, and, increasingly, minimally invasive approaches [35]. Esophageal resection should be considered for all physiologically fit patients with resectable esophageal cancer (>5 cm from cricopharyngeus). In patients with advanced tumors, clinical T3 or N+ disease should be considered for laparoscopic staging with peritoneal washings as positive peritoneal cytology indicates M1 disease and poor prognosis. The extent of local extension and nodal stage defines the resectability of the tumor (**Table 4**).

#### *6.3.1 Esophagectomy*

The type of resection depends on the location of the tumor, the available choices for conduit, as well as by the surgical expertise and patient's preference [45]. Since

| Resectable esophageal cancer | Unresectable esophageal cancer |
|---|---|
| • T1a tumors, defined as tumors involving the mucosa but not invading the submucosa, may be considered for EMR + ablation or esophagectomy in experienced centers.<br>• Tumors in the submucosa (T1b) or deeper.<br>• T1–T3 tumors with regional nodal metastases (N+), although bulky.<br>• Multi-station lymphatic involvement is a relative contraindication.<br>• T4a tumors with involvement of pericardium, pleura, or diaphragm. | • cT4b tumors with involvement of the heart, great vessels, trachea, or adjacent organs including liver, pancreas, and lung.<br>• Multi-station, bulky lymphadenopathy with other factors, including age, performance status, and response to therapy indicating poor outcome.<br>• Supraclavicular lymph node involvement should be considered unresectable.<br>• Distant metastases (stage IV) and non-regional lymph node metastasis. |

**Table 4.**
*Resectability of esophageal cancer.*

dysphagia secondary esophageal neoplasm results in poor nutritional status, preoperative nutritional rehabilitation with esophageal dilatation or a feeding jejunostomy tube (J-tube) may be required. Gastrostomy is avoided as the reconstruction may require a gastric conduit. Esophagectomy incorporates various surgical approaches ranging from open thoracotomy and laparotomy (Ivor Lewis esophagogastrectomy and McKeown esophagogastrectomy) to minimally invasive techniques. Robotic minimally invasive esophagogastrectomy is also an acceptable operative approach for esophageal cancer. The stomach, colon, and jejunum can be reconstructed as the conduit. At least 15 lymph nodes should be removed while lymph node dissection for the achievement of adequate nodal staging [46]. Minimally invasive techniques are associated with decreased postoperative mortality, earlier recovery, and increased long-term survival [47].

### *6.3.2 Combined trimodal therapy*

Combined modality therapy has been shown to significantly increase survival in patients with esophageal locoregional disease compared to resection alone. Surgery alone can adequately eradicate early-stage, small (<3 cm), and well-differentiated carcinomas. For management of locally advanced disease, trimodal therapy with neoadjuvant chemoradiation followed by esophagectomy has the most favorable outcome [48]. Intensity-modulated radiation therapy (IMRT) is beneficial in reducing cardiac and pulmonary complications [49].

The European Organization for Research and Treatment of Cancer (EORTC) also demonstrated a lower rate of local failure with the addition of radiotherapy to 46 from 67% but failed to establish survival benefits [50]. Even though the imbalance of lower-stage tumors conflicts with the interpretation of the results, the recent studies that reported improved survival in patients that received chemotherapy [51]. The multicenter phase III randomized CROSS trial compared surgery alone in esophageal carcinoma with preoperative chemoradiation consisting of paclitaxel and carboplatin followed by surgery. The results demonstrated significant improvement in overall survival (OS) and disease-free survival (DFS) with chemoradiation followed by surgery compared to surgery alone in patients with resectable lesions. Median OS improved from 24 month in surgery alone to 49 months with neoadjuvant therapy (hazard ratio: 0.657; $P = 0.003$). The complete R0 resection rate was achieved in 92% of patients receiving neoadjuvant therapy while the resection rate diminished to 69% in surgery alone group. ($P < 0.001$) [52]. The efficacy and safety of preoperative fluorouracil and oxaliplatin (FOLFOX) combined with radiotherapy were evaluated in a single-arm phase II SWOG trial. Complete resection was achieved in 28% (95% CI, 19.1–38.2) of patients. Median and 3-year OS were 28.3 months and 45.1%, respectively at a median follow-up of 39.2 months [53].

## 6.4 Management of metastatic cancer

### *6.4.1 Systemic therapy*

Locally advanced and metastatic EC is not subjected to surgical resection. Hence, the objective of systemic therapy is to provide palliation, improve overall survival, and enhance the quality of life. A combination of 5 -Fluorouracil (5-FU) and platinum is considered the standard of care first-line therapy while other regimens including paclitaxel with platinum regimen and irinotecan plus 5-FU are recommended as well. Three drug combinations (Docetaxel, Cisplatin, 5-FU) are appropriate for high volume disease, young age, and good performance status. Low-volume disease or poor performance status indicates a single-agent treatment [35]. The ToGA trial was a randomized phase III trial that demonstrated that chemotherapy with trastuzumab had better overall survival in Her-2 expressing tumors, leading to the approval of this combination in this patient population [54].

Results of the phase III CheckMate- 648 trial approved nivolumab as the first-line treatment of patients with advanced or metastatic esophageal SCC. The participants received nivolumab combined with platinum and fluoropyrimidine-based chemotherapy along with ipilimumab. The trial demonstrated that median OS is significantly longer with nivolumab plus chemotherapy than with chemotherapy alone (15 vs. 9 months) with tumors in which PD-L1 expression of 1% or greater. OS was also significantly prolonged from 9 to 14 months in the nivolumab plus ipilimumab group with tumor cell PD-L1 expression of 1% or greater [55].

Pembrolizumab in combination with fluoropyrimidine and platinum-based chemotherapy has been approved as first-line treatment for patients with locally advanced or metastatic esophageal tumors. The phase III KEYNOTE-590 trial compared pembrolizumab plus chemotherapy and placebo plus chemotherapy in patients with previously untreated, locally advanced, or metastatic esophageal SCC, and EAC [56]. The incorporation of pembrolizumab in chemotherapy depicted improved OS from 9.8 months to 12.4 months and prolonged progression-free survival (PFS) from 5.8 months to 6.3 months over the follow-up period of 22.6 months which was statistically significant.

#### *6.4.2 Palliative therapy*

In patients with advanced or metastatic EC, palliative/best supportive care aims for the provision of symptom relief and improvement in overall quality of life. A multimodality interdisciplinary approach should be adopted. Palliative management of dysphagia can be achieved through the placement of permanent or temporary self-expandable metallic stents (SEMS). Membrane-covered stents have decreased rates of tumor ingrowth and are associated with lower rates of endoscopic reintervention for dysphagia secondary to restenosis [57]. Severe esophageal obstruction can be treated with endoscopy- or fluoroscopy-guided placement of SEMS as well as endoscopic lumen enhancement (wire-guided dilation or balloon dilation). Dilation of malignant strictures may be associated with an increased risk of perforation [58]. In case the endoscopic interventions are unsuccessful, surgical or radiologic placement of a jejunostomy or gastrostomy tube may be required for adequate hydration and nutrition. Bleeding from the tumor surface may be controlled with endoscopic electrocoagulation using bipolar electrocoagulation or argon plasma coagulation. However, endoscopic intervention may lead to precipitous exsanguination and a high rate of recurrent bleeding [59]. Pain, nausea, and vomiting should be addressed aggressively.

Palliative radiotherapy is commonly delivered for esophageal obstruction, severe pain, chronic blood loss, or nausea due to the tumor mass effect. Brachytherapy may be considered if a lumen can be restored that allows for the use of appropriate applicators [60]. Newer literature supports the use of intraluminal brachytherapy for durable palliation with caution for fistulation or stenosis [35].

Pembrolizumab has been approved for the treatment of unresectable and metastatic high-tumor mutational burden solid tumors that are unresponsive to prior treatment. This was based on the findings by KEYNOTE-158 trial which included

102 patients for analysis. The trial demonstrated objective response rate in 29% and complete response rate in 4% of participants [61].

## 7. Conclusion

Dysphagia is the most common presenting complaint with patient with esophageal carcinoma. Dysphagia associated with alarming features like advanced age, weight loss, anorexia, upper gastrointestinal bleeding and past history of BE should be investigated for esophageal malignancy. Currently, the multimodality therapy that is the combination of neoadjuvant chemoradiation followed by esophagectomy is the standard of care for resectable tumors consisting of either locally advanced EAC or SCC. In addition, early mucosal lesions can be managed definitively by endoscopic resections. The majority of patients progress to distant metastatic disease, which is presently incurable. Newer novel agents have been introduced as the targeted therapies for this cancer and the results are promising.

## Conflict of interest

The author declares no conflict of interest.

## Author details

Lilamani Rajthala
Department of Surgery, Patan Academy of Health Sciences, Lalitpur, Nepal

*Address all correspondence to: lilamanirajthala@gmail.com

## References

[1] Then EO, Lopez M, Saleem S, Gayam V, Sunkara T, Culliford A, et al. Esophageal cancer: An updated surveillance epidemiology and end results database analysis. World Journal of Oncology. 2020;**11**(2):55

[2] He S, Xu J, Liu X, Zhen Y. Advances and challenges in the treatment of esophageal cancer. Acta Pharmaceutica Sinica B. 2021;**11**(11):3379-3392

[3] Uhlenhopp DJ, Then EO, Sunkara T, Gaduputi V. Epidemiology of esophageal cancer: Update in global trends, etiology and risk factors. Clinical Journal of Gastroenterology. 2020;**13**(6):1010-1021

[4] Mansour NM, Groth SS, Anandasabapathy S. Esophageal adenocarcinoma: Screening, surveillance, and management. Annual Review of Medicine. 2017;**68**(1):213-227

[5] Townsend CM, Beauchamp RD, Evers BM, Mattox KL. Sabiston Textbook of Surgery: The Biological Basis of Modern Surgical Practice. Philadelphia, PA: Elsevier Health Sciences; 2016

[6] Ferlay J, Soerjomataram I, Dikshit R, Eser S, Mathers C, Rebelo M, et al. Cancer incidence and mortality worldwide: Sources, methods and major patterns in GLOBOCAN 2012. International Journal of Cancer. 2015;**136**(5):E359-EE86

[7] Siegel RL, Miller KD, Jemal A. Cancer statistics, 2019. CA: A Cancer Journal for Clinicians. 2019;**69**(1):7-34

[8] Yang CS, Chen X, Tu S. Etiology and prevention of esophageal cancer. Gastrointestinal Tumors. 2016;**3**(1):3-16

[9] Cook M, Chow W, Devesa S. Oesophageal cancer incidence in the United States by race, sex, and histologic type, 1977-2005. British Journal of Cancer. 2009;**101**(5):855-859

[10] Meves V, Behrens A, Pohl J. Diagnostics and early diagnosis of esophageal cancer. Viszeralmedizin. 2015;**31**(5):315-318

[11] Brown LM, Devesa SS, Chow W-H. Incidence of adenocarcinoma of the esophagus among white Americans by sex, stage, and age. Journal of the National Cancer Institute. 2008;**100**(16):1184-1187

[12] Pandeya N, Williams G, Green AC, Webb PM, Whiteman DC, Study AC. Alcohol consumption and the risks of adenocarcinoma and squamous cell carcinoma of the esophagus. Gastroenterology. 2009;**136**(4):1215-1224. e2

[13] Anderson LA, Cantwell MM, Watson RP, Johnston BT, Murphy SJ, Ferguson HR, et al. The association between alcohol and reflux esophagitis, Barrett's esophagus, and esophageal adenocarcinoma. Gastroenterology. 2009;**136**(3):799-805

[14] Van der Veen A, Dees J, Blankensteijn J, Van Blankenstein M. Adenocarcinoma in Barrett's oesophagus: An overrated risk. Gut. 1989;**30**(1):14-18

[15] Ronkainen J, Aro P, Storskrubb T, Johansson SE, Lind T, Bolling-Sternevald E, et al. Prevalence of Barrett's esophagus in the general population: An endoscopic study. Gastroenterology. 2005;**129**(6):1825-1831

[16] Dam AN, Klapman J. A narrative review of Barrett's esophagus in 2020, molecular and clinical update. Annals of Translational Medicine. 2020;**8**(17):1107-1122

[17] Daly JM, Fry WA, Little AG, Winchester DP, McKee RF, Stewart AK, et al. Esophageal cancer: Results of an American College of Surgeons patient care evaluation study. Journal of the American College of Surgeons. 2000;**190**(5):562-572

[18] Brooks PJ, Enoch MA, Goldman D, Li TK, Yokoyama A. The alcohol flushing response: An unrecognized risk factor for esophageal cancer from alcohol consumption. PLoS Medicine. 2009;**6**(3):e1000050

[19] Rice TW, Patil DT, Blackstone EH. AJCC/UICC staging of cancers of the esophagus and esophagogastric junction: Application to clinical practice. Annals of Cardiothoracic Surgery. 2017;**6**(2):119

[20] Rice TW, Kelsen D, Blackstone EH, Ishwaran H, Patil DT, Bass AJ, et al. Esophagus and esophagogastric junction. AJCC Cancer Staging Manual. 2017;**8**:185-234

[21] Pouw RE, Heldoorn N, Herrero LA, Ten Kate FJ, Visser M, Busch OR, et al. Do we still need EUS in the workup of patients with early esophageal neoplasia? A retrospective analysis of 131 cases. Gastrointestinal Endoscopy. 2011;**73**(4):662-668

[22] Kelly S, Harris K, Berry E, Hutton J, Roderick P, Cullingworth J, et al. A systematic review of the staging performance of endoscopic ultrasound in gastro-oesophageal carcinoma. Gut. 2001;**49**(4):534-539

[23] Puli SR, Reddy JB, Bechtold ML, Antillon D, Ibdah JA, Antillon MR. Staging accuracy of esophageal cancer by endoscopic ultrasound: A meta-analysis and systematic review. World Journal of Gastroenterology: WJG. 2008;**14**(10):1479

[24] Thakkar S, Kaul V. Endoscopic ultrasound staging of esophageal cancer. Gastroenterology & Hepatology. 2020;**16**(1):14

[25] Rice TW. Clinical staging of esophageal carcinoma. CT, EUS, and PET. Chest Surgery Clinics of North America. 2000;**10**(3):471-485

[26] Schmidlin EJ, Gill RR. New frontiers in esophageal radiology. Annals of Translational Medicine. 2021;**9**(10):904-913

[27] Stawinski PM, Dziadkowiec KN, Kuo LA, Echavarria J, Saligram S. Barrett's esophagus: An updated review. Diagnostics. 2023;**13**(2):321

[28] Kramer JR, Fischbach LA, Richardson P, Alsarraj A, Fitzgerald S, Shaib Y, et al. Waist-to-hip ratio, but not body mass index, is associated with an increased risk of Barrett's esophagus in white men. Clinical Gastroenterology and Hepatology. 2013;**11**(4):373-381. e1

[29] Shaheen NJ, Falk GW, Iyer PG, Souza RF, Yadlapati RH, Sauer BG, et al. Diagnosis and management of Barrett's esophagus: An updated ACG guideline. Official Journal of the American College of Gastroenterology|ACG. 2022;**117**(4):559-587

[30] Qumseya BJ, Wani S, Desai M, Qumseya A, Bain P, Sharma P, et al. Adverse events after radiofrequency ablation in patients with Barrett's esophagus: A systematic review and meta-analysis. Clinical Gastroenterology and Hepatology. 2016;**14**(8):1086-1095. e6

[31] Shaheen NJ, Sharma P, Overholt BF, Wolfsen HC, Sampliner RE, Wang KK,

et al. Radiofrequency ablation in Barrett's esophagus with dysplasia. New England Journal of Medicine. 2009;**360**(22):2277-2288

[32] Mohan BP, Krishnamoorthi R, Ponnada S, Shakhatreh M, Jayaraj M, Garg R, et al. Liquid nitrogen spray cryotherapy in treatment of Barrett's esophagus, where do we stand? A systematic review and meta-analysis. Diseases of the Esophagus. 2019;**32**(6):doy130

[33] Kodashima S, Fujishiro M. Novel image-enhanced endoscopy with i-scan technology. World Journal of Gastroenterology: WJG. 2010;**16**(9):1043

[34] Singh R, Shahzad MA, Tam W, Goda K, Yu LHK, Fujishiro M, et al. Preliminary feasibility study using a novel narrow-band imaging system with dual focus magnification capability in B arrett's esophagus: Is the time ripe to abandon random biopsies? Digestive Endoscopy. 2013;**25**:151-156

[35] Cummings D, Wong J, Palm R, Hoffe S, Almhanna K, Vignesh S. Epidemiology, diagnosis, staging and multimodal therapy of esophageal and gastric tumors. Cancers. 2021;**13**(3):582

[36] Rastogi A, Puli S, El-Serag HB, Bansal A, Wani S, Sharma P. Incidence of esophageal adenocarcinoma in patients with Barrett's esophagus and high-grade dysplasia: A meta-analysis. Gastrointestinal Endoscopy. 2008;**67**(3):394-398

[37] Pech O, May A, Manner H, Behrens A, Pohl J, Weferling M, et al. Long-term efficacy and safety of endoscopic resection for patients with mucosal adenocarcinoma of the esophagus. Gastroenterology. 2014;**146**(3):652-660 e1

[38] Han C, Sun Y. Efficacy and safety of endoscopic submucosal dissection versus endoscopic mucosal resection for superficial esophageal carcinoma: A systematic review and meta-analysis. Diseases of the Esophagus. 2021;**34**(4):doaa081

[39] Ning B, Abdelfatah MM, Othman MO. Endoscopic submucosal dissection and endoscopic mucosal resection for early stage esophageal cancer. Annals of Cardiothoracic Surgery. 2017;**6**(2):88

[40] Ishihara R, Arima M, Iizuka T, Oyama T, Katada C, Kato M, et al. Endoscopic submucosal dissection/endoscopic mucosal resection guidelines for esophageal cancer. Digestive Endoscopy. 2020;**32**(4):452-493

[41] Ahmed Y, Othman M. EMR/ESD: techniques, complications, and evidence. Current Gastroenterology Reports. 2020;**22**:1-12

[42] Sharma P, Shaheen NJ, Katzka D, Bergman JJ. AGA clinical practice update on endoscopic treatment of Barrett's esophagus with dysplasia and/or early cancer: Expert review. Gastroenterology. 2020;**158**(3):760-769

[43] Dumoulin FL, Hildenbrand R, Oyama T, Steinbrück I. Current trends in endoscopic diagnosis and treatment of early esophageal cancer. Cancers. 2021;**13**(4):752

[44] Mizrak Kaya D, Wang X, Harada K, Blum Murphy MA, Das P, Minsky BD, et al. 101 long-term survivors who had metastatic gastroesophageal cancer and received local consolidative therapy. Oncology. 2017;**93**(4):243-248

[45] Ng T, Vezeridis MP. Advances in the surgical treatment of esophageal cancer. Journal of Surgical Oncology. 2010;**101**(8):725-729

[46] Rizk NP, Ishwaran H, Rice TW, Chen L-Q, Schipper PH, Kesler KA, et al. Optimum lymphadenectomy for esophageal cancer. Annals of Surgery. 2010;**251**(1):46-50

[47] Luketich JD, Pennathur A, Franchetti Y, Catalano PJ, Swanson S, Sugarbaker DJ, et al. Minimally invasive esophagectomy: Results of a prospective phase II multicenter trial—The eastern cooperative oncology group (E2202) study. Annals of Surgery. 2015;**261**(4):702-707

[48] Tepper J, Krasna MJ, Niedzwiecki D, Hollis D, Reed CE, Goldberg R, et al. Phase III trial of trimodality therapy with cisplatin, fluorouracil, radiotherapy, and surgery compared with surgery alone for esophageal cancer: CALGB 9781. Journal of Clinical Oncology. 2008;**26**(7):1086-1092

[49] Kole TP, Aghayere O, Kwah J, Yorke ED, Goodman KA. Comparison of heart and coronary artery doses associated with intensity-modulated radiotherapy versus three-dimensional conformal radiotherapy for distal esophageal cancer. International Journal of Radiation Oncology* Biology* Physics. 2012;**83**(5):1580-1586

[50] Gignoux M, Roussel A, Paillot B, Gillet M, Schlag P, Favre JP, et al. The value of preoperative radiotherapy in esophageal cancer: Results of a study of the EORTC. World Journal of Surgery. 1987;**11**(4):426-432

[51] Nygaard K, Hagen S, Hansen HS, Hatlevoll R, Hultborn R, Jakobsen A, et al. Pre-operative radiotherapy prolongs survival in operable esophageal carcinoma: A randomized, multicenter study of pre-operative radiotherapy and chemotherapy. The second Scandinavian trial in esophageal cancer. World Journal of Surgery. 1992;**16**:1104-1109

[52] van Hagen P, Hulshof M, Van Lanschot J, Steyerberg E, Henegouwen MVB, Wijnhoven B, et al. Preoperative chemoradiotherapy for esophageal or junctional cancer. New England Journal of Medicine. 2012;**366**(22):2074-2084

[53] Leichman LP, Goldman BH, Bohanes PO, Lenz HJ, Thomas CR, Billingsley KG, et al. S0356: A phase II clinical and prospective molecular trial with oxaliplatin, fluorouracil, and external-beam radiation therapy before surgery for patients with esophageal adenocarcinoma. Journal of Clinical Oncology. 2011;**29**(34):4555-4560

[54] Bang Y-J, Van Cutsem E, Feyereislova A, Chung HC, Shen L, Sawaki A, et al. Trastuzumab in combination with chemotherapy versus chemotherapy alone for treatment of HER2-positive advanced gastric or gastro-oesophageal junction cancer (ToGA): A phase 3, open-label, randomised controlled trial. The Lancet. 2010;**376**(9742):687-697

[55] Doki Y, Ajani JA, Kato K, Xu J, Wyrwicz L, Motoyama S, et al. Nivolumab combination therapy in advanced esophageal squamous-cell carcinoma. New England Journal of Medicine. 2022;**386**(5):449-462

[56] Sun J-M, Shen L, Shah MA, Enzinger P, Adenis A, Doi T, et al. Pembrolizumab plus chemotherapy versus chemotherapy alone for first-line treatment of advanced oesophageal cancer (KEYNOTE-590): A randomised, placebo-controlled, phase 3 study. The Lancet. 2021;**398**(10302):759-771

[57] Vakil N, Morris AI, Marcon N, Segalin A, Peracchia A, Bethge N, et al. A prospective, randomized, controlled trial of covered expandable metal stents in the palliation of

malignant esophageal obstruction at the gastroesophageal junction. Official Journal of the American College of Gastroenterology|ACG. 2001;**96**(6):1791-1796

[58] Fan Y, Song H-Y, Kim JH, Park J-H, Kim J, Jung H-Y, et al. Evaluation of the incidence of esophageal complications associated with balloon dilation and their management in patients with malignant esophageal strictures. American Journal of Roentgenology. 2012;**198**(1):213-218

[59] Sheibani S, Kim J, Chen B, Park S, Saberi B, Keyashian K, et al. Natural history of acute upper GI bleeding due to tumours: Short-term success and long-term recurrence with or without endoscopic therapy. Alimentary Pharmacology & Therapeutics. 2013;**38**(2):144-150

[60] Homs MY, Steyerberg EW, Eijkenboom WM, Tilanus HW, Stalpers LJ, Bartelsman JF, et al. Single-dose brachytherapy versus metal stent placement for the palliation of dysphagia from oesophageal cancer: Multicentre randomised trial. The Lancet. 2004;**364**(9444):1497-1504

[61] Marabelle A, Fakih M, Lopez J, Shah M, Shapira-Frommer R, Nakagawa K, et al. Association of tumour mutational burden with outcomes in patients with advanced solid tumours treated with pembrolizumab: Prospective biomarker analysis of the multicohort, open-label, phase 2 KEYNOTE-158 study. The Lancet Oncology. 2020;**21**(10):1353-1365

Chapter 10

# Swallowing Disorders after Laryngectomy

*Ljiljana Širić, Marinela Rosso and Aleksandar Včev*


## Abstract

Laryngectomy is a surgical procedure that leaves mutilating functional consequences for the patient, one of which is often a swallowing disorder. Swallowing disorders after laryngectomy can be of varying degrees and can occur at any time in the postoperative period. Some consequences that interfere with swallowing difficulties after laryngectomy are: edema, pain in the soft tissues of the cheeks and neck, dental problems, xerostomia, hyposalivation or fibrosis of masticatory muscles, and odynophagia. The diagnostic processing of dysphagia includes detailed anamnestic data collection, instrumental and clinical evaluation of swallowing, and self-assessment of swallowing. Swallowing rehabilitation is individual and carried out by an interdisciplinary team within a healthcare facility that has the necessary medical equipment and aids to care for patients with dysphagia and the consequences of dysphagia. The purpose of rehabilitation is to provide the patient with safe oral feeding that will meet his nutritional needs and prevent the possible consequences of dysphagia. Detecting early clinical signs of dysphagia enables timely therapeutic intervention and prevention of secondary consequences of dysphagia, which is especially important in oncology patients.


**Keywords:** dysphagia, laryngectomy, odynophagia, swallowing, swallowing disorders

## 1. Introduction

Swallowing (deglutition) is a function that takes place in the upper part of the alimentary tract, and the purpose of swallowing is the intake of water and food into the body to ensure the supply of necessary nutrients, electrolytes, and water. In addition to the possibility of food intake, the speed of movement of the bolus through the alimentary tract is also important for the development of all digestive and absorption processes. Swallowing is a complex mechanism, even when the function itself is preserved and undisturbed, because it requires good coordination of more than twenty muscles, as well as appropriate coordination with the breathing function, while part of the anatomical spaces and structures that participate in the swallowing process also serve other purposes, and the central nervous swallowing control is very complex. Successive phases of swallowing are controlled for the most part automatically in a precisely determined order from the deglutition center (areas of neurons of the reticular formation in the lower part of the pons and medulla oblongata), while motor impulses from the center to the peripheral organs are transmitted by eight cranial nerves (from the 5th to the 12th nerve) and several peripheral (upper cervical) nerves [1].

The function of deglutition is divided into three main phases [1]:

1. Oral phase—voluntary phase in which a person takes, retains a certain amount of liquid or food, chews a morsel, manipulates the bolus, and in the final part begins the process of swallowing in the narrower sense.

2. Pharyngeal phase—a largely involuntary, reflex phase that only begins with a voluntary movement, and it is this movement that causes the swallowing reflex. In this phase, the bolus passes through the pharynx and enters the esophagus.

3. Esophageal phase—an involuntary phase in which the bolus passes through the esophagus to the stomach with the help of primary and secondary peristaltic movements of the esophagus.

Disturbances and disorders of swallowing can occur in one, two or all stages at the same time. Given that laryngectomy is a mutilating surgical procedure that removes a part of the larynx or the entire larynx with the hyoid bone and infrahyoid muscles (**Figures 1** and **2**) for the purpose of treatment, most often of a malignant process of the larynx and surrounding structures [2], and the pharynx is consequently reconstructed, the physiology and biomechanics of swallowing are changed in laryngectomized patients. In the early postoperative period, no laryngectomized patient will be able to feed orally, but will receive food through a nasogastric tube, while some laryngectomized patients will have difficulty swallowing even later.

Residual disturbances and swallowing disorders are more common in patients who have undergone a partial laryngectomy, especially if a supraglottic laryngectomy has

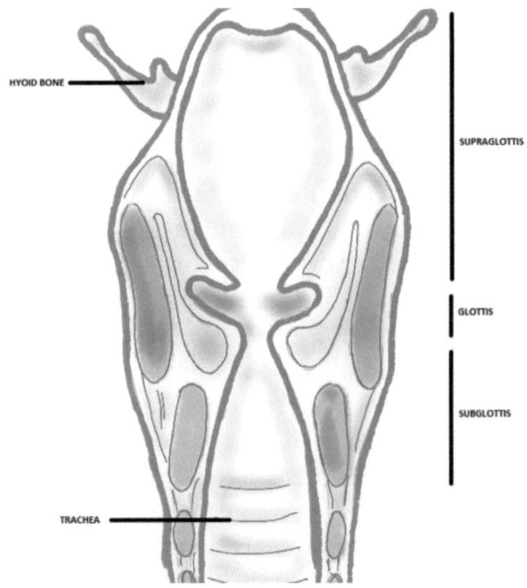


**Figure 1.**
*Anatomical structures.*

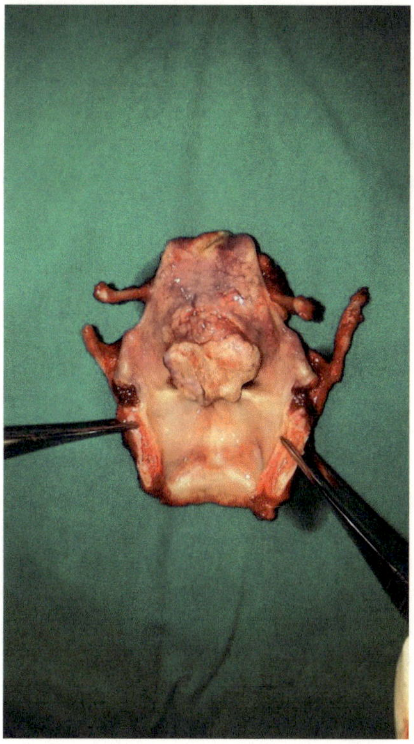

**Figure 2.**
*Larynx and hyoid bone removed by laryngectomy.*

been performed. In general, the prevalence of swallowing disorders after laryngectomy is highly variable and, according to different studies, is 17–72%. In addition to the occurrence, swallowing disorders also vary in the intensity of the dysfunction and can occur at any time during the postoperative period [2–4]. As feeding is one of the existential functions, untreated swallowing disorders represent a significant medical problem resulting in conditions that can be vitally threatening (dehydration, malnutrition, and aspiration pneumonia) for humans. However, swallowing disorders are not only a medical problem if we take into account that in many communities and cultures significant social events are necessarily accompanied by the consumption of food and drink, and then swallowing disorders also represent a psychosocial problem. Swallowing disorders and disturbances that persist result in a number of other consequences and impair a person's quality of life. The aim of this chapter is to show the types of swallowing disorders after laryngectomy and the surgical consequences that interfere with them, along with the presentation of diagnostic assessment and rehabilitation methods in patients with dysphagia.

## 2. Swallowing problems following laryngectomy

Immediately after the laryngectomy, a nasogastric tube through which the operated patient is fed is placed. The time of use of the nasogastric tube is of individual duration while the wound is healing, usually 3–12 days if the early postoperative recovery goes smoothly and without complications. Unlike partially laryngectomized patients and patients exposed to radiotherapy, most totally laryngectomized patients who are not irradiated will not have major difficulties with feeding and swallowing in the later stages, but any change in anatomical relationships in the body affects functions and requires adaptation. Thus, laryngectomized patients will initially find it easier to consume food that is softer, smoother, and mushy in consistency, and later only a part of the patients will adjust their eating habits by taking smaller bites, chewing and swallowing more carefully, and consuming liquids more often while swallowing solid food. After complete recovery, some patients will be able to eat food of different consistency as before the operation [5].

In laryngectomized patients who have difficulty swallowing (dysphagia), depending on the localization and extension of the malignant disease, the condition is manifested by a clinical picture in the form of general and specific symptomatology (**Table 1**). In the literature, the consequences of dysphagia, such as dehydration, malnutrition, and aspiration pneumonia [6] are included in the general symptomatology, while the "real" symptoms such as aspiration with consequent cough, changes in the quality of voice timbre (moist, raspy voice), bolus regurgitation, and postglutitional residues in the oral cavity or pharynx [6, 7] are included in the specific symptomatology. According to data from clinical practice, several authors in their studies [8–10] state that patients most often complain of difficult bolus propulsion and slow swallowing, i.e., prolonged duration of meals, retention of food in the throat, regurgitation, multiple attempts to swallow, and feeling of tightness in the throat. The cause of the aforementioned disorders is precisely the altered anatomy and physiology of the reconstructed pharynx (neopharynx) [8, 11].

Edema, which will contribute to difficulty swallowing, may occur after surgery or after radiotherapy, but it tends to decrease over time. In laryngectomized patients who have undergone oncological treatment, more precisely, radiotherapy, the range of dysphagia symptoms is wider in the form of trismus, difficulty in taking and chewing food due to changes in the surrounding structures (edema, pain in the soft tissues of the cheeks and neck, dental problems, etc.) and because xerostomia, hyposalivation or fibrosis of masticatory muscles and odynophagia may occur as a result of radiotherapy. Odynophagia is painful swallowing that should be distinguished from dysphagia, and often odynophagia and dysphagia occur simultaneously in this population. Also, part of the laryngectomized patients whose pharynx and upper esophagus were reconstructed using a skin-muscle (myocutaneous) flap will have narrowing and reduced peristalsis of the esophagus. The manifestation of dysphagia symptoms is enhanced by the patient's inadequate behavioral pattern during feeding, such as insufficient chewing and eating too quickly. It is estimated that up to 50% of laryngectomized patients notice swallowing disorders in their full extent only after discharge from hospital treatment [12]. Patients who have temporary or long-term

| **General symptomatology (consequences of dysphagia)** | **Specific symptomatology (symptoms of dysphagia)** |
|---|---|
| dehydration | aspiration |
| malnutrition | cough |
| aspiration pneumonia | bolus regurgitation |
| | postglutitional residues |

**Table 1.**
*General and specific symptomatology of dysphagia.*

aphagia (complete inability to swallow) or profound dysphagia will undergo rehabilitation of the deglutition function by a speech therapist who specializes in the assessment, diagnosis, and rehabilitation of swallowing disorders. The incidence of aphagia is more frequent after partial operations on the larynx, especially after supraglottic laryngectomy, in which the epiglottis and supraglottis are removed. In this way, the patient is left without two of the three levels of protection of the lower respiratory tract when swallowing a bolus.

### 2.1 Reasons for the appearance of dysphagia

From the etiological aspect, the primary causes of swallowing disorders after laryngectomy differ depending on the type of laryngectomy performed and the patient's comorbidities. However, in general, some of the reasons for the appearance of dysphagia, as a result of surgery, are the following [11–14]:

- lack of elevation of the laryngohyoid complex;
- dysfunction of the neopharynx and pharyngeal muscle dysmotility;
- reduction of tongue movement amplitude and tongue dysmotility;
- prolonged duration of palatopharyngeal occlusion as a result of a slower increase in intraoral pressure;
- narrowing of the esophagus;
- reduction of static and dynamic strength of muscles involved in swallowing;
- occurrence of pseudoglottis (the localization of origin of the esophageal or tracheoesophageal voice (after the loss of the laryngeal voice) in the narrowed area of the pharyngoesophageal segment);
- esophageal stricture;
- submucosal fibrosis of the oropharynx or the upper part of the esophagus;
- development of diverticulum in the area of the pharyngoesophageal segment;
- cricopharyngeal spasm resulting in delayed opening of the pharyngoesophageal sphincter;
- lack of certain anatomical structures after partial operations on the larynx (e.g., lack of epiglottis after supraglottic laryngectomy);
- tracheoesophageal fistula;
- pharyngocutaneous fistula;
- tumor recurrence.

With total laryngectomy, in addition to removing the larynx, the hyoid bone is also removed, which results in prolonged swallowing time due to [15]:

- changes in pressure values in individual anatomical structures;
- slower velopharyngeal occlusion;
- a slower increase in pressure in the oropharynx, which affects the contraction of the muscles of the pharynx and the propulsion of the bolus;
- by increasing the pressure in the area of the pharyngoesophageal sphincter, which also increases the resistance.

According to a review of the literature, the most common reasons include the formation of a pseudodiverticulum in the bed of the oropharynx and the formation of a tracheoesophageal fistula, both in 42–60% of cases, while cricopharyngeal spasm occurs in 22–36% of cases, narrowing of the pharyngoesophageal segment in 15–19% of cases, and tumor recurrence in 7–13% of cases [14]. The appearance of narrowing of the pharyngoesophageal segment and the formation of a pseudoventricle are associated with a certain surgical technique (especially the tissue suturing method), such complications occur more often after primary reconstruction, and about 80% of stenosis appear within the first year after the operation [14]. Hypertonicity of pharyngeal constrictors, as well as pharyngoesophageal spasm that can occur after laryngectomy cause an increase in intraesophageal pressure, which hinders the passage of the bolus through the upper part of the alimentary tract. Esophageal stricture is a narrowing of the esophagus in one part in the shape of an hourglass, which makes it difficult for a bolus to pass. Esophageal stricture after laryngectomy is most often the result of radiotherapy or hypertonicity/rigidity of the neopharynx, although it can also occur due to the formation of scar tissue (fibrosis).

Some authors associate the occurrence of submucosal fibrosis in the pharyngoesophageal segment with the deposition of fibrinogen and collagen in ulcers in the tissue and inflammation of the mucous membrane. One of the complications of surgical treatment is pharyngocutaneous fistula, which usually occurs seven to ten days after surgery. In addition to surgical technique, exposure to chemoradiotherapy is also considered a risk factor for the formation of pharyngocutaneous fistula [14–17]. It is recommended to avoid attempts at oral feeding until the fistula is healed or repaired surgically, which in these cases prolongs nasogastric tube feeding. In laryngectomized patients who underwent reconstruction of part of the esophagus using one of the musculocutaneous (myocutaneous) flaps, swallowing takes a long time (5–10 seconds) in the esophageal phase, because the bolus takes longer to pass through the esophagus, given that the reconstructed part of the esophagus does not have peristalsis but the food descends down the esophagus under the influence of gravity [12]. This also applies to reconstruction of the pharynx with a tubular flap in cases where part or majority of the pharynx is required to be resected due to tumor extension. The pharyngeal phase may be disrupted.

### 2.2 Disorders and dysfunctions correlated with swallowing problems

The pharyngoesophageal sphincter, i.e., the cricopharyngeal muscle, whose physiological function is to prevent the bolus from returning to the pharynx or oral cavity, is resected during laryngectomy and pharynx reconstruction, which results in flaccidity and openness of the upper part of the esophagus and consequently facilitates regurgitation of contents. A cricomyotomy is performed in some clinical centers to relax the cricopharyngeous muscles to allow for primary or secondary trachea-esophageal punctures for postlaryngectomy vocalization. But, for this reason, laryngectomized patients are more susceptible to gastroesophageal reflux (GER), and most of them develop gastroesophageal reflux disease (GERD) in the postoperative period. Patients with an implanted voice prosthesis are even more at risk for this problem, because the production of the tracheoesophageal voice requires a strong expiration that additionally stimulates the opening of the pharyngoesophageal sphincter. Also, laryngectomized persons who have been placed with a voice prosthesis are unable or have difficulty producing voice while eating, which is best seen at the moment when the bolus passes through the esophagus at the level of the tracheoesophageal fistula where the voice prosthesis lies. At the same time, difficult production of the alaryngeal voice and difficult swallowing are caused by weaker coordination of muscle movements that participate in both functions and the entry of a larger amount of air into the esophagus through the voice prosthesis, so the air mixes with the bolus.

Part of the laryngectomized patients had premorbidly poor dental hygiene and problems with teeth, and postmorbidly, part of the patients will also have problems with teeth that were not present before. Patients who have undergone radiotherapy are particularly at risk for this problem. Radiotherapy promotes hyposalivation of the salivary glands, changes in the chemical composition of saliva, reduced blood supply in the area of the maxilla and mandible, and an imbalance of microorganisms ("good" bacteria) in the oral cavity, which increases the risk of gingivitis, dental caries, periodontosis, and osteoradionecrosis. Given that most laryngectomized patients have gastroesophageal reflux disease, they are more susceptible to tooth erosion and tooth loss [12].

By breathing through the nose, the air is naturally warmed, purified, and moistened before entering the upper and lower respiratory tract. In totally laryngectomized persons (who are permanently tracheotomized), the airway is shortened and begins in the area of the tracheostomy. In this way, the essential function of the upper airways is lost. Breathing through a tracheostomy causes changes in the respiratory epithelium, increased production of mucus, chronic inflammation of the lamina propria, and more frequent infections of the lower respiratory tract. The lack of physiological stimulation of olfactory receptors leads to clinical, histological, and cytological changes of the nasal mucosa, i.e., to atrophy of the olfactory neuroepithelium, so patients have a significantly reduced (hyposmia) or completely disabled sense of smell (anosmia) [18, 19]. Conducted studies show that reduction or loss of olfactory function occurs in 35–78% of laryngectomized patients [20, 21].

Dysfunction of the sense of smell in a certain number of patients proportionally causes a reduction in the sense of taste (dysgeusia). Disturbance of the sense of taste can also occur as a result of radiotherapy. Dysgeusia contributes to swallowing difficulties after laryngectomy. The primary and secondary listed consequences of surgical and oncological treatment of these patients, and especially those that interfere together, are responsible for the occurrence of dysphagia and odynophagia in a large percentage of cases after laryngectomy and radiotherapy [18, 22].

### 2.3 Secondary consequences of swallowing disorders

Dysphagia is a swallowing disorder due to which the patient certainly has a reduced intake of liquid and food in the body, so this places him in the group of the population at risk for dehydration and malnutrition. When patients are laryngectomized for the purpose of treating a malignant process of the larynx, they, as oncology patients, are even more at risk of developing dehydration and malnutrition. The daily need for fluid depends on several factors, such as chronological age, and body weight, but the required daily hydration intake is estimated at 35 ml/kg, while in the population over 65 years old it is 30 ml/kg [23].

The patient's hydration status is assessed by recording daily fluid intake and loss, certain laboratory parameters, and clinical examination of the patient (assessment of mucosal and skin dryness, skin turgor, orthostatic hypotension, and oliguria). Given that enteral preparations contain only 60–70% of liquid, it is necessary to correct the total daily liquid intake of the patient when nutrition takes place exclusively through a nasogastric tube [23].

One of the leading symptoms of dysphagia is the aspiration of contents, which causes the patient to cough, but the reflex reaction of coughing does not ensure complete expectoration, which can lead to aspiration pneumonia, especially if it is silent aspiration. The incidence of aspiration pneumonia in patients with dysphagia in the postoperative period ranges from 1.42–26.2% [24].

## 3. Assessment and diagnosis of swallowing disorders

Any care, treatment, and rehabilitation of certain diseases and conditions, including swallowing disorders, require a preliminary assessment and diagnosis in order to determine with certainty which disorder it is, what is the cause of the disorder (if it can be determined), and what are the other active factors which contribute to the manifestation of the patient's clinical picture. This information enables an appropriate prognosis, a detailed rehabilitation plan, the setting of rehabilitation goals, and enables a higher success rate of rehabilitation. Assessment and diagnosis of swallowing disorders is performed by taking anamnestic data and subjective and objective assessment of swallowing function. Subjective assessment includes a clinical examination and subjective assessment of the act of swallowing liquid and food of different consistency, as well as questionnaires for self-assessment of swallowing, while the objective assessment includes instrumental diagnostic processing of the act of swallowing using medical techniques and objective methods.

### 3.1 Anamnestic data

Taking the patient's personal history is simpler, faster and more efficient if a structured interview is used with pre-prepared questions related to the occurrence, time of occurrence, duration and course of certain symptoms, information on other conditions and diseases that are or may be related to the occurrence of disturbances of swallowing. Structured questionnaires also ensure that the clinician takes the anamnestic data of all patients in the same way and does not forget any of the important information if the patients do not remember to mention it themselves. The anamnestic data collected in this way can be reliably processed for professional and scientific research purposes.

Available questionnaires for assessment and self-assessment of the degree of swallowing disorders are as follows [14, 25, 26]:

- Eating Assessment Tool 10 (EAT 10);
- Modified Swallowing Assessment (MSA);
- Sydney Swallow Questionnaire (SSQ);
- Dysphagia Handicap Index (DHI);
- M.D. Anderson Dysphagia Inventory (MDADI);
- The Performance Status Scale for Head and Neck Cancer Patients (PSS).

According to data from clinical practice, laryngectomized patients often complain of aspiration of contents with consequent cough and inability to expectorate completely, oral regurgitation or regurgitation of contents on the tracheostomy, multiple dysfunctional swallows, prolonged swallowing and duration of meals, lack of saliva and dryness of the oral cavity, feeling of food sticking in the oral cavity or pharynx, painful swallowing, and inability to consume solid food. The presence of these symptoms is usually noticed by patients a few days after the operation when they try oral feeding, while the intensity, duration, and course of the mentioned symptoms are individual and depend on a number of other factors.

### 3.2 Instrumental assessment

Instrumental assessment of the swallowing function is necessary for objectifying the assessment, making an accurate diagnosis, determining further rehabilitation procedures and counseling the patient. The diagnostic tests that are available for the evaluation of (disorders of) swallowing are the following [6, 12, 14]:

- videofluoroscopy (VFSS);
- flexible endoscopic evaluation of swallowing (FEES);
- flexible endoscopic evaluation of swallowing with sensation testing (FEEST);
- fiberoptic nasopharyngeal laryngoscopy;
- radiograph of swallowing and esophageal passage;
- multifrequency manometry of the pharynx and esophagus (HRM);
- endoscopic ultrasound;
- scintigraphy.

Not all of the listed available methods of instrumental assessment are performed, but the choice of a specific test depends on the clinical status and needs of the individual patient. Videofluoroscopy and fiberoptic endoscopic evaluation of swallowing are complementary diagnostic examinations that are usually performed in clinical practice in parallel, with the fact that videofluoroscopy offers the possibility of a more detailed assessment of the oral phase, including the assessment of lingual motility, pharyngeal, and partially esophageal phases of swallowing, while with fiberoptic endoscopic evaluation of swallowing, where the patient is not exposed to ionizing radiation, it is possible to evaluate the shape of the operating bed, and the pharyngeal phase of swallowing is more visible [27]. Multifrequency manometry is a useful test for evaluating esophageal motility and in the diagnosis of cricopharyngeal spasm. Endoscopic ultrasound is non-invasive and enables better visibility of submucosal changes and is good for observing the oral phase of swallowing [6].

### 3.3 Subjective assessment

Subjective clinical assessment of swallowing disorders is performed by a multidisciplinary team of experts that includes speech therapists, otorhinolaryngologists, and neurologists who deal with the diagnosis of swallowing disorders. The otorhinolaryngologist will perform a laryngological examination that includes pressure measurement in the area of the pharyngoesophageal sphincter and assessment of changes after chemoradiotherapy. The neurologist will perform a neurological examination and pay special attention to the functions of the V, VII, IX, and XII cranial nerves, sensation on the skin of the face and in the oral cavity, and strength and functionality of the facial and oropharyngeal musculature [14].

The speech therapy diagnostic treatment protocol includes an assessment of the patient's current general status, assessment of the act of swallowing when consuming food of different consistency (if possible), application of various scales and tests for clinical assessment of swallowing, and assessment of the risk of aspiration. The literature also mentions obtaining useful information during palpation of the neck during the pharyngeal phase of swallowing (PPFR), cervical auscultation, and the use of pulse oximetry, although these parameters are not fully scientifically based [28].

The available tests that can be used for the clinical evaluation of the act of swallowing are the following [29, 30]:

- Volume viscosity swallow test (V-VST);
- 100-ml water swallowing test.

After the tests, the severity of dysphagia is determined using [31]:

- Functional oral intake scale (FOIS);
- Dysphagia severity score (DSS).

## 4. Rehabilitation of deglutition function

Swallowing rehabilitation is carried out by an interdisciplinary team within a healthcare facility that has the necessary medical equipment and aids to care for patients with dysphagia and the consequences of dysphagia. The interdisciplinary team includes specialists of different profiles: otolaryngologist, speech therapist, gastroenterologist, neurologist, infectious disease specialist, physiotherapist, nurse, nutritionist, and if necessary, in an individual case, doctors from other specialties and a psychologist. The purpose of rehabilitation is to provide the patient with safe oral feeding that will meet his nutritional needs and prevent the possible consequences of dysphagia. The otolaryngologist and speech therapist, after the evaluation and diagnosis, will determine the way of feeding the patient, that is, the type of intake of contents into the body (usually determined according to the scale of Prosiegel et al. [32]). Then they will determine the modification of the consistency and viscosity of food and liquid, they will adjust the amount of individual sips, that is, the size of bites when feeding, they will educate the patient about the correct position of the head, neck, and body when feeding, and they will apply certain compensatory motor techniques and modify patient's inadequate behavioral patterns during food and liquid consumption [33]. In the direct conservative rehabilitation of the deglutition function, the speech therapist will apply predefined methods and rehabilitation operators according to the rehabilitation plan made individually for each patient depending on their basic diagnosis, symptoms, and other characteristics. Rehabilitation operators are intended to increase the amplitude of movement, static and dynamic strength of all muscles involved in the function of swallowing, and generally improve coordination of movements to ensure safe swallowing and successful feeding. Certain rehabilitation operators for the oropharyngeal musculature, postural and compensatory techniques, and specific maneuvers for swallowing are available in the rehabilitation process, such as:

- Masako maneuver;
- Mendelsohn maneuver;
- Shaker maneuver;
- Supraglottic maneuver;
- Super-supraglottic maneuver;
- Effortful swallow maneuver;
- Double swallow exercise;
- Chin tuck exercise;
- Elevator pitch exercise and others.

It is also possible to use a medical technique that is applied in the rehabilitation of the oro-motor abilities of the articulator, such as VitalStim Plus Electrotherapy and the Iowa Oral Performance Instrument, as well as the use of the Novel Swallowing Exercise Aid (SEA 2.0) [8, 34].

When determining the individual rehabilitation plan and program, the speech therapist must take into account the anthropological status of the patient (health status, morphological characteristics, current motor and functional abilities, cognitive abilities, and conative characteristics) while determining the main goals and tasks of rehabilitation, rehabilitation conditions, rehabilitation operators, and periodization of the rehabilitation. In rehabilitation programming, it is necessary to pay attention to the type of rehabilitation operators and props (aids) that will be used, load, modeling (distribution and arrangement of operators), optimization and dosage, rehabilitation methods, and duration of recovery, because otherwise the rehabilitation carried out can lead to biological hypercompensation, be counterproductive and without the desired result, or the rehabilitation time until the patient's status improves will be prolonged.

Nutritional therapy is oriented toward nutritional support for the purpose of satisfying energy needs and improving the nutritional status of the patient, as well as preventing dehydration and malnutrition, and thus also preventing the deterioration of the general health status. Nutritional therapy plays an important role in the course of treatment and rehabilitation of patients with dysphagia, as it reduces the morbidity rate and shortens the duration of hospitalization, thereby improving the patient's quality of life. This form of therapy is indicated by an otolaryngologist, and it is carried out and monitored by a multidisciplinary team of experts in the care of patients with dysphagia. Preparations with a modified consistency and texture using available thickeners facilitate the oral intake of liquid and food, do not change the taste of the contents, enable safer swallowing, and reduce the patient's fear of aspiration. When it is not possible to establish oral feeding in this way, artificial nutrition is applied. Preparations for enteral nutrition have different chemical composition, energy value, density, composition (e.g., proportion of proteins, macro- and micro-nutrients, and osmolarity), and viscosity, so care should be taken about the purpose of introducing a certain preparation into the patient's diet [33, 35].

## 5. Conclusion

Anatomical and functional changes after laryngectomy cause a number of problems, and one of them is a swallowing disorder of varying degrees with a variable incidence of a high upper limit. As swallowing is a physiological function of existential importance, dysphagia is a potentially life-threatening disorder for the laryngectomized patient. Therefore, it requires early detection and recognition of symptoms, immediate diagnosis of the disorder, and timely and appropriate professional multidisciplinary rehabilitation intervention based on modern knowledge and recognized professional methods. Early intervention and appropriate rehabilitation under professional guidance will prevent secondary medical and psychosocial consequences of dysphagia.

## Acknowledgements

We would like to thank Ms. Mirna Brunčić for translating this text.

## Conflict of interest

The authors declare no conflict of interest.

## Notes/other declarations

The figures and the table are from the author's own source.

## Author details

Ljiljana Širić[1]*, Marinela Rosso[1] and Aleksandar Včev[2]

1 Faculty of Education, J. J. Strossmayer University of Osijek, Osijek, Croatia

2 Faculty of Dental Medicine and Health, J. J. Strossmayer University of Osijek, Osijek, Croatia

*Address all correspondence to: ljsiric@foozos.hr

## References

[1] Guyton AC. Medicinska fiziologija. 2nd ed. Beograd, Zagreb: Medicinska knjiga; 1965. pp. 779-793

[2] Obid R, Redlich M, Tomeh C. The treatment of laryngeal cancer. Oral and Maxillofacial Surgery Clinics of North America. 2019;**31**:1-11. DOI: 10.1016/j.coms.2018.09.001

[3] Maclean J, Cotton S, Perry A. Post-laryngectomy: it's hard to swallow: An Australian study of prevalence and self-reports of swallowing function after a total laryngectomy. Dysphagia. 2009;**24**:172-179

[4] Hrvat Radunković M, Lj Š, Grabovac S. Possibility of deglutition function after laryngectomy: Correlation analysis of physiological condition and consequences. Medica Jadertina. 2022;**52**(1):51-56

[5] Širić L. Rehabilitacija glasa i govora nakon operacije grla. In: Bajtl V, Lj P, editors. Vodič kroz karcinom grla. 1st ed. Osijek: Klub laringektomiranih osoba Osijek, Gradska liga protiv raka Osijek, KBC Osijek; 2020. pp. 35-45

[6] Prgomet D et al. Tumori glave i vrata. 1st ed. Zagreb: Medicinska naklada; 2019. 421 p

[7] Murry T, Carrau RL. Clinical Management of Swallowing Disorders. 3rd ed. San Diego: Plural Publishing Inc.; 2012. pp. 69-99

[8] Neijman M, Hilgers F, van den Brekel M, van Son R, Stuiver M, van der Molen L. Dysphagia after total laryngectomy: An exploratory study and clinical phase II rehabilitation trial with the novel swallowing exercise aid (SEA 2.0). Dysphagia. 1 Apr 2024. DOI: 10.1007/s00455-024-10673-7. [Epub ahead of print]. Erratum in: Dysphagia. 2024 May 8. DOI: 10.1007/s00455-024-10711-4. PMID: 38558177

[9] Pernambuco Lde A, Oliveira JH, Regis RM, Lima LM, Araujo AM, Balata PM, et al. Quality of life and deglutition after total laryngectomy. International Archives of Otorhinolaryngology. 2012;**16**:460-465. DOI: 10.7162/S1809-97772012000400006

[10] Ward EC, Bishop B, Frisby J, Stevens M. Swallowing outcomes following laryngectomy and pharyngolaryngectomy. Archives of Otolaryngology Head Neck Surgery. 2002;**128**:181-186. DOI: 10.1001/archotol.128.2.181

[11] Maclean J, Szczesniak M, Cotton S, Cook I, Perry A. Impact of a laryngectomy and surgical closure technique on swallow biomechanics and dysphagia severity. Otolaryngology Head Neck Surgery. 2011;**144**:21-28. DOI: 10.1177/0194599810390906

[12] Brook I. Vodič za laringektomirane osobe. Zenica: Udruženje laringektomiranih osoba Glas; 2020. 132 p

[13] Zhang T, Szczesniak M, Maclean J, Bertrand P, Wu PI, et al. Biomechanics of pharyngeal deglutitive function following total laryngectomy. Otolaryngology Head Neck Surgery. 2016;**155**(2):295-302. DOI: 10.1177/0194599816639249

[14] Terlingen LT, Pilz W, Kuijer M, Kremer B, Baijens LW. Diagnosis and treatment of oropharyngeal dysphagia after total laryngectomy with or without

pharyngoesophageal reconstruction: Systematic review. Head & Neck. 2018;**40**:2733-2748. DOI: 10.1002/hed.25508

[15] Bua BA, Pendletonc H, Westinb U, Rydellc R. Voice and swallowing after total laryngectomy. Acta Otolaryngologica. 2018;**138**(2):170-174. DOI: 10.1080/00016489.2017.1384056

[16] Stoner PL, Fullerton AL, Freeman AM, Chheda NN, Estores DS. Endoscopic dilation of refractory postlaryngectomy strictures: A case series and literature review. Gastroenterology Research and Practice. 28 May 2019;**2019**:8905615. DOI: 10.1155/2019/8905615. PMID: 31275367; PMCID: PMC6558613

[17] Hone RWA, Rahman E, Wong G, Annan Y, Alexander V, et al. Do salivary bypass tubes lower the incidence of pharyngocutaneous fistula following total laryngectomy? A retrospective analysis of predictive factors using multivariate analysis. European Archives of Otorhinolaryngology. 2017;**274**:1983-1991. DOI: 10.1007/s00405-016-4391-9

[18] Širić Lj. Utjecaj vrste alaringealne fonacije na akustičke parametre glasa i prozodijske elemente govora [PhD thesis]. Osijek: Medicinski fakultet Osijek; 2018

[19] Mumović G, Hočevar-Boltezar I. Olfaction and gustation abilities after total laryngectomy. Radiology and Oncology. 2014;**48**(3):301-306

[20] Van Dam FS, Hilgers FJM, Emsbroek G, Tuow FI, Van As JC, de Jong N. Deterioration of olfaction and guestation as a consequence of total laryngectomy. Laryngoscope. 1999;**109**:1150-1155

[21] Morales-Puebla JM, Morales-Puebla AF, Jimenaz-Antolin JA, Munoz-Platon E, Padilla-Parrado M, Chacon-Martinez J. Olfactory rehabilitation after total laryngectomy. Acta Otorhinolaryngologica Espanola. 2010;**61**:128-134

[22] Balfe DM, Koehler RE, Setzen M, Weyman PJ, Baron RL, Ogura JH. Barium examination of the esophagus after total laryngectomy. Radiology. 1982;**143**(2):501-508

[23] Vivanti AP, Campbell KL, Suter MS, Hannan-Jones MT, Hulcombe JA. Contribution of thickened drinks, food and enteral and parenteral fluids to fluid intake in hospitalised patients with dysphagia. Journal of Human Nutrition and Dietetics. 2009;**22**(2):148-155

[24] Mitsuhata T, Teramoto S. Epidemiology of aspiration pneumonia: How frequently does aspiration pneumonia occur in older adults? In: Teramoto S, Komiya K, editors. Aspiration Pneumonia. Respiratory Disease Series: Diagnostic Tools and Disease Managements. Singapore: Springer; 2020. pp. 3-13

[25] Belafsky PC, Mouadeb DA, Rees CJ, Pryor JC, Postma GN, et al. Validity and reliability of the eating assessment tool (EAT-10). Annals of Otology, Rhinology and Laryngology. 2008;**117**(12):919-924. DOI: 10.1177/000348940811701210

[26] Sibergleit AK, Schulz L, Jacobson BH, Beardsley T, Johnson AF. The dysphagia handicap index: Development and validation. Dysphagia. 2012;**27**:46-52

[27] Jamróz B, Chmielewska-Walczak J, Milewska M. Dysphagia among patients after total laryngectomy: Diagnostic and therapeutic procedures. Polish Otorhinolaryngology

Review. 2020;**9**(4):23-28. DOI: 10.5604/01.3001.0014.5705

[28] Zupan M. Preventiva aspiracijske pljučnice s cervikalno avskultacijo in pulzno oksimetrijo pri moždanski kapi. In: Zupanc Isoski V, Pražnikar A, editors. Disfagija in možganska kap. Ljubljana: Nevrološka klinika, UKC; 2011. p. 257

[29] Suiter DM, Leder SB. Clinical utility of the 3-ounce water swallow test. Dysphagia. 2008;**23**:244-250

[30] Wu MC, Chang YC, Wang TG, Lin LC. Evaluating swallowing dysfunction using a 100-ml water swallowing test. Dysphagia. 2004;**19**:43-47

[31] O'Neil KH, Purdy M, Falk J, Gallo L. The dysphagia outcome and severity scale. Dysphagia. 1999;**14**:139-145

[32] Prosiegel M, Heintze M, Wagner-Sonntag W, Hannig C, Wuttge-Hannig A, Yassouridis A. Schluckstörungen bei neurologischen Patienten: Eine prospective Studie zu Diagnostik, Störungsmustern, Therapie und outcome. Nervenarzt. 2002;**73**:364-370

[33] Poljaković Z, Vodanović D, Vranešić Bender D, Ljubas Kelečić D, Starčević K, Kolundžić Z, et al. Smjernice za rano prepoznavanje, dijagnostiku i terapiju neurogene orofaringealne disfagije. Liječnički Vjesnik. 2017;**139**:118-135

[34] Frost J, Robinson HF, Hibberd J. A comparison of neuromuscular electrical stimulation and traditional therapy, versus traditional therapy in patients with longstanding dysphagia. Current Opinion Otolaryngology & Head and Neck Surgery. 2018;**26**(3):167-173

[35] Krznarić Ž, Vranešić D. Pripravci u enteralnoj prehrani danas (praktične smjernice). Medicina. 2003;**42**(4):269-273

Chapter 11

# Post-Radiation Dysphagia and Its Prevention

*Prachi Upadhyay and Piyush Kumar*

## Abstract

Radiotherapy has become a primary treatment modality for head and neck cancers (HNC), aimed at organ and functional preservation. Despite its effectiveness, conventional radiotherapy often leads to severe side effects, notably swallowing dysfunction, or dysphagia, which is a common and distressing complication. This condition greatly impacts the quality of life (QoL) of patients, causing issues such as aspiration pneumonia, malnutrition, and difficulties with speaking and eating. Advancements in radiotherapy, particularly intensity modulated radiotherapy (IMRT), offer the potential to reduce these adverse effects while maintaining or even improving therapeutic efficacy. One key advantage of IMRT is its ability to shape the radiation beams to precisely match the contours of the tumour, allowing for optimal targeting while sparing critical swallowing-related structures such as the pharyngeal muscles, base of the tongue, larynx, and upper oesophageal sphincter. Together, these structures are referred to as dysphagia aspiration-related structures (DARS). This level of precision can lead to lower rates of swallowing dysfunction and other complications commonly associated with traditional radiation therapy methods. In conclusion, IMRT represents a significant advancement in radiation therapy technology and has the potential to reduce swallowing dysfunction and other side effects seen with conventional radiotherapy.

**Keywords:** head and neck cancer, radiation-induced dysphagia, intensity modulated radiotherapy, swallowing exercise, quality of life

## 1. Introduction

For decades, the true bottleneck in the treatment of HNC organ preservation has been radiation-associated dysphagia. Patients undergoing radiation therapy, either in conjunction with or apart from concurrent chemotherapy (RTCT), report varying degrees of dysphagia both during and immediately after treatment. This dysphagia, which may result from oral mucositis and laryngeal edema, which typically resolves within 3–4 months. However, in certain individuals, the healing process may lead to neurological impairment, lymphoedema, scarring, and soft tissue fibrosis. This can result in a swallowing disorder after the course of treatment is completed. This chapter explores how IMRT reduces swallowing dysfunction compared to conventional radiotherapy, examining the underlying mechanisms, clinical evidence, patient implications, and its prevention.

## 1.1 Understanding swallowing dysfunction in radiotherapy

### *1.1.1 Structures involved in swallowing*

Thirty pairs of muscles and six cranial nerves—the XI nerve being less significant than the others—plays a crucial role in the swallowing process. These nerves include the trigeminal, facial, glossopharyngeal, vagus, accessory, and hypoglossal nerves (V, VII, IX, X, XI, XII) [1–3]. These structures involved in swallowing include:

*Oral cavity and pharynx*:

- *Tongue:* Critical for moving food and initiating swallowing.
- *Soft palate:* Closes off the nasal passages during swallowing.
- *Pharyngeal muscles:* Propel the food bolus from the mouth into the oesophagus.
- *Epiglottis:* Prevents food from entering the trachea (windpipe) by covering it.
- Larynx:
    - *Vocal cords:* Close during swallowing to protect the airway; this represents the principle mechanism to prevent aspiration.
    - *Arytenoid cartilages:* Assist in closing the vocal cords.
- *Upper oesophageal sphincter (UES):* Assist food to pass from the pharynx into the oesophagus when open.

### *1.1.2 Normal physiology of swallowing*

Two paradigmatic models typically describe the physiology of normal eating and swallowing: the four-stage model for drinking and swallowing liquids and the process model for eating and swallowing solid food. The normal human swallowing model was first described using a three-staged sequential model. The four-stage model was originally split into three phases based on the swallowing process and the bolus's location [4, 5]—the mouth, throat, and oesophagus phases. The four-stage model was eventually established after the oral phase was further spilt into two stages, i.e., oral preparatory and oral propulsive stage.

*Oral phase*:

*Oral preparatory stage:* The bolus is mixed with saliva and pressed against the hard palate in the anterior part of the tongue to form a seal, preventing the bolus from migrating into the oropharynx before swallowing.

*Oral propulsive stage:* Base of the tongue descends to widen the space between the tongue and palate, and the tongue tip rises to make contact with the hard palate's alveolar ridge.

*Pharyngeal phase:* This phase is the shortest but the most complex because there is no pharyngeal activity until the bolus reaches the UES and triggers the swallowing reflux. This phase is entirely involuntary and involves cranial nerves that supply both motor and sensory functions, primarily the glossopharyngeal (IX) and vagus (X). The two crucial components of this phase are food passage and airway protection. Airway protection involves preventing food from entering the trachea and larynx from the pharynx during food passage, while food passage refers to moving the food bolus down the pharynx, UES, and oesophagus. Several protective mechanisms ensure airway safety during this phase. The mechanisms that prevent aspiration include:

- The arytenoid cartilages bend forward to make contact with the vocal cords and epiglottis, closing the larynx before the UES opens.
- The thyrohyoid and suprahyoid muscles contract, pulling the hyoid bone and propelling the larynx posteriorly. Eventually, the laryngeal vestibule closes as the epiglottis tilts backwards.
- The UES opens to allow the bolus to enter the oesophagus due to the action of the proximal oesophagus, the inferior group of constrictor muscles, and the relaxation of the cricopharyngeal muscles.

*Oesophageal phase:* True peristalsis, regulated by the autonomic nervous system, controls bolus transport in the lower oesophagus, distinguishing it from the upper oesophagus. The UES helps the bolus enter the upper oesophagus. The oesophagus then experiences peristaltic waves, which assist in pushing the bolus past the lower oesophageal sphincter and into the stomach.

#### *1.1.3 Neural pathway*

The neural pathway is crucial to the act of swallowing. Temperature palpation, pressure, taste, and nociceptive somatic stimuli from the larynx and oropharynx are among the physicochemical properties of the bolus that are transmitted to the central pattern in the nucleus tractus solitarius through cranial nerves V, VII, IX, and X. There, data from the cortex is integrated with these inputs. The somatic sensory input required for normal swallowing is perceived by the pharyngeal branches of the X and IX nerves, the lingual branches of the V and IX nerves, and the laryngeal branches of the X nerve. The swallow response is initiated by the brainstem swallowing centre, which receives significant modulating inputs from both the oropharynx and the cortex [3].

### 1.2 Pathophysiology of radiation-induced dysphagia

Swallowing dysfunction, or dysphagia, resulting from radiotherapy is multifactorial. The intricate coordination of muscles and nerves responsible for swallowing can be disrupted by radiation. This can involve both acute and chronic changes to the structures involved in swallowing. The key factors include:

- Acute (Early) Effect:

  This phase occurs during or shortly after radiation and generally lasts for a few months but can be severe.

  a. *Inflammation (Mucositis):* During and after radiotherapy, patients often experience mucositis, which is inflammation and ulceration of the mucous membranes lining the mouth and throat. This inflammation causes pain and swelling, making the act of swallowing painful (odynophagia) and more difficult.

b. *Oedema:* Radiation can cause swelling (oedema) in the structures involved in swallowing. This swelling can narrow the passageway, creating an obstruction that makes it harder for food and liquids to pass through.

c. *Dysgeusia (taste dysfunction):* This may have negatively impact the QoL. A decrease in oral intake caused by taste dysfunction may compromise nutrition.

d. *Fatigue and weakness*: Radiation therapy-related general fatigue can weaken and impair the coordination and strength of the swallowing muscles.

- Chronic (Late) Effects:

a. *Tissue fibrosis:* Radiotherapy can lead to fibrosis, which is the formation of excessive connective tissue and scarring. This fibrosis affects the muscles and connective tissues in the head and neck, reducing their flexibility and strength. Consequently, the coordinated movements required for effective swallowing are impaired. These progressive and irreversible effects may become noticeable between 6 months and 5 years following radiotherapy.

b. *Nerve damage*: Radiation can damage the nerves that control the muscles involved in swallowing. This damage can disrupt the signalling pathways necessary for initiating and coordinating the swallowing process, leading to weakened or uncoordinated muscle contractions. Increased sensory impairment of the upper aerodigestive tract mucosa due to tissue loss or modifications after radiation therapy appears to be one of the primary causes of swallowing disorders, particularly aspiration.

c. *Muscle atrophy*: Prolonged inflammation and disuse of the swallowing muscles due to pain or difficulty can lead to muscle atrophy. The function of swallowing is further compromised by decreased muscle mass and strength. The underlying constrictors muscles are also affected by the acute inflammation of the pharyngeal mucosa, which covers these muscles. This suggests that inflammation of the pharyngeal constrictors is a significant cause of inflammation.

d. *Chronic xerostomia:* Radiotherapy has the potential to harm the salivary glands, resulting in a significant reduction in saliva production (xerostomia). Saliva is essential for moistening and lubricating food, aiding in its formation into a cohesive bolus, and facilitating its smooth passage through the throat. A lack of saliva makes swallowing dry and solid foods particularly challenging.

e. *Oesophageal stricture*: Radiation can cause the oesophagus to narrow (stricture), leading to persistent and progressive difficulty in swallowing solid foods, which may require medical or surgical intervention to dilate the oesophagus.

f. *Structural changes:* Radiotherapy can induce structural changes in the tissues and organs involved in swallowing, including the larynx and throat, as well as strictures, which are narrowing of the oesophagus. These changes can create physical barriers to effective swallowing.

g. *Combined impact:* The combination of these factors results in multifaceted swallowing dysfunction, which includes difficulty initiating a swallow, pain during swallowing, a sensation of food sticking in the throat, choking, and an increased risk of aspiration (food or liquids entering the airway). The cumulative effect significantly impacts the patient's ability to eat and drink, potentially leading. To dietary deficiencies and a lower QoL.

### 1.3 Consequences of radiation-induced dysphagia

Patients frequently experience swallowing dysfunction and its potentially fatal complications (malnutritional and aspiration pneumonia), which are brought on by both primary cancer (baseline dysphagia) and treatment due to the close proximity of tumour location and structures related to dysphagia and aspiration [6–8]. Dysphagia has impacts on the patient, their family, and the healthcare system.

The consequences of radiation-induced dysphagia include:

1. *Aspiration pneumonia*: Aspiration, in which food or liquid enters the lungs rather than the stomach, is a risk factor for dysphagia. This can cause pneumonia, a serious lung infection that can be life-threatening, particularly in immunocompromised patients.

2. *Nutritional deficiency*: Difficulty swallowing can lead to reduced food intake, resulting in malnutrition and weight loss. This can weaken the immune system, reduce muscle mass, and affect overall health.

3. *Chronic pain*: Some patients may experience chronic pain and discomfort in the throat or chest due to inflammation and fibrosis (scarring) of the tissues affected by radiation.

4. *Dehydration*: Trouble swallowing liquids can lead to inadequate fluid intake, causing dehydration, which can affect various bodily functions such as low blood pressure, deranged kidney function, and exacerbate other health issues.

5. *Decline in QoL*: Eating and drinking can be challenging and uncomfortable, which can significantly lower one's QoL. Patients may feel depressed, anxious, or frustrated due to their inability to socialise or enjoy meals.

6. *Social isolation:* The inability to eat normally can lead to social isolation, as patients might avoid social gatherings that involve food, further impacting their emotional wellbeing.

## 2. Advantages of IMRT over conventional radiotherapy

A high rate of radiotherapy-associated dysphagia has historically been associated with radiation-related dysphagia, which affects over 50% of patients and frequently results in pharyngo-oesophageal strictures, aspiration pneumonia, malnutrition, and prolonged reliance on percutaneous endoscopic gastrostomy (PEG) tube dependence [6, 9–11]. Therefore, over the past 30 years, radiotherapy has evolved from being based on two-dimensional (2D), or conventional, to three-dimensional (3D). Incorporating

3D images, and advanced computer algorithms has reduced radiation-related side effects, and IMRT is a form of 3D conformal radiotherapy (3DCRT) that allows for precise targeting of tumours while minimising exposure to surrounding healthy tissues. Numerous studies have shown that IMRT lowers the risk of swallowing dysfunction because, in contrast to 3DCRT, it can produce concave dose distributions that better avoid a number of significant dose-limiting structures, including DARS. This could result in better functional outcomes [12–15]. Key features of IMRT include:

- *Modulated radiation beams*: IMRT is an optimal method for allocating non-uniform intensities, or weights, to small subdivisions of beams, referred to as "beamlets" or "rays." The greatly enhanced control over the radiation fluence results from the ability to optimally manipulate the intensities of individual rays within each beam, allowing for the customised design of ideal dose distributions. These better dose distributions could result in less toxicity to normal tissue as well as better tumour control.

- *3D imaging:* Advanced imaging techniques (e.g., computed tomography, magnetic resonance imaging) guide the precise delivery of radiation, optimising tumour targeting and sparing normal tissues.

- *Multiple angles of delivery:* IMRT can deliver radiation from multiple angles, further refining the distribution of the dose and reducing the risk to non-target tissues.

- *Dose escalation:* Higher doses can be delivered to the tumour with fewer side effects.

- *Dose distribution optimisation:* Algorithms that calculate the optimal radiation dose distribution to maximise tumour control and minimise side effects.

## 3. Prevention of radiation-induced dysphagia

### 3.1 IMRT in reducing swallowing dysfunction

#### *3.1.1 Evidence*

Numerous studies on parotid sparing have demonstrated the potential of IMRT to lower doses to the parotid glands as well as reduce the risk of developing xerostomia. This leads to a shift in focus to the most debilitating effect on a patient's daily life, i.e., swallowing dysfunction, which can even result in life-threatening complications such as aspiration pneumonia. Regardless of the primary tumour site, radiated patients typically experience similar swallowing dysfunction. For instance, nasopharyngeal tumours have been shown to cause issues with both the oral stage of swallowing and the pharyngeal stage, even though the primary tumour is limited to the nasal cavity [16, 17]. Recent research indicates that long-term dysphagia may negatively affect QoL even more than xerostomia [18–21]. Following the disclosure that radiation-induced dysphagia impairs QoL and increases the risk for silent aspiration in patients, various studies have been conducted to identify structures that may be responsible for swallowing dysfunction and to evaluate the potential of dose constraints of these structures [22–24].

Eisbruch et al. have conducted a research to determine which structures have anatomical or functional abnormalities that cause dysphagia, aspiration, or impaired swallowing. Additionally, they investigated the viability of sparing these structures with specific IMRT techniques, taking care to preserve the target tumour volume [25]. Eisbruch et al. were the first to raise doubts about a relationship between dose-volume parameters and dysphagia. Thirty-two patients with locally advanced HNC had a high incidence of dysphagia after two chemoradiation protocols. The researchers observed a significant increase in the thickness of the supraglottic larynx (SGL), glottic larynx, and pharyngeal constrictors. This allowed the authors to designate these organs as dose-limiting structures, and they recommended a 50 Gy starting dose limit for the pharynx to prevent stricture at this site [12]. The contouring guidelines proposed by Eisbruch et al. and the anatomical swallowing organ at risk have been used in later studies to provide more evidence for reducing dysphagia. These structures were identified as the pharyngeal constrictors, larynx, and SGL. Unlike 3DCRT and conventional methods, IMRT preserved these structures through the use of optimised and customised IMRT plans. IMRT decreased DARS V50 (the percentage of volume that received a dose of 50 Gy) by 7–10% on average, which led several centres to examine the effect of the dose given to DARS on different late dysphagia measures [12]. A study conducted at our institute by Upadhyay et al. also revealed that low-volume DARS could be significantly spared by using IMRT as opposed to 3DCRT [26].

Felix et al., conducted a prospective longitudinal investigation that included patients with oropharyngeal and nasopharyngeal cancers in stages I–IV. All these patients were treated with a definitive chemo-IMRT regimen to spare the pharyngeal constrictors, glottis, SGL, and other dysphagia-related structures. Sparing of DARS is very challenging in nasopharyngeal carcinomas because the retropharyngeal nodes are always contoured in high-risk volumes, i.e., >50 Gy and are in close approximation to the constrictor's muscles. The novel IMRT approach resulted in swallowing outcomes that were marginally worse than baseline over the long term, indicating the possibility of functional improvements [27].

Van der Molen et al., assessed the dose-effect relationship for swallowing difficulties following concurrent chemotherapy in locally advanced HNC. They found that the likelihood of developing dysphagia increased with each 1 Gy mean dose increase to the inferior constrictor muscle, with an odds ratio of 1.11. Other DARS structures that were known to be important in the dysphagia status but had not yet been studied include the base of the tongue, larynx, oesophagus, and cricopharyngeus muscle [28].

Nutting et al., in comparison to standard IMRT (st IMRT), examined whether a dysphagia-optimised IMRT (do-IMRT) could lower the dose to DARS as well as improve swallowing function in a randomised multicentre trial. They It was discovered that at 3, 12, and 24 months, participants who received do-IMRT reported normalcy in their diet and eating in public—more than 75% or more than 90%—compared to those who received stIMRT. IMRT reduces V50 (volume receiving a dose of 50 Gy) of pharyngeal constrictors by 10%, and do-IMRT reduces these volumes further by an average of 10% [29].

### *3.1.2 Delineation guidelines for DARS*

Following the identification of DARS, efforts were made to implement new strategies into practice with the goal of lowering the dosage to these structures. Guidelines have been developed in various literatures based on normal anatomy and function, and consensus from various literature has been summarised in **Table 1** and **Figure 1** depicting contoured DARS on a contrast-enhanced computed tomography scan using these guidelines.

| **Delineation of individual dars** | | | | | | |
|---|---|---|---|---|---|---|
| | **Cranial** | **Caudal** | **Anterior** | **Posterior** | **Middle** | **Lateral** |
| SCM | Caudal tip of pterygoid plate or occipital condyle | Upper edge of hyoid bone | Anterior edge of pterygoid plate | Cervical vertebrae or longus capitis muscle | Pharynx | Palatine tonsil or parapharyngeal space |
| MCM | Upper edge of hyoid bone | Lower edge of hyoid bone | Oropharynx | Cervical vertebrae or longus capitis muscle | Pharynx | Parapharyngeal space |
| ICM | Lower edge of hyoid bone | Lower edge of cricoid cartilage | Arytenoid, first tracheal ring | Vertebral body or longus capitis muscle | Pharynx | Parapharyngeal space |
| BOT | Below the soft palate (uvula) | Upper edge of hyoid bone | Posterior third of tongue | Pharynx | Pharynx | Palatine tonsils |
| LARYNX | Upper edge of epiglottis | Lower edge of cricoid cartilage | Anterior tip of thyroid cartilage | Inferior constrictor muscle | Thyroid cartilage | Pharyngeal lumen |
| UES | Lower edge of cricoid cartilage | Upper edge of trachea or sternal notch | Tracheal lumen | Vertebral body | — | — |

*Abbreviations: SCM, superior constrictor muscles; MCM, middle constrictor muscles; ICM, inferior constrictor muscles; BOT, base of tongue; UES, upper oesophageal sphincter.*

**Table 1.**
*Summarised delineation guidelines for individual DARS.*

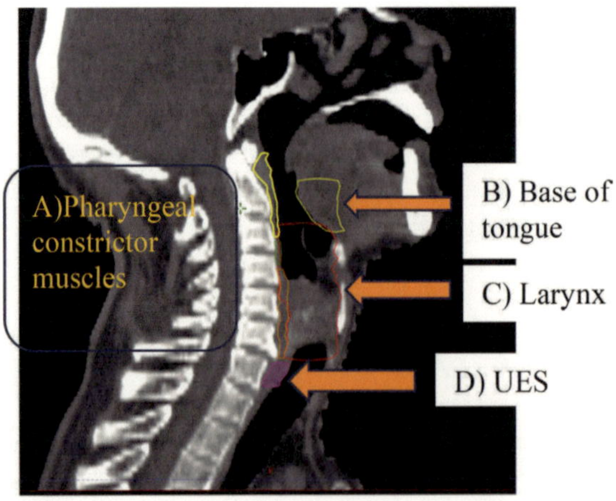


**Figure 1.**
*Contoured individual DARS in a sagittal section of a contrast-enhanced computed tomography scan of neck; (A) pharyngeal constrictor muscles [yellow-superior, green-middle, orange-inferior]; (B) base of tongue (dark yellow); (C) larynx (red); (D) upper oesophageal sphincter (UES) (pink).*

### *3.1.3 Relation of dose and dysphagia*

Numerous dose-volume constraints linked to dysphagia have been proposed. As per the study by Dirix et al., there is a correlation between late dysphagia and V50, Dmean for SGL, and the middle pharyngeal constrictor muscle (MPCM) [30].

Caudell et al. showed that aspiration and PEG tube dependence were related to Dmean (more than 41 Gy), V60 [volume receiving a dose of 60 Gy] (more than 24%) for the inferior pharyngeal constrictor muscle (IPCM), and the larynx's V60 (greater than 12%) [31].

Li et al., state that the recommended dose constraints of less than 55 Gy to the IPCM and a maximum dose of less than 60 Gy to UES to minimise the risk of long-term use of percutaneous endoscopic gastrostomy (PEG) [32].

Feng et al., [27] examined 73 patients with stage III/IV oropharyngeal cancers to determine the effectiveness of swallow-sparing chemotherapy-IMRT. By imposing a dosimetric constraint of less than 50 Gy, the IMRT technique spared the supraglottic larynx (SGL) and pharyngeal constrictor muscles (PCM) surrounding the infrequently affected medial retropharyngeal lymph nodes (RPLN). The entire organ system received mean doses of 58 and 48 Gy, respectively; the mean doses to the spared portions of PCM and SGL were 48 and 42 Gy. Significantly, no relapses were found inside or close to the spared structures, indicating that this dosimetric sparing did not raise the risk of locoregional recurrence. The novel IMRT approach resulted in swallowing outcomes that were marginally worse than baseline over the long term, indicating the possibility of functional improvements.

Improved swallowing outcomes were significantly correlated with mean doses to the entire PCM and its constituent parts, the oesophagus, superior constrictor, and SGL, according to subsequent dosimetric analysis [33]. Comparing the mean doses and partial volumes of these structures (PCM and SGL) receiving 50–65 Gy to the video-fluoroscopy-based aspirations revealed significant correlations; the strongest correlations were observed with the superior pharyngeal constrictor ($p = 0.005$). Furthermore, the volume of PCM receiving 65 Gy was higher than 50% in all aspiration patients, the volume of SGL receiving more than 50 Gy was greater than 50%, and the mean dose to the pharyngeal constrictors was higher than 60 Gy.

Van der Molen et al., [28], evaluated that when the dose-effect relationship for swallowing dysfunction following concurrent chemotherapy in locally advanced HNC was examined, it was discovered that aspiration at 10-weeks was significantly predicted by the mean IPCM dosage and the volume of IPCM receiving 60 Gy (V60). Swallowing problems were found to be significantly correlated with masseter dose parameters (mean, volume receiving 20 Gy {V20}, volume receiving 40 Gy {V40}, and V60) 1 year after treatment. For the IPCM's V60, there was also an inverse relationship (lower dose related to a higher probability). They only had constrictor muscles. The incidence of aspiration or laryngeal penetration can be significantly predicted by the mean dose of 1 Gy, resulting in an odds ratio of 1.11. An additional important predictor is the dose-volume V60 to the inferior constrictor. Other DARS structures that were known to be important in the dysphagia status but had not yet been studied included the base of the tongue, larynx, and oesophagus with the cricopharyngeus muscle.

In an investigation done by Prameela et al., [34] concluded that there were clear-cut statistical and subjective correlations between dosages of the swallowing structures, particularly the base of the tongue, larynx, as well as constrictor muscles. The patient's ability to swallow is correlated statistically and clinically with the probable mean dose constraints. IMRT outperformed 3DCRT statistically significantly in terms of volume receiving a dose of 30 Gy (V30) ($P = 0.051$), V50 ($P = 0.002$), V60

(P = 0.002), and dose of 80 Gy receiving how much volume (D80) (P = 0.023) for swallowing structures taken together.

A statistical cut-off dose of 65.18 Gy in IMRT and 62.76 Gy in 3DCRT was determined for the base of the tongue. It was found that 3/8 (37.5%) of the patients who had undergone radiation therapy greater than 63 Gy were in need of feeding tubes. A mean dose to the larynx exceeding 41 Gy [31] or above 50 Gy, [35] was linked to PEG tube dependence. According to their analysis, patients in the 3DCRT group who received a dose higher than 55.10 Gy to the larynx experienced significant dysphagia and feeding tube dependence. This dose was shown to have both subjective and statistical significance. According to the study, 63 and 55 Gy are the likely limiting doses for the occurrence of dysphagia in the base of the tongue and larynx, respectively.

Hedge RA et al., determined the tolerance limits for dysphagia in HNC and noted that the range of the Dmean to the combined constrictor volume was 16.59–71.31 Gy. The ability to swallow only liquids and to take semisolids but not solids (Grade 3 and 4 late toxicity, respectively) is statistically significant, and it is correlated with a threshold mean dose of 63 Gy to the superior constrictors muscles. Higher doses to the base of the tongue and superior constrictor muscles independently contribute to late toxicity with grade 3 and 4 late toxicities (p = 0.013 and 0.005, respectively). They also found that a significant parameter for expected grade 3 and 4 toxicities was V60 of the inferior constrictor. Given that it is the longest constrictor, this may imply a volume correlation [36].

Sharma A et al., studied the possibility of using IMRT to lower the risk of post-treatment dysphagia in HNC and found that lowering the V50 of these structures or lowering the mean dose below 50 Gy may help lower the incidence of aspiration and dysphagia. There may be a steep dose-effect relationship following a 55 Gy DARS dose, with a 19% rise in the likelihood of dysphagia for each 10 Gy [14]. It seems that the most significant dosimetric predictor of late swallowing dysfunction is the mean dose that PCM received. Additionally, patients with mean doses to PCM of 61–64 Gy and mean doses to the larynx of 48–54 Gy exhibit worsening aspiration and swallowing in comparison to mean doses of 52–55 Gy and 36–38 Gy, respectively, in 3DCRT and IMRT to these structures [37].

Two studies done in our institute: The first study done by Upadhyay et al., compared 3DCRT and IMRT without giving any dose constraints to structures related to dysphagia and found that there is a significant advantage with IMRT in comparison to 3DCRT in terms of the pharyngeal constrictor mean dosage (66.03 vs. 68.7 Gy; p = 0.003) and the mean dose to combined DARS has also been statistically significantly lower in IMRT i.e. (66.15 vs. 70.09 Gy, p = 0.001). Furthermore, the IMRT group experienced a decreased rate of clinical worsening of dysphagia (48 vs. 80%, p = 0.003) [26]. After realising there is a relative reduction in doses in IMRT in comparison to 3DCRT, another study done in our institute by Agarwal et al., aimed to see how feasible IMRT is in achieving dose constraints for DARS and concluded that V60 and V70 of the inferior constrictor and larynx are statistically significant in preventing swallowing dysfunction in the do-IMRT group [38].

#### *3.1.4 How feasible is IMRT in achieving dose constraints*

Radiation-induced acute and late dysphagia can be predicted by T and N stage, primary site, treatment volume, and patient characteristics (baseline swallowing function, performance status (PS), any history of addiction, age, lean mass). The following question arises: Is the primary site an important factor that results in an increased incidence of late dysphagia? According to a series of reports by Logemann et al., the most common disorders that are observed are those that affect pressure during swallowing and protect the airway (reduced tongue base retraction and reduced tongue strength) [39]. Patients with oropharyngeal and laryngeal cancer were reported to exhibit a reduction in the base of tongue movement more frequently. The posterior tongue is most likely to receive the maximum radiation dose when treating oropharyngeal and laryngeal cancers because it is situated between them. A similar result was found by Langius et al., who discovered that at 3 months following radiation therapy, patients with oropharyngeal tumours had a statistically significant worsening in their ability to handle semisolids [40]. In a study by Caudell et al., patients with pharyngeal carcinoma (oropharynx, hypopharynx, larynx) showed grade 3 or more dysphagia, i.e., 28.6% of cases, compared to 7.5% for oral cavity and nasopharynx cases [31]. The author's study showed similar findings, whereby dysphagia is commoner in patients with pharyngeal carcinoma, i.e., 48% (n = 24), followed by hypopharynx with 28% (n = 7), larynx 20% (n = 5) and least common in patients with oral cavity carcinoma, i.e., 12% (n = 3) [26].

Because a significant portion of DARS was observed to lie within the treating volume in cases of oro-larynopharynx carcinoma, being challenging to spare, dose constraints to DARS cannot be achieved in all HNC cases. A study conducted by Adan et al., noticed that when the volume of the planning target volume (PTV) is more than 150 cc, DARS overlaps with PTV, which makes achieving dose constraints below 60 Gy difficult [41]. **Figure 2** illustrates that 73% of the 70 Gy dose covers DARS. Therefore, patient selection and tumour site are important factors in providing better swallowing function and therapeutic results.

Other predicted factors affecting radiation-induced dysphagia is age as an important risk factor because radiation-induced fibrosis and atrophy have a contributing effect on dysphagia, as explained previously, and worsen in older age groups [42].

### 3.2 Swallowing exercise

Preventive evidence is mounting that patients with HNC should start proactive swallowing exercises before receiving radiation therapy. Numerous compensatory

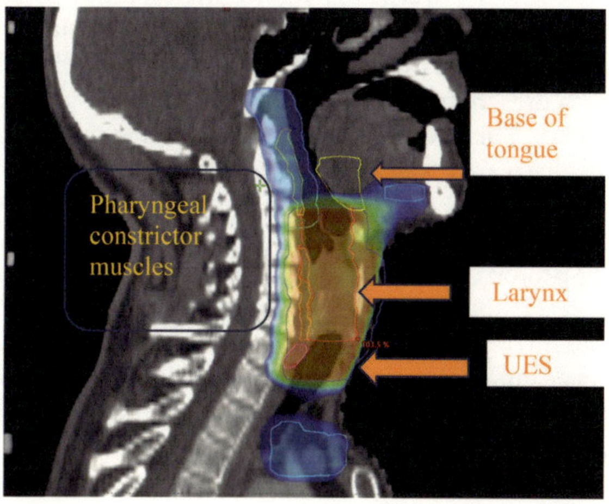


**Figure 2.**
*Ca Supraglottic Larynx (cT3N2aM0) Stage IVa, showing the dose wash of radiotherapy plan without applying any dose constraints to DARS. The red dose wash indicates a dose of more than 95% of 70 Gy; the blue indicates less than 50% of 70 Gy. It is well appreciated that most of the DARS are within the PTV.*

strategies exist, such as postural adjustments and manoeuvres. Most people agree that even if a patient has a feeding tube, these exercises should begin before cancer treatment and continue both during and after treatment [7, 43–45]. While swallowing rehabilitation can be beneficial if it is initiated soon after treatment, it can also help prevent swallowing episodes from occurring less frequently and enhance the patient's QoL. Therefore, it is widely believed that prevention should be prioritised [7, 44–46]. Some swallowing functions may be improved by preventive swallowing exercises following radiotherapy [45–50], but treatment compliance issues limit their effectiveness. The prophylactic swallowing exercises consist of

- *Effortful swallow:* Patients are instructed to swallow hard, squeezing all the muscles involved in swallowing.

- *Mendelsohn manoeuvre:* This involves holding the larynx (voice box) at its highest point during a swallow for a few seconds before releasing.

- *Masako manoeuvre:* Accomplished by swallowing with the tongue wedged between the teeth.

- *Shaker exercise*: This involves lifting the head while lying down to strengthen the muscles involved in swallowing.

- *Tongue hold swallow*: To strengthen and coordinate the tongue, hold it against the roof of the mouth while swallowing.

- *Supraglottic swallow*: Includes clearing the airway of any leftover food or liquid by coughing, holding one's breath, and swallowing.

## 4. Future directions

By offering a better toxicity profile than conventional radiotherapy, IMRT has demonstrated that it is safe in terms of oncological outcomes and can prevent dysphagia. These results have paved the way for an even more conformal method, i.e., proton therapy, which uses intensity modulated proton therapy (IMPT) to further refine its treatment plan. The advantage of IMPT is that the majority of the energy is concentrated in a localised area, and as it travels through the medium there is minimal energy, very little energy loss in the process—a phenomenon is referred to as the Bragg peak. As a result, the distal side of the tumour receives less radiation. As IMPT gains popularity and more proton centres open globally, clinical trials are being conducted to demonstrate the effectiveness of IMPT in preventing post-radiation dysphagia.

When using more intricate treatment methods, it is crucial to accurately identify the organ at risk and administer the medication. Small changes in the tumour's volume brought on by tumour shrinkage or anatomical changes in the patient, such as weight loss or sarcopenia, may pose a risk for dosimteric changes that could lead to treatment failure or an increase in toxicity. Adaptive radiotherapy (ART) might offer a remedy for this issue. During radiotherapy, RT plans are modified according to anatomical changes and tumour volume using sequential CT scans. However, it is unlikely that every patient receiving IMRT will require ART. Because ART requires significant time and resources, it should only be used for patients who will benefit clinically. Brown et al., created ART risk profiles that could serve as a roadmap for clinical judgement for nasopharyngeal and oropharyngeal cancers. This would enable the identification of patients who would benefit from ART prior to the initiation of therapy [51]. Most likely, the use of ART in conjunction with IMPT will become even more crucial than IMRT alone.

## 5. Conclusions

Swallowing issues should be considered when assessing the aggressiveness of cancer-directed treatment and evaluating the potential benefits of post-treatment care in HNC patients to prevent swallowing dysfunction and lower the risk of aspiration. Therapeutic interventions, along with routine diagnostic swallowing assessments before, during, and after radiation therapy, should be part of the new standard of care for HNC patients. This will enable accurate supportive care to be provided during treatment to prevent dysphagia and allow for proper prediction of late dysphagia.

## Conflict of interest

The authors declare no conflict of interest.

## Author details

Prachi Upadhyay* and Piyush Kumar
SRMS IMS Hospital, Bareilly, India

*Address all correspondence to: prachiupadhyay20@gmail.com

## References

[1] Jean A. Brain stem control of swallowing: Neuronal network and cellular mechanisms. Physiological Reviews. 2001;**81**:929-969. DOI: 10.1152/physrev.2001.81.2.929

[2] Rofes L, Cola P, Clavé P. The effects of sensory stimulation on neurogenic oropharyngeal dysphagia. Journal of Gastroenterology and Hepatology Research. 2014;**3**:1066-1072. DOI: 10.1136/gutjnl-2011-300753

[3] Alvarez-Berdugo D, Rofes L, Casamitjana JF, Padrón A, Quer M, Clavé P. Oropharyngeal and laryngeal sensory innervation in the pathophysiology of swallowing disorders and sensory stimulation. Annals of the New York Academy of Sciences. 2016;**1380**(1):104-120. DOI: 10.1111/nyas.13150

[4] Dodds WJ, Stewart ET, Logemann JA. Physiology and radiology of the normal oral and pharyngeal phases of swallowing [see comments]. AJR. American Journal of Roentgenology. 1990;**154**(5):953-963. DOI: 10.2214/ajr.154.5.2108569

[5] Logemann JA. Dysphagia: evaluation and treatment. Folia Phoniatr Logop. 1995;**47**(3):140-164. DOI: 10.1159/000266348

[6] Caudell JJ, Schaner PE, Meredith RF, Locher JL, Nabell LM, Carroll WR, et al. Factors associated with long-term dysphagia after definitive radiotherapy for locally advanced head-and-neck cancer. International Journal of Radiation Oncology, Biology, Physics. 2009;**73**:410-415. DOI: 10.1016/j.ijrobp.2008.04.048

[7] Rosenthal DI, Lewin JS, Eisbruch A. Prevention and treatment of dysphagia and aspiration after chemoradiation for head and neck cancer. Journal of Clinical Oncology. 2006;**24**:2636-2643. DOI: 10.1200/JCO.2006.06.0079

[8] Robbins KT. Barriers to winning the battle with head-and- neck cancer. International Journal of Radiation Oncology, Biology, Physics. 2002;**53**:4-5. DOI: 10.1016/s0360-3016(02)02713-x

[9] Nguyen NP, Sallah S, Karlsson U, Antoine JE. Combined chemotherapy and radiation therapy for head and neck malignancies: Quality of life issues. Cancer. 2002;**94**:1131-1141. DOI: 10.1002/cncr.10257

[10] Nguyen NP, Moltz CC, Frank C, Vos P, Smith HJ, Karlsson U, et al. Dysphagia following chemoradiation for locally advanced head and neck cancer. Annals of Oncology. 2004;**15**:383-388. DOI: 10.1093/annonc/mdh101

[11] Batth SS, Caudell JJ, Chen AM. Practical considerations in reducing swallowing dysfunction following concurrent chemoradiotherapy with intensity-modulated radiotherapy for head and neck cancer. Head and Neck. 2014;**36**:291-298. DOI: 10.1002/hed.23246

[12] Eisbruch A, Schwartz M, Rasch C, et al. Dysphagia and aspiration after chemoradiotherapy for head-and-neck cancer: Which anatomic structures are affected and can they be spared by IMRT? International Journal of Radiation Oncology, Biology, Physics. 2004;**60**:1425-1439. DOI: 10.1016/j.ijrobp.2004.05.050

[13] Mazzola R, Ferrera G, Alongi F, Mannino M, Abbate B, Cucchiara T, et al. Organ sparing and clinical outcome with step-and- shoot IMRT for head and neck

cancer: A mono-institutional experience. La Radiologia Medica. 2015;**120**:753-758. DOI: 10.1007/s11547-015-0512-6

[14] Levendag PC, Teguh DN, Voet P, van der Est H, Noever I, WJM d K, et al. Dysphagia disorders in patients with cancer of the oropharynx are significantly affected by the radiation therapy dose to the superior and middle constrictor muscle: A dose-effect relationship. Radiotherapy and Oncology. 2007;**85**:64-73. DOI: 10.1016/j.radonc.2007.07.009

[15] Bhide SA, Gulliford S, Kazi R, El-Hariry I, Newbold K, Harrington KJ, et al. Correlation between dose to the pharyngeal constrictors and patient quality of life and late dysphagia following chemo-IMRT for head and neck cancer. Radiotherapy and Oncology. 2009;**93**:539-544. DOI: 10.1016/j.radonc.2009.09.017

[16] Ku PK, Yuen EH, Cheung DM, et al. Early swallowing problems in a cohort of patients with nasopharyngeal carcinoma: Symptomatology and videofluoroscopic findings. Laryngoscope. 2007;**117**:142-146. DOI: 10.1097/01.mlg.0000248738.55387.44

[17] Logemann JA, Rademaker AW, Pauloski BR, et al. Site of disease and treatment protocol as correlates of swallowing function in patients with head and neck cancer treated with chemoradiation. Head and Neck. 2006;**28**:64-73. DOI: 10.1002/hed.20299

[18] Jensen K, Lambertsen K, Grau C. Late swallowing dysfunction and dysphagia after radiotherapy for pharynx cancer: Frequency, intensity and correlation with dose and volume parameters. Radiotherapy and Oncology. 2007;**85**:74-82. DOI: 10.1016/j.radonc.2007.06.004

[19] Langendijk JA, Doornaert PA, Verdonck-de Leeuw IM, Leemans CR, Aaronson NK, Slotman BJ. Impact of late treatment-related toxicity on quality of life among patients with head and neck cancer treated with radiotherapy. Journal of Clinical Oncology. 2008;**26**:3770-3776. DOI: 10.1200/JCO.2007.14.6647

[20] Goguen LA, Posner MR, Norris CM, et al. Dysphagia after sequential chemoradiation therapy for advanced head and neck cancer. Otolaryngology and Head and Neck Surgery. 2006;**134**:916-922. DOI: 10.1016/j.otohns.2006.02.001

[21] List MA, Siston A, Haraf D, et al. Quality of life and performance in advanced head and neck cancer patients on concomitant chemoradiotherapy: A prospective examination. Journal of Clinical Oncology. 1999;**17**:10208. DOI: 10.1200/JCO.1999.17.3.1020

[22] Smith RV, Kotz T, Beitler JJ, Wadler S. Long-term swallowing problems after organ preservation therapy with concomitant radiation therapy and intravenous hydroxyurea: Initial results. Archives of Otolaryngology—Head and Neck Surgery. 2000;**126**:384-389. DOI: 10.1001/archotol.126.3.384

[23] Wu CH, Hsiao TY, Ko JY, Hsu MM. Dysphagia after radiotherapy: Endoscopic examination of swallowing in patients with nasopharyngeal carcinoma. The Annals of Otology, Rhinology, and Laryngology. 2000;**109**(320):325. DOI: 10.1177/000348940010900315

[24] Nguyen NP, Moltz CC, Frank C, et al. Dysphagia severity following chemoradiation and postoperative radiation for head and neck cancer. European Journal of Radiology. 2006;**59**:453-459. DOI: 10.1016/j.ejrad.2006.03.019

[25] Eisbruch A, Lyden T, Bradford CR, Dawson LA, Haxer MJ, Miller AE, et al.

Objective assessment of swallowing dysfunction and aspiration after radiation concurrent with chemotherapy for head and neck cancer. International Journal of Radiation Oncology, Biology, Physics. 2002;**53**:23-28. DOI: 10.1053/srao.2002.32435

[26] Upadhyay P Sr, Kumar P, Chauhan AK, Kumar P, Nigam J, S N. Comparison of dosimetric parameters in dysphagia aspiration- related structures and clinical correlation in head and neck cancer patients treated with radiotherapy. Cureus. 2022;**14**(7):e26765. DOI: 10.7759/cureus.26765

[27] Feng FY, Kim HM, Lyden TH, et al. Intensity-modulated radiotherapy of head and neck cancer aiming to reduce dysphagia: Early dose–effect relationships for the swallowing structures. International Journal of Radiation Oncology, Biology, Physics. 2007;**68**:1289-1298. DOI: 10.1016/j.ijrobp.2007.02.049

[28] Van der Molen L, Heemsbergen WD, de Jong R, van Rossum MA, Smeele LE, Rasch CR, et al. Dysphagia and trismus after concomitant chemo-intensity-modulated radiation therapy (chemo-IMRT) in advanced head and neck cancer; dose-effect relationships for swallowing and mastication structures. Radiotherapy and Oncology. 2013;**106**:364-369. DOI: 10.1016/j.radonc.2013.03.005

[29] Nutting C et al. Dysphagia-optimised intensity modulated radiotherapy versus standard intensity-modulated radiotherapy in patients with head and neck cancer (DARS): A phase 3, multicentre, randomised, controlled trial. The Lancet. Oncology. 2023;**24**(8):868-880. DOI: 10.1016/S1470-2045(23)00265-6

[30] Dirix P, Abbeel S, Vanstraelen B, et al. Dysphagia after chemoradiotherapy for head-and-neck squamous cell carcinoma: Dose–Effect relationships for the swallowing structures. International Journal of Radiation Oncology, Biology, Physics. 2009;**75**:385-392. DOI: 10.1016/j.ijrobp.2008.11.041

[31] Caudell JJ, Schaner PE, Desmond RA, Meredith RF, Spencer SA, Bonner JA. Dosimetric factors associated with long-term dysphagia after definitive radiotherapy for squamous cell carcinoma of the head and neck. International Journal of Radiation Oncology, Biology, Physics. 2010;**76**:403-409. DOI: 10.1016/j.ijrobp.2009.02.017

[32] Li B et al. Clinical-dosimetric analysis of measures of dysphagia including gastrostomy-tube dependence among head and neck cancer patients treated definitively by intensity-modulated radiotherapy with concurrent chemotherapy. Radiation Oncology. 2009;**4**:52. DOI: 10.1186/1748-717X-4-52

[33] Schwartz DL et al. Candidate dosimetric predictors of long-term swallowing dysfunction after oropharyngeal intensity-modulated radiotherapy. International Journal of Radiation Oncology, Biology, Physics. 2010;**78**(5):1356-1365. DOI: 10.1016/j.ijrobp.2009.10.002

[34] Prameela CG, Ravind R, Renil Mon PS, Sheejamol VS, Dinesh M. Radiation dose to dysphagia aspiration-related structures and its effect on swallowing: Comparison of three-dimensional conformal radiotherapy and intensity- modulated radiation therapy plans. Journal of Cancer Research and Therapeutics. 2016;**12**:845-851. DOI: 10.4103/0973-1482.163676

[35] Caglar HB, Tishler RB, Othus M, Burke E, Li Y, Goguen L, et al. Dose to larynx predicts for swallowing complications after intensity-modulated

radiotherapy. International Journal of Radiation Oncology, Biology, Physics. 2008;**72**:1110-1118. DOI: 10.1016/j.ijrobp.2008.02.048

[36] Hegde A, Vishwanath L. Dysphagia Associated Organ Sparing Radiotherapy: Defining the Limits of Tolerance for Late Toxicity. 2019. DOI:10.30564/amor.v4i5.189

[37] Sharma A, Bahl A. Intensity-modulated radiation therapy in head- and neck- carcinomas: Potential beyond sparing the parotid glands. Journal of Cancer Research and Therapeutics. 2020;**16**(3):425-433. DOI: 10.4103/jcrt.JCRT_880_18

[38] Agarwal K, Kumar P, Navitha S, et al. Feasibility of achieving dose constraints for dysphagia aspiration related structures and its clinical significance in intensity-modulated radiotherapy planning of head and neck cancer. Cureus. 2024;**16**(2):e53769. DOI: 10.7759/cureus.53769

[39] Logemann JA. Update on clinical trials in dysphagia. Dysphagia. 2006;**21**(2):116-120. DOI: 10.1007/s00455-006-9017-8

[40] Langius JA, Bakker S, Rietveld DH, Kruizenga HM, Langendijk JA, Weijs PJ, et al. Critical weight loss is a major prognostic indicator for disease-specific survival in patients with head and neck cancer receiving radiotherapy. British Journal of Cancer. 2013;**109**(5):1093-1099. DOI: 10.1038/bjc.2013.458

[41] Calcuttawala A, Shinghal A, Budrukkar AN, et al. Can dysphagia aspiration related structures (DARS) be spared in patients with oropharyngeal cancers? Dosimetric evaluation in a prospective study of DARS optimized intensity modulated radiation therapy. Journal of Cancer Research and Therapeutics. 2024;**20**(5):1499-1506. DOI: 10.4103/jcrt.jcrt_166_23

[42] Ramia P, Bodgi L, Mahmoud D, Mohammad MA, Youssef B, Kopek N, et al. Radiation-induced fibrosis in patients with head and neck cancer: A review of pathogenesis and clinical outcomes. Clinical Medicine Insights: Oncology. 2022;**16**:11795549211036898. DOI: 10.1177/11795549211036898

[43] Hutcheson KA, Bhayani MK, Beadle BM, et al. Eat and exercise during radiotherapy or chemoradiotherapy for pharyngeal cancers: Use it or lose it. JAMA Otolaryngology. Head and Neck Surgery. 2013;**139**:1127-1134. DOI: 10.1001/jamaoto.2013.4715

[44] Murphy BA, Gilbert J. Dysphagia in head and neck cancer patients treated with radiation: Assessment, sequelae, and rehabilitation. Seminars in Radiation Oncology. 2009;**19**(1):35-42. DOI: 10.1016/j.semradonc.2008.09.007

[45] Paleri V, Roe JWG, Strojan P, et al. Strategies to reduce long-term postchemoradiation dysphagia in patients with head and neck cancer: An evidence based review. Head and Neck. 2014;**36**(3):431-443. DOI: 10.1002/hed.23251

[46] Kraaijenga SA, van der Molen L, van den Brekel MWM, Hilgers FJM. Current assessment and treatment strategies of dysphagia in head and neck cancer patients: A systematic review of the 2012/13 literature. Current Opinion in Supportive and Palliative Care. 2014;**8**:152-163. DOI: 10.1097/SPC.0000000000000050

[47] Mittal BB, Pauloski BR, Haraf DJ, et al. Swallowing dysfunction—Preventative and rehabilitation strategies in patients with head-and-neck cancers treated with surgery, radiotherapy,

and chemotherapy: A critical review. International Journal of Radiation Oncology. 2003;**57**:1219-1230. DOI: 10.1016/s0360-3016(03)01454-8

[48] Cnossen IC, van Uden-Kraan CF, Rinkel RNPM, et al. Multimodal guided self-help exercise program to prevent speech, swallowing, and shoulder problems among head and neck cancer patients: A feasibility study. Journal of Medical Internet Research. 2014;**16**:e74. DOI: 10.2196/jmir.2990

[49] Kotz T, Federman AD, Kao J, et al. Prophylactic swallowing exercises in patients with head and neck cancer undergoing chemoradiation: A randomized trial. Archives of Otolaryngology – Head & Neck Surgery. 2012;**138**:376-382. DOI: 10.1001/archoto.2012.187

[50] Van der Molen L, van Rossum MA, Burkhead LM, Smeele LE, Rasch CRN, Hilgers FJM. A randomized preventive rehabilitation trial in advanced head and neck cancer patients treated with chemoradiotherapy: Feasibility, compliance, and short-term effects. Dysphagia. 2011;**26**:155-170. DOI: 10.1007/s00455-010-9288-y

[51] Brown E, Owen R, Harden F, Mengersen K, Oestreich K, Houghton W, et al. Predicting the need for adaptive radiotherapy in head and neck cancer. Radiotherapy and Oncology. 2015;**116**:57-63. DOI: 10.1016/j.radonc.2015.06.025

**Chapter 12**

# Dysphagia: Nutritional Management and Implications

*Donnette Alicia Wright*

## Abstract

Dysphagia is a public health concern, which is strongly associated with undernutrition impacting serum levels of both macro- and micro nutrient intake levels. Nearly 40% of all dysphagia patients are at risk of malnutrition. The link between malnutrition and quality of life increases the importance of optimal nutritional management of dysphagia. A comprehensive multi-team individualized therapy, including assessment, diagnosis (of the related nutritional risks), intervention and follow-up, is necessary to ensure optimization of nutritional status and general well-being. Nutritional standards have been presented as traditional approaches, which present risks and gaps to ideal nutritional status when compared to conventional recommendations, which individualize therapies for the best outcomes in the nutritional standards of patients with dysphagia. A review of the current evidence will provide contemporary guidance and best practice for nutritional wellness in this unique group of patients.

**Keywords:** nutritional optimization, dysphagia, nutritional status, swallowing, deglutition, nutritional assessment

## 1. Introduction

Dysphagia is a gastrointestinal dysfunction mainly affecting the upper gastrointestinal system. It may be a symptom of an underlining condition or a primary physiological dysfunction. It involves the pathophysiological dysregulation of the deglutition of foods. Nutritional impairment presents as a strong risk factor, approximately 32% of all dysphagia patients experience malnutrition and negative outcome of dysphagia [1, 2]. Older and infirm people present as having higher risk of developing dysphagia. Due to the limitations in healthcare resources that lead to a lack of assessment and diagnosis of non-communicable disease, developing countries have a higher disease burden. These conditions increase the risk of dysphagia. Stroke, for example, is one of the risk factors of dysphagia. The current evidence suggests that the bulk of stroke burden (80% of all incident strokes, 77% of all stroke survivors, 87% of all deaths from stroke and 89% of all stroke-related disability-adjusted life years (DALYs)) in 2017 was in low- and middle-income countries (LMICs) [3]. Health outcomes related to dysphagia include malnutrition, weight loss, muscle wasting, increased risk of infections and increased length of hospital stay that are linked

 IntechOpen

to dysphagia [4]. These conditions have been clearly documented to influence the quality of life, particularly influencing morbidity and in extremes, mortality risks. These outcomes can be modified with multi-specialty team management, focusing on detailed assessment, accurate diagnosis, individualized interventions, continuous follow-up and personalized adjustments throughout therapy. The treatment of dysphagia is recommended to be comprehensive with the principal goal of nutritional optimization. It is also imperative that research, examination and evidence-based treatment form the platform for the therapeutic management of dysphagia to optimize health outcomes. This chapter aims to examine the current epidemiological context of dysphagia, risks and clinical outcomes of dysphagia. It summarizes the contemporary strategies to diagnose dysphagia and comprehensively examines the contemporaneous standards to treat and manage dysphagia, especially its nutritional requirements.

## 2. Incidence

Dysphagia is the medical term for an umbrella group of swallowing disorders, which may be structural, neurological or psychogenic, as it affects quality of life and physiological outcomes. Internationally, dysphagia has an estimated prevalence rate of 20% in the general population; however, it disproportionally affects the elderly when compared to young adults and children. The estimates are documented to affect approximately 50–66% of people over 60 years of age [5]. In the United States of America, the number of people affected is lower. The reported prevalence data are one in 17 (6%) adults and similar sources have reported that mean affected age has increased from 46.6 to 48.1 years [6]. Contradictory evidence exists, suggesting that the prevalence data were as high as 16% among Americans [7]. The disparity in the reported prevalence data has been explained by the difference in the subset of Americans sampled, the timing of the studies, the criteria used to define and the tools used to test for dysphagia. While the recorded prevalence of dysphagia in America is only 6% (1 in 17), the rates in Asia are closer to that described for the general international population. Asian prevalence of dysphagia in the geriatric population living in the community ranges from 13.8 to 33.7%, while the international rates of institutional dysphagia were documented to be between 26 and 60% [8]. In South African countries, the prevalence of dysphagia following stroke was 56% [9]. Caution must be exercised when interpreting the prevalence of dysphagia in [9] study. This is due to the use of very conservative measurement/assessment practices they employed in the study to evaluate dysphagia cases in the targeted population. The patient's history and bedside subjective tests were used as the primary means to diagnose the disease, rather than confirmatory diagnostic and radiological tests. This limited evidence does not fully capture the disproportional disease and disability burden of the continent. Moreover, no current evidence is available on the general prevalence of dysphagia in Africa, which is partly accounted for by the under-resourced healthcare system [10]. However, due to the potential for poor quality of life and increased disease burden associated with dysphagia, urgent and comprehensive healthcare interventions are critical globally, particularly in Africa. Though the prevalence data vary by region, the elderly are predominantly affected and there is a greater concentration of the condition among those who are institutionalized, with hospitalized patients having higher incidence when compared to community-dwelling individuals. This rate balloons when individuals are admitted to tertiary care facilities and nursing homes. In addition to the disproportionate impact of dysphagia on the elderly, it substantially affects more women when compared to men. The current incidence suggests 52.9% females compared with 47.1% of males who were diagnosed with dysphagia. The same study reported an unusual finding with respect to the difference in health-seeking behaviors by gender [7]. They found that older age, male gender, having insurance, having comorbidities and more severe dysphagia symptoms were associated with increased odds for seeking care for dysphagia. In view of the statistics and the impact on functionality, health and maintenance, it is clear that dysphagia affects quality of life and the magnitude of its impact is directly related to early comprehensive multi-disciplinary but individualized care.

## 3. Definition and classification

Contemporary evidence points to a lack of consensus on the actual levels of population data for dysphagia. The pundits suggest that the dissonance surrounding the statistical evidence rests in the definition, assessment and ultimately diagnosis of dysphagia. To define the condition, it is imperative that the first step be the examination of the normal physiology of deglutition. Swallowing is a process requiring the coordination of a complex series of motor, sensory and psychological activities that are voluntary and involuntary [11]. This complex process begins with lip closure and the formation of the bolus and terminates with the admittance of the bolus through the esophageal sphincter and its subsequent closure [12]. Several authorities have defined dysphagia and definitions recorded include concepts that express a change in the normal physiology and consider that there is a normal structural decline with aging, which predisposes the elderly to dysphagia. One of the most well-defined meanings stems from an articulation of normal swallowing advanced by The International Classification of Functioning, Disability and Health (ICF), which classifies swallowing as "the function of clearing food and drink through the oral cavity, pharynx, and oesophagus (gullet) with an appropriate rate." They propose that dysphagia is defined as: the difficulty in transferring food from the mouth to the stomach at an appropriate rate [11]. Importantly, dysphagia is a condition that involves the difficulty in the transition of both liquid and solid bolus through the esophagus and into the stomach. It spans both intermittent, transient and chronic forms [13].

Moreover, dysphagia may also be classified as psychogenic. This form of dysphagia is described as lacking structural, organic or physiological cause but is a perception of difficulty swallowing with associated avoidance in swallowing certain foods and liquids. To avoid misdiagnosis, a multi-disciplinary team of medical practitioners should be enlisted and the diagnosis should be suspected in patients with strong psychological history of mental disability, such as paranoia, anxiety and delusions [14]. Organic dysphagia can be classified into two groups, oropharyngeal dysphagia (OD) and esophageal dysphagia. The time and anatomical health impact differs between the categories of organic dysphagia. In oropharyngeal dysphagia (OD), the patient experiences the difficulty immediately upon swallowing. Additionally, the affected patient undergoes physiological abnormalities in the upper gastrointestinal tract due to physical changes, which may include an imbalance in the coordination between the respiratory and nutritional systems [11]. In the elderly, OD is described as being associated with decline in functional capacity, increase in frailty, polymedication and multimorbidity [15]. In the younger population, dysphagia is more likely to be linked with underlying systemic illnesses, such as autoimmune diseases, gastroesophageal reflux disease (GERD) or eosinophilic esophagitis [5]. In the general population, other conditions, such as radiation, peptic ulcer disease, as well as improper esophageal contraction in achalasia, increase the risk of dysphagia (see **Figure 1**).

Alternatively, esophageal dysphagia occurs moments after swallowing is initiated and is usually described as the perception of food being lodged in the throat. Medical professionals suggest that it occurs when there is difficulty with the passage of solid or liquid material through the gullet, anatomically this is the region between the pharynx and the inlet (esophageal/cardiac sphincter) to the cardia of the stomach [13, 17]. Both forms of organic dysphagia may be caused or affected by structural, neuromuscular, infectious and inflammatory diseases and are broadly classified as mechanical or motility factors. Mechanical factors within the esophagus that predisposes a patient to dysphagia include cancers, strictures, lesions, inflammation and muscular damage and usually only affect the deglutition of solids. Alternatively, motility-related factors include spasms, achalasia and systemic sclerosis and are thought to impair the swallowing of both liquids and solids.

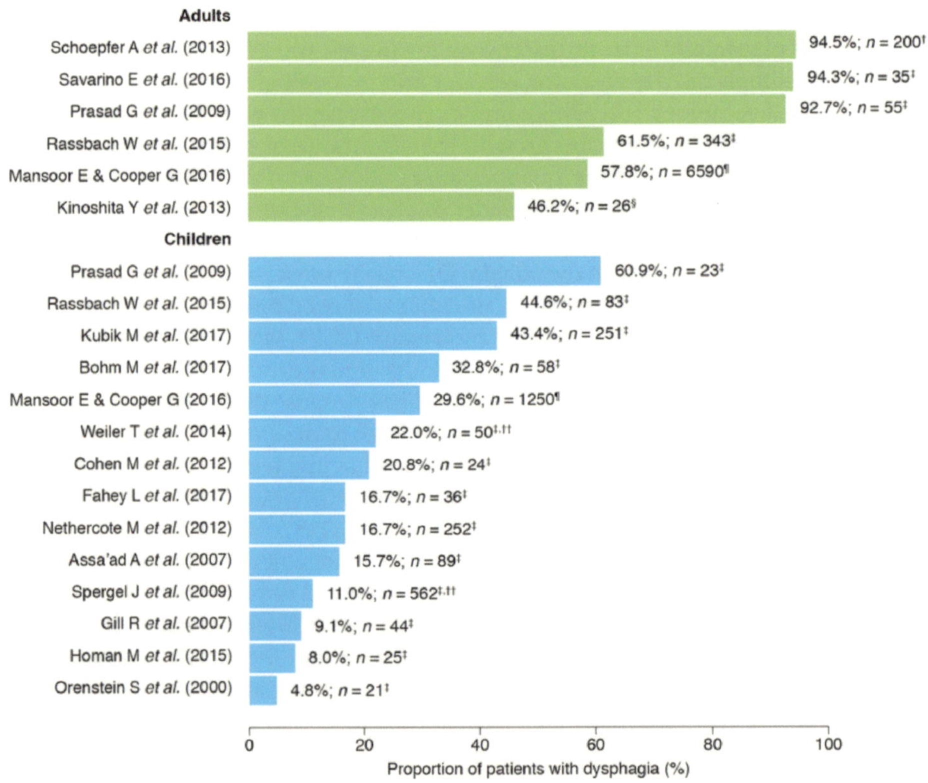


**Figure 1.**
*Epidemiology of dysphagia. Available from: [16]. Republished through creative common license. Licensed under CC BY 4.0 (Prevalence of dysphagia in adults and children. Sample sizes (n) are shown to the right of each bar. Please note that the denominators of at-risk populations from the studies presented in this figure may have different definitions, i.e., some populations may be highly symptomatic or selected. † Diagnostic criteria based on esophageal dysfunction or esophageal eosinophilia. ‡ Diagnostic criteria based on eosinophil count per high-power field. § Diagnostic criteria based on 2007 guidelines. 2 Diagnostic criteria based on SNOMED-CT diagnosis; no diagnostic codes were reported for any other study. † † Data refer to dysphagia or food impaction. SNOMED-CT, Systematized Nomenclature of Medicine-Clinical Term).*

## 4. Diagnosing dysphagia

The diagnosis of dysphagia is inconsistent and the related prevalence and incidence data are to be interpreted with caution due to the variation within the scientific community with respect to its established definition and defining features. Accurate diagnosis of dysphagia is critical to the acceptance of research findings and the available statistical evidence. Diagnostic accuracy also guides intervention and individualization of treatment. Contemporary evidence points to a multi-team specialist approach in diagnosing the condition. The multi-disciplinary team includes the following professionals; doctors, physiotherapists, speech therapists, rehabilitators, nurses, auxiliary nursing care technicians and some jurisdictions recognize the role of the lactation specialists in diagnosing neonatal and infantile dysphagia [18]. This multi-disciplinary team approach is thought to be effective in identifying nuanced changes, especially with respect to nutrition in at-risk and specific populations [19, 20].

There exist a number of assessment measures that can be employed in the diagnosis of dysphagia and that incorporate standards of history taking, physical assessment and diagnostic tests/procedures. There is scientific consensus that history taking is important in diagnosing and guiding the diagnostic process for dysphagia. Questions concerning the onset, duration and severity of the dysphagia, and a variety of associated symptoms may help to distinguish between the organic forms of dysphagia and guide the need for other diagnostic procedures. In addition to the timing and duration of swallowing difficulty, doctors routinely ask about coughing, weakness, weight loss, heartburn, pain and regurgitation [21, 22]. Contemporary scientists support these seminal views and suggest that most (80%) of all dysphagia-afflicted patients may be diagnosed by detailed targeted history taking [23]. Moreover, scientists suggest that a detailed examination of the respiratory and upper gastrointestinal tract be examined to determine structural factors that may contribute to dysphagia. Each structure in these shared systems should be assessed, as presented in **Figure 2**.

Data gathered from anamnesis (history taking) will also determine whether the subsequent diagnostic procedure should be an endoscopy, a barium swallow or esophageal manometry. Targeted questions about the onset, timing and severity of swallowing impairments and the associated symptoms such as coughing and breathing may help to narrow the differential diagnosis. Instances of swallowing impairment immediately after ingestion may lead to the suspicion of oropharyngeal dysphagia and the report of challenges with only solid foods may lead to the impression that there may be mechanical impairments (See **Figure 3**). In some difficult cases, all three diagnostic techniques may need to be performed to establish an accurate diagnosis [21].

- Barium swallow is an imaging study that includes a fluorescent dye to detect structural changes in the mucosal lining of the throat and esophagus. It is often performed first.

- Endoscopy is minimally invasive and provides imagery of the upper gastrointestinal tract using an endoscope camera.

Esophageal manometry examines gullet motility, esophageal musculature and the functionality of the upper and lower esophageal sphincters. This diagnostic evaluation is customarily performed after the barium meal and endoscopic evaluations. North American practice identifies additional diagnostic strategies in evaluation of dysphagia. They include dysphonia assessment, abnormal pharyngeal sensation

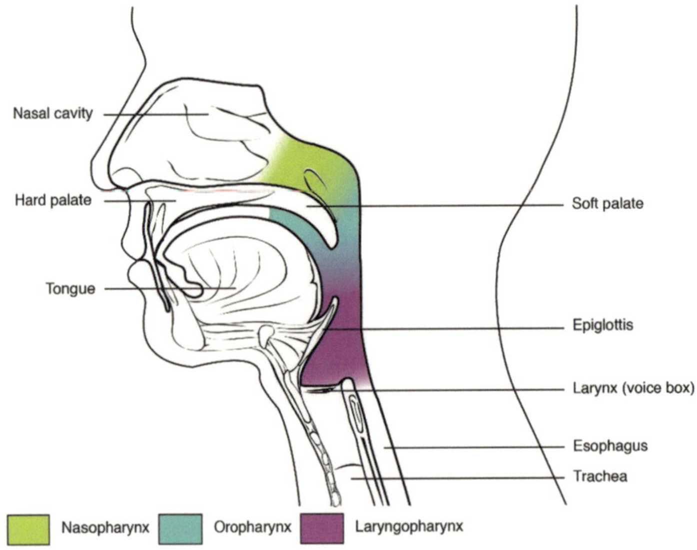


**Figure 2.**
*Anatomical structures affected by dysphagia. Available from: LOUIS: The Louisiana library network (September, 2022). Medical terminology: an interactive approach. https://louis.pressbooks.pub/medicalterminology/chapter/respiratory-anatomy-physiology/. Republished through creative common license. Licensed under CC BY 4.0.*

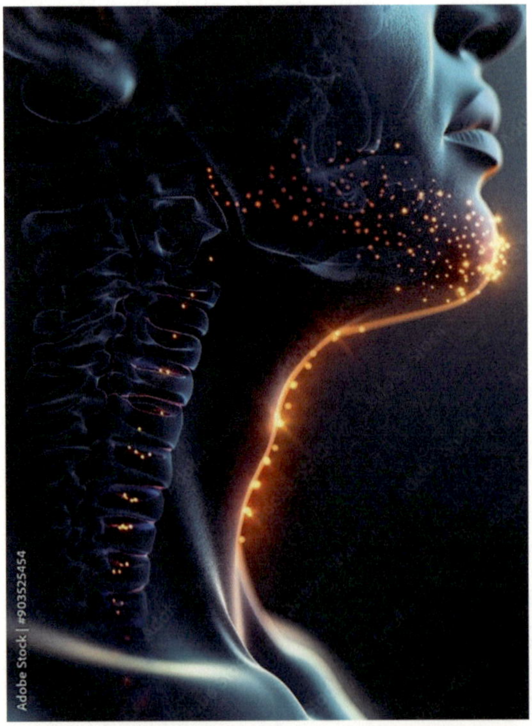


**Figure 3.**
*Image of throat with dysphagia diagnosis and medical markers. Available from: Adobe stock, difficulty swallowing (September 7, 2024). https://stock.adobe.com/jm/search?k=&token_type=bearer&expires_in=86399&asset_id=903525454. Republished through standard license with permission.*

| Factors of positive beside water swallow test (BWST) | Positive sign |
|---|---|
| Water intake | Taking more than one swallow to finish the 10 mL water |
| Drooling | Drooling of water from the mouth |
| Laryngeal movement | The absence of laryngeal movement while drinking the water (10 mL) and up to 10 minutes after drinking |
| Oxygen saturation | A 2% and above decrease in oxygen saturation while drinking |
| Coughing | Coughing after drinking water |
| Voice | Presence of voice change |

**Table 1.**
*Positive signs of BWST.*

assessments and water swallow test. These procedures are described as probative and valuable in dysphagia detection but have an overarching caution that they are collectively inconsistently sensitive [24].

There is also a vibrant discourse concerning the application of the bedside water swallow test (BWST) in the evaluation of dysphagia. This procedure is well documented and involves the administration of 10 mL of water to the affected patient and a subsequent medical examination including pulse oximetry. The patient who is found to have a positive test demonstrates most of the following symptoms (**Table 1**).

The patient receives a numeric score from 0 to 6, where 1 is assigned for every symptom observed. Scores of 0–2 are categorized as normal and 3–6 as being positive for dysphagia [25].

In addition to the described diagnostic procedures and assessments, practitioners may utilize videofluoroscopic swallow study or a fiberoptic endoscopic evaluation of swallowing (FEES) in the evaluation of oropharyngeal dysphagia [23].

In summary, dysphagia diagnosis is dynamic and relies on several processes including history taking, clinical assessment and diagnostic procedures. There is scientific consensus surrounding the value of history taking in diagnosing dysphagia. Furthermore, where history taking is insufficient in determining swallowing difficulties, it is critical in guiding the other investigative procedures that may provide definitive diagnosis. The diagnostic protocols that exist to evaluate impairments in deglutition include barium esophagography, endoscopy and manometry. More expansive evidence has examined the value of the beside water swallow test (BWST) and described the sensitivity of videofluoroscopy. Research authorities also agree that evaluation of dysphagia is critical to support research and population statistics. More importantly, diagnosis contextualizes the disease and provides guidance for dietitians to maintain nutritional wellness.

## 5. Health impact

In the last 30 years, the prevalence of dysphagia has increased significantly. In North America and United States in particular, the data concerning dysphagia show that prevalence has increased from 408,035 (2.5% of admissions) in 2009 to 656,655 (3.3%) in 2013 [4]. Other sources point to an increase in the incidence of dysphagia increased from 7.14 in 2006 to 15.64 in 2016 in Korea [8]. Dysphagia has several associated health outcomes that impact quality of life. Moreover, there has been a significant general increase in the global burden of illness and disease and related disability over the same period. Support services for dysphagia include a range of specialized resources, such as access to speech therapists, dietary modification tools, support products, caregivers for the patients and community support. Unfortunately, developing low- and middle-income countries have lower access and availability of these resources, which limit the quality of life of people affected by dysphagia in their jurisdiction [10].

The normal physiology of respiration and deglutition shares similar structural sites (pharynx), which may result in pathophysiological changes when either is affected. The evidence suggests that patients diagnosed with dysphagia, who are unable to control the passage of bolus, may not be able to control the opening and the closure of the epiglottis. The movement of the bolus along the esophagus through the cardiac sphincter may have several upper respiratory and gastrointestinal disorders and symptoms. Common respiratory symptoms associated with dysphagia include dysphonia, pneumonia, lower respiratory tract infection (LRTI), aspiration, chronic coughing and wheezing [26, 27]. Conversely, the gastrointestinal symptoms and conditions that may arise as a result of dysphagia include halitosis, belching, globus (perception of food stuck in the throat) sensation, regurgitation, pyrosis (heartburn) and odynophagia. Several of the symptoms arise with incomplete or dysfunctional closure of the lower esophageal sphincter and mechanical (anatomic) features of dysphagia [26]. The consequence of these symptoms leads to iatrogenic and organic malnutrition and/or dehydration where the patient is either medically prohibited from eating normally or has physical impairment that limits adequate dietary intake [23].

Patients diagnosed with dysphagia may also experience increased rates of mortality, rehospitalization and long-term care admission leading to increased risk of concomitant disease and financial costs [23, 28, 29]. Additionally, elderly individuals who experience unresolved chronic dysphagia are often discharged to nursing homes from hospitals rather than their own homes [23]. These circumstances impact the quality of life of the afflicted patients.

Patients with intractable dysphagia with dietary intake less than 50% for more than 7 days often require enteral nutrition or tube feeding to meet nutritional needs. Consequently, these patients may require longer institutionalization to ensure nutritional adequacy [28, 30]. Patients who required tube or enteral feeding may be managed acutely in secondary or tertiary care facilities, such as hospitals and hospices. Stable patients with no additional comorbidities may be discharged home and continue with independent or supported tube feeding in their respective homes. Healthcare workers, in particular nurses and dietitians, are responsible for discharge teaching concerning the management and delivery of enteral nutrition as well as the assessment of the signs and symptoms of the complications, such as diarrhea, constipation, infections, metabolic complications and mechanical complications (dislocation of the tube). The nutritional support for enteral feeding should be based ideally on calorimetric assessments. In under-resourced settings, energy may be computed using a recommendation of 25 kcal/g [30]. The recommendations for macronutrient intake are as follows:

- Carbohydrate intake—4 gm/kg daily with a target serum glucose level below 180 mg/dl.
- Lipid intake—0.7 to 1.5 gm/kg per day.
- Protein (consumed as amino acid in enteral feeds) should be adjusted to 1–1.8 g/kg per day increased from normal 0.8–1 g/kg with an adequate supply of carbohydrate and fat [30].

Other schools of thought suggest that there is significant morbidity risk that may arise as a consequence of dysphagia and may impact both the respiratory and the gastrointestinal systems. They document conditions including aspiration, asphyxiation, and eventually, premature death. Importantly, the authorities described some physiological and pathological changes that increase individual risk of dysphagia, such as loss of muscle mass, changes of the cervical spine, impaired dentition and xerostomia (reduction of saliva production) [11]. In the elderly, aging causes structural changes in the anatomy, such as xerostomia, loss of muscle mass, impairment in dentition and reduction in gastric motility. Consequently, dysphagia risk is higher in older individuals due to the normal structural decline of aging [11].

In summary, the global disease profile has changed in the last two decades. The related disease prevalence and disability burden inequitably affect low- and middle-income countries (LMICs) when compared to developed countries. The quality of life of an affected person worsens with several physiological changes affecting the gastrointestinal and respiratory systems. In order to improve clinical outcomes, healthcare practitioners should include symptomatic management, examination of underlying contributory factors and diagnostic evaluation as part of the strategic management of the condition.

## 6. Treatment

Dysphagia has been documented to significantly impact the quality of life, health, recovery and healthcare costs. Similar to the diagnostic process, the treatment of dysphagia is a multi-specialty team approach that requires each patient being ordered an individualized nutrition treatment plan. Based on the patient's health status and physiological needs, varying nutritional interventions may be employed; primarily including dietary adjustments by mouth or tube as shown in **Figure 4**.

Jukic Peladic et al. [31]. For the best clinical outcomes with nutritional management, texture-modified diets (TMDs) are standardized into levels according to the level of modification and are recommended to be individualized based on the clinical/functional capacity of the patient. The recommended texture of the diet was classified according to the International Dysphagia Diet Standardization Initiative (IDDSI). The framework consists of eight levels of modification based on liquid viscosity and form adjustment (see **Figure 5**). The ratings are on a numerical scale from 0 to 7, where drinks are measured from Levels 0 (thin) to 4 (extremely thick) and foods are measured from Levels 3 (liquidized) to 7 (regular) [31].

Dysphagia increases the risk and prevalence of malnutrition in the affected population. Malnutrition occurs in patients affected by dysphagia due to disease-related

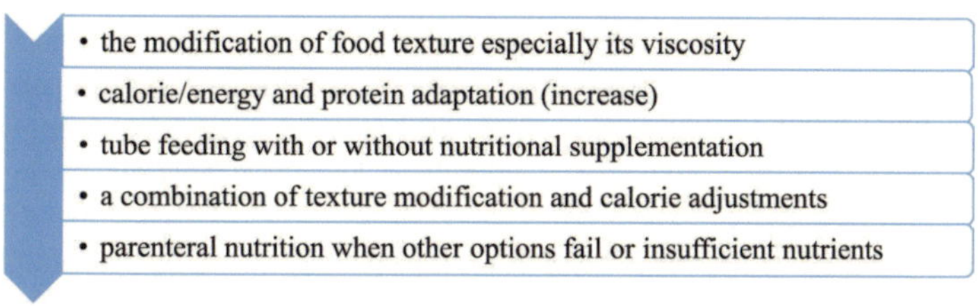


**Figure 4.**
*Nutritional interventions in dysphagia management.*

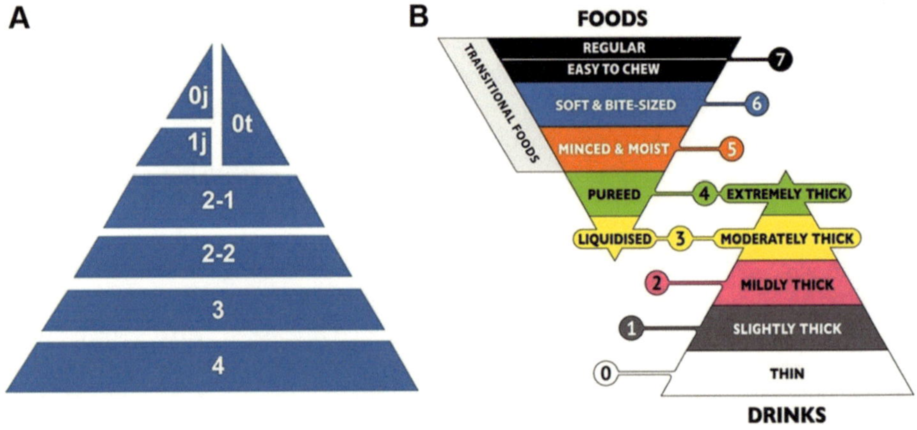


**Figure 5.**
*Texture modification classifications for foods. Available from: [29].*

factors and iatrogenic consequences. Dysphagia impairs the volume and the quality of nutritional intake, leading to calorie and micronutrient deficiencies. Alternatively, therapeutic orders of *nil per os* (NPO) are often included as part of the treatment to prevent aspiration and related conditions. This treatment option limits dietary intake, which contributes to macro- and micro nutrient deficiencies. Therefore, malnutrition recognition and management are essential for patients with dysphagia. The relationship between malnutrition and dysphagia is cyclical. On the one hand, dysphagia limits dietary intake and increases the risk of malnutrition. Alternatively, malnourished states increase the risk of dysphagia because malnutrition leads to a decrease in fat-free mass including lean mass and striated muscle mass, which include swallowing-related muscles. This is further compounded in the elderly who are likely to experience sarcopenia as a feature of aging. This condition results in global decline in muscle mass and increases the risk of dysphagia development in sarcopenia, especially in the elderly and dependent populations [29]. This demonstrates the direct cyclical relationship between dysphagia and malnutrition. In the first instance, dysphagia restricts dietary intake quality and volume resulting in malnutrition, while malnutrition impairs the strength and functionality of the muscles of the body and in particular those that support deglutition potentiating dysphagia. Texture modification has been practiced as the standard nutritional management strategy for dysphagia; however, there are many associated disadvantages to this therapy. Texture-modified diets (TMDs) have lower nutrient content than regular diets. Both micro- and macro nutrient alterations' restrictions have been documented as side effects of texture modifications. To modify a regular meal to achieve texture manipulation, chopping, mincing, grinding or blending is done. For some foods, there are adequate fluids including in the product to facilitate the manipulation and the intake. For other foods such as meats, fluid or liquid must be added to achieve the intended viscosity [32]. This results in alteration in the nutrient density dependent on the product used to liquefy the TMD. Consequently, calorie and protein intake was lower in patients receiving a TMD than in patients receiving a regular diet. Dietary analysis comparing textured (regular) and TMD has shown a variation of 400–600 kcal/d and protein difference of 20 g/d between dietary types [32]. Several cross-sectional and retrospective observational studies have reported malnutrition and muscle mass loss in patients on TMDs [29].

Other nutritional deficiencies have been associated with texture modifications. The evidence suggests that modifications closer to 0 or thin on the texturization scale are associated with lower levels of micronutrients where foods that are more viscous are more likely to be nutrient dense. Due to the high risk of iatrogenic malnutrition associated with dysphagia management, the healthcare team must take all precautions to prevent dietary deficiency. Notably, nutrient quality can be preserved and enhanced in texturization with the introduction of nutrient-dense liquids and constituents, such as skimmed milk, egg albumin, protein-based infant cereals and carbohydrate thickeners [32]. It is important that standard recipes and modification standards are recorded and utilized in institutional settings. Both fat-soluble and water-soluble vitamins have been linked to texture modification, including ascorbic acid, retinal, folate, pantothenic acid, tocopherol and cyanocobalamin. These deficiencies, overt and subclinical, may be treated with fortification or supplementation. It is important that nutritional intervention be personalized and target the specific needs of the patient rather than rote practiced therapy with global dietary challenges. It is also imperative a multi-specialty team, including the speech-language therapist, responsible for assessment, the medical doctor for diagnostic and therapeutic orders, the phlebotomist, the occupational therapist, the nurse and the dietitian, participate in a comprehensive management and support of the patient with dysphagia.

Despite the value of detailed initial and ongoing follow-up assessments, there is still no gold standard for nutritional assessment indicators for adult patients with dysphagia [29]. Nevertheless, the value of continuous evaluation cannot be overemphasized in this population for best health outcomes including early detection of deficiency, deviations and improvements to guide individualized adjustments in therapy.

In the multi-specialty team approach to the therapeutic management of dysphagia, all members of the team are valuable at varying points in the management, assessment, diagnosis, intervention, evaluation and referral. Nevertheless, the literature makes reference to a group of specialists who are critical of achieving the best outcomes in dysphagia management. They are especially valuable in the assessment and diagnostic phases of dysphagia management. Speech-language pathologists use various tests ranging from bedside assessment to instrumented swallowing studies to determine specific deficits, the patient's prognosis and probability of improvement, and the most appropriate dietary modifications and swallow therapies [33]. These professionals are widely available in developed countries; however, they are limited and sometimes non-existent in developing countries. One of the principal collaborative treatments that is instituted is thickened liquids and foods with specific textures to assist in reducing aspiration risk. Medical specialists who treat dysphagia also teach patients rehabilitative strategies, such as maneuvers of the head, neck and chin, capable of promoting safer swallowing [33].

Speech-language pathologists are trained to offer therapy grouped as dietary modifications with mindful eating involving—careful chewing, avoidance of offensive foods, resizing food, eating slowly, minimal liquid intake to soften bolus, including lubricating sauces and smaller bites [33]. The specialists may also offer a second approach that targets swallowing rehabilitation—structural and muscular strengthening of the mouth, tongue and jaw. Additionally, the speech-language pathologists may introduce dysphagia patients to compensatory safe swallowing techniques such as eating upright and specialized techniques such as chin-tuck in stroke patients and head turn technique in patients with unilateral weakness. If patients continue to decline and have a poor response to other strategies, the management team may recommend enteral feed (tube feeding) and

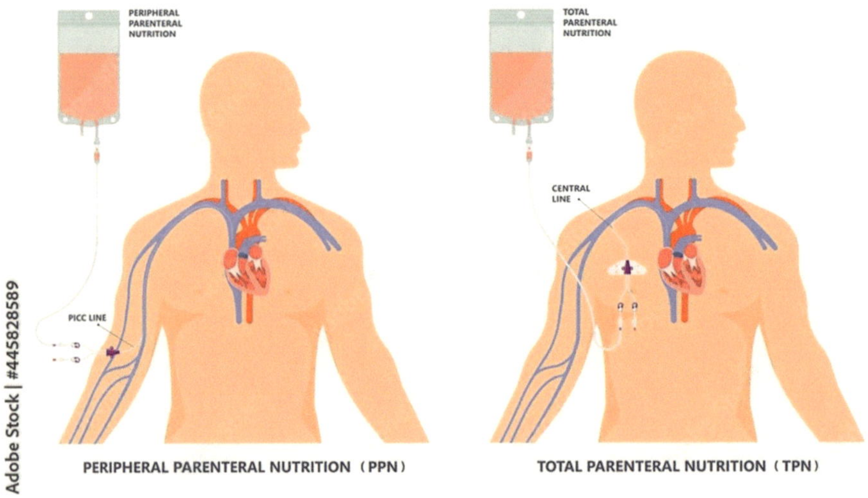


**Figure 6.**
*Image of total parenteral and partial parenteral nutrition. Available from: Adobe stock, TPN (September 11, 2024). https://stock.adobe.com/search?k=tpn&asset_id=445828589. Republished through standard license with permission.*

in the later phase parenteral nutrition where benefits outweigh risks [33]. Importantly, for patients receiving tube feeding as well as patients receiving modified oral intake, the estimation of energy requirement is integral to the adequacy of their dietary supply. Formulae including the Harris-Benedict and Mifflin St. Jeor are beneficial in determining basal requirements. Additional needs for full support include accounting for stress using the appropriate stress multipliers such as 1.1 or 1.4 for weight loss and cancer weight loss [34]. Enteral formulation is prescribed in patients who have lost the voluntary capacity to swallow or have non-functional upper gastrointestinal structures such as strictures or blockage. In such instances, the insertion is placed below the level of the stricture or blockage. The formula that is used is dependent on nutritional status and underlining or concomitant disease such as having normal levels of glucose in persons with diabetes, high protein and high calorie levels in weight loss. Parenteral nutrition is the last resort that is used in the dietary management of dysphagia and should only be used when benefits of life preservation and restriction of malnutrition outweigh the risk of thrombus formation, sepsis, hyperglycemia, among others [35]. This involves the process of hyperalimentation or the administration of dietary products outside of the gastrointestinal tract in a high volume vein such as the subclavian or jugular veins (see **Figure 6**). Total parental nutrition is the intravenous administration of nutrients as the sole source of nutrition [36].

## 7. Recommendations

Dysphagia is a condition, which affects nutritional status, length of hospitalization, financial burden and the risk of infection and primarily includes the structural/mechanical or sensory impairment in the deglutition process. It preferentially affects older persons due to the physiological decline in the gastrointestinal system with more significant disease-related disability in developing countries. Community-based dysphagia has lower recorded prevalence when compared to institutional-based levels and global incidence is recorded to be one in every five adults. There is a strong link between dysphagia and malnutrition where the relationship is characterized as vicious and cyclical. There are a range of assessment strategies including history taking, bedside assessment of the clinical presentation and a variation of diagnostic procedures including imagery, manometry and fluoroscopic assessments. For best outcomes, a multi-specialty team approach is advised. While medical therapies, such as withholding food (NPO), excision and correction of strictures and physical blockades, are valuable, a significant element of the management includes therapeutic nutritional care principally involving texture modification. Though this is the primary care strategy, there are several associated poor outcomes including micro- and macro nutrient deficiencies.

Given this context, it is essential that nutritional optimization and health maintenance serve as the main goals of therapy. Therefore, the recommendations for care should include:

1. Detailed and continuous physical assessment from multiple members of the healthcare team to accurately diagnose and track improvements or deterioration in the nutritional and health status of the patient

2. Prescription and administration of texture-modified diets based on the assessment findings at admission and modified throughout care based on improvements or physiological decline

3. Formulation of the dietary offerings in keeping with an established dietary standard and with as little modification as individually required for the patients

4. The inclusion of nutrient-dense texturized constituents, such as skimmed milk, egg albumin thickeners, infant cereals and carbohydrate thickeners, to preserve macronutrient and micronutrient nutritional status

5. Biochemical assessments of the patient to direct meal fortification and micronutrient supplementation, especially targeting fat miscible and water-soluble vitamins, such as ascorbic acid, pantothenic acid, tocopherol, folate and cyanocobalamin.

6. Continuous physical assessment and targeted nutritional assessment are essential to guiding the need for tube feeding or enteral nutrition or in the event of failed attempts of artificial or parenteral nutrition.

These strategies along with research and evaluation of current evidence are essential to guide the most strategic and beneficial approach to nutrition and therapeutic optimization in dysphagia.

## 8. Conclusion

The impact of dysphagia ranges from mild symptoms such as coughing and wheezing to severe symptoms such as malnutrition, aspiration, pneumonia and death. Due to the implications and the variations of presentation, diagnostic procedures should be guided by symptomology and detailed history taking. Following diagnosis, health care is primarily focused on nutritional management. The nutrition therapy should be individualized and patient centered to promote optimal health recovery and outcomes. The main nutritional support includes texture modification where the greatest modification should be offered to the patient with the most severe swallowing challenge and the least modification to the patient with the least significant swallowing deviation. The healthcare team should institute the highest level of nutrition support to promote nutritional adequacy with the inclusion of thickeners that have higher macronutrient values and micronutrient supplementation. Furthermore, continuous patient assessment using biochemical and anthropometric tests is critical to optimizing nutritional status and for early intervention where deficiencies exist. Cost-benefit analysis is important in determining the need for enteral and parenteral nutrition support for patients with the most severe forms of dysphagia.

**Author details**

Donnette Alicia Wright
The University of the West Indies, Mona, Kingston, Jamaica

*Address all correspondence to: donnette.wright02@uwimona.edu.jm

## References

[1] Gallegos C, Brito-De La Fuente E, Clavé P, Costa A, Assegehegn G. Nutritional aspects of dysphagia management. Advances in Food and Nutrition Research. 2017;**81**:271-318

[2] Ueshima J, Momosaki R, Shimizu A, Motokawa K, Sonoi M, Shirai Y, et al. Nutritional assessment in adult patients with dysphagia: A scoping review. Nutrients. 2021;**13**(3):778

[3] Krishnamurthi RV, Ikeda T, Feigin VL. Global, regional and country-specific burden of ischaemic stroke, intracerebral haemorrhage and subarachnoid haemorrhage: A systematic analysis of the global burden of disease study 2017. Neuroepidemiology. 2020;**54**(2):171-179

[4] Patel DA, Krishnaswami S, Steger E, Conover E, Vaezi MF, Ciucci MR, et al. Economic and survival burden of dysphagia among inpatients in the United States. Diseases of the Esophagus. 2018;**31**(1):dox131

[5] Chilukuri P, Odufalu F, Hachem C. Dysphagia. Missouri Medicine. 2018;**115**(3):206-210

[6] Hong I, Bae S, Lee HK, Bonilha HS. Prevalence of dysphonia and dysphagia among adults in the United States in 2012 and 2022. American Journal of Speech-Language Pathology. 2024;**33**(4):1868-1879. DOI: 10.1044/2024_AJSLP-23-00407

[7] Adkins C, Takakura W, Spiegel BM, Lu M, Vera-Llonch M, Williams J, et al. Prevalence and characteristics of dysphagia based on a population-based survey. Clinical Gastroenterology and Hepatology. 2020;**18**(9):1970-1979

[8] Kwon S, Cha S, Kim J, Han K, Paik NJ, Kim WS. Trends in the incidence and prevalence of dysphagia requiring medical attention among adults in South Korea, 2006-2016: A nationwide population study. PLoS One. 2023;**18**(6):e0287512

[9] Blackwell Z, Littlejohns P. A review of the management of dysphagia: A south African perspective. Journal of Neuroscience Nursing. 2010;**42**(2):61-70

[10] Jayes M, Madima V, Marshall J, Pillay M. Dysphagia management in community/home settings: A scoping review investigating practices in Africa. International Journal of Speech-Language Pathology. 2024;**21**:1-12. DOI: 10.1080/17549507.2023.2287992

[11] Rajati F, Ahmadi N, Naghibzadeh ZAS, Kazeminia M. The global prevalence of oropharyngeal dysphagia in different populations: A systematic review and meta-analysis. Journal of Translational Medicine. 2022;**20**(1):175. DOI: 10.1186/s12967-022-03380-0

[12] Dziewas R, Michou E, Trapl-Grundschober M, Lal A, Arsava EM, Bath PM, et al. European stroke organisation and European society for swallowing disorders guideline for the diagnosis and treatment of post-stroke dysphagia. European Stroke Journal. 2021;**6**(3):LXXXIX-CXV

[13] Azer SA, Kanugula AK, Kshirsagar RK. Dysphagia. In: StatPearls. Treasure Island (FL): StatPearls Publishing; 2023. Available from: https://www.ncbi.nlm.nih.gov/books/NBK559174/

[14] Bülow M. Psychogenic dysphagia. In: Principles of Deglutition: A Multidisciplinary Text for Swallowing and its Disorders. New York, NY: Springer; 2013. pp. 771-776. DOI: 10.1007/978-1-4614-3794-9_52

[15] Baijens LW, Clavé P, Cras P, Ekberg O, Forster A, Kolb GF, et al. European society for swallowing disorders–European union geriatric medicine society white paper: Oropharyngeal dysphagia as a geriatric syndrome. Clinical Interventions in Aging. 2016;**11**:1403-1428. DOI: 10.2147/CIA.S107750

[16] Shaheen NJ, Mukkada V, Eichinger CS, Schofield H, Todorova L, Falk GW. Natural history of eosinophilic esophagitis: a systematic review of epidemiology and disease course. Diseases of the Esophagus. 2018;**31**(8):doy015. Available from: https://academic.oup.com/dote/article/31/8/doy015/4958126

[17] Walker HK, Hall WD, Hurst JW. Clinical Methods: The History, Physical, and Laboratory Examinations. 3rd ed. Boston: Butterworths; 1990. Available from: https://www.ncbi.nlm.nih.gov/books/NBK408/

[18] Sánchez-Sánchez E, Avellaneda-López Y, García-Marín E, Ramírez-Vargas G, Díaz-Jimenez J, Ordonez FJ. Knowledge and practice of health professionals in the management of dysphagia. International Journal of Environmental Research and Public Health. 2021;**18**(4):2139

[19] Wright D. Nutrition and hospital mortality, morbidity and health outcomes. In: Strategies to Reduce Hospital Mortality in Lower and Middle Income Countries (LMICs) and Resource-Limited Settings. London, UK: IntechOpen; 2019

[20] Wright DA. Nutritional care and intervention in spinocerebellar ataxia. In: Ataxia-Practice Essentials and Interventions. London, UK: IntechOpen; 2023. DOI: 10.5772/intechopen.111734

[21] Cook IJ. Diagnostic evaluation of dysphagia. Nature Clinical Practice Gastroenterology and Hepatology. 2008;**5**(7):393-403

[22] Spieker MR. Evaluating dysphagia. American Family Physician. 2000;**61**(12):3639-3648

[23] Thiyagalingam S, Kulinski AE, Thorsteinsdottir B, Shindelar KL, Takahashi PY. Dysphagia in older adults. In: Mayo Clinic Proceedings. Vol. 96, No. 2. Amsterdam: Elsevier; 2021. pp. 488-497

[24] O'Horo JC, Rogus-Pulia N, Garcia-Arguello L, Robbins J, Safdar N. Bedside diagnosis of dysphagia: A systematic review. Journal of Hospital Medicine. 2015;**10**(4):256-265

[25] Parlak MM, Tokgöz SA, Bizpınar Ö, Saylam G, Köse A. Investigation of cognition, nutrition, independence and swallowing difficulty, relationship with quality of life, and effect levels in elderly people with Alzheimer's disease living with their families. Neurology Asia. 2022;**27**(3):701-708

[26] Lind CD. Dysphagia: Evaluation and treatment. Gastroenterology Clinics. 2003;**32**(2):553-575

[27] Matsuo K, Palmer JB. Anatomy and physiology of feeding and swallowing: Normal and abnormal. Clinics in Integrated Care. 2023;**16**:100139

[28] Rivelsrud MC, Hartelius L, Bergström L, Løvstad M, Speyer R. Prevalence of oropharyngeal dysphagia in adults in different healthcare settings:

A systematic review and meta-analyses. Dysphagia. 2023;**38**(1):76-121. DOI: 10.1007/s00455-022-10465-x

[29] Ueshima J, Shimizu A, Maeda K, Uno C, Shirai Y, Sonoi M, et al. Nutritional management in adult patients with dysphagia: Position paper from Japanese working group on integrated nutrition for dysphagic people. Journal of the American Medical Directors Association. 2022;**23**(10):1676-1682

[30] Adeyinka A, Rouster A, Valentine M. Enteric feedings. In: StatPearls. Treasure Island (FL): StatPearls Publishing; 2022. p. 2024. Available from: https://www.ncbi.nlm.nih.gov/books/NBK532876/

[31] Jukic Peladic N, Orlandoni P, Di Rosa M, Giulioni G, Bartoloni L, Venturini C. Multidisciplinary assessment and individualized nutritional management of dysphagia in older outpatients. Nutrients. 2023;**15**(5):1103

[32] Keller H, Chambers L, Niezgoda H, Duizer L. Issues associated with the use of modified texture foods. The Journal of Nutrition, Health and Aging. 2012;**16**(3):195-200

[33] Wilkinson JM, Codipilly DC, Wilfahrt RP. Dysphagia: Evaluation and collaborative management. American Family Physician. 2021;**103**(2):97-106

[34] Reeves MM, Capra S. Variation in the application of methods used for predicting energy requirements in acutely ill adult patients: A survey of practice. European Journal of Clinical Nutrition. 2003;**57**(12):1530-1535

[35] Cleveland Clinic. Parenteral Nutrition. 2022. Available from: https://my.clevelandclinic.org/health/treatments/22802-parenteral-nutrition

[36] Hamdan M, Puckett Y. Total parenteral nutrition. In: StatPearls. Treasure Island (FL): StatPearls Publishing; 2023; 2024. Available from: https://www.ncbi.nlm.nih.gov/books/NBK559036/